Nothing About Us Without Us

Developing Innovative Technologies
For, By and With Disabled Persons

David Werner
with the PROJIMO team
and many friends

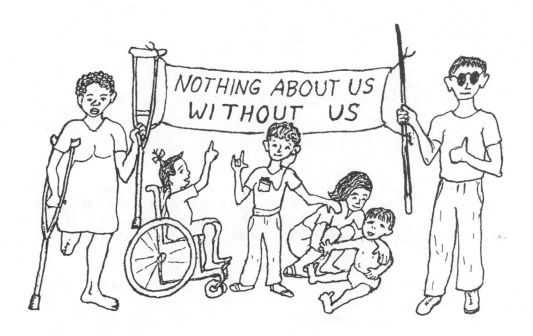

Drawings and photos by the author

Nothing About Us Without Us
Developing Innovative Technologies
For, By and With Disabled Persons
by David Werner

Library of Congress Cataloging in Publication Data
Includes Index
1. Medicine, Popular—Handbooks, manuals, etc.
2. Rehabilitation—Handbooks, manuals, etc.
3. Community Health Aids—Handbooks, manuals, etc.
4. Appropriate Technology—Handbooks, manuals, etc.

Library of Congress Catalog Card No: 97-073594
Werner, David, 1934–
      Nothing About Us Without Us: Developing Innovative Technologies
      For, By and With Disabled Persons / David Werner
      360 pages
      ISBN 0–9655585–3–3

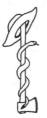

Published by

HEALTHWRIGHTS
Workgroup for People's Health and Rights

Post Office Box 1344
Palo Alto, CA 94302, USA

Copyright © 1998 by David Werner
10 9 8 7 6 5 4 3 2 1

Printed in the United States of America on recycled paper

This book is dedicated to those people
everywhere who, because they are different,
are looked down upon or are not given
an equal chance. . .

and to my friends at PROJIMO
who continue to show us that persons
who are different can make a difference.

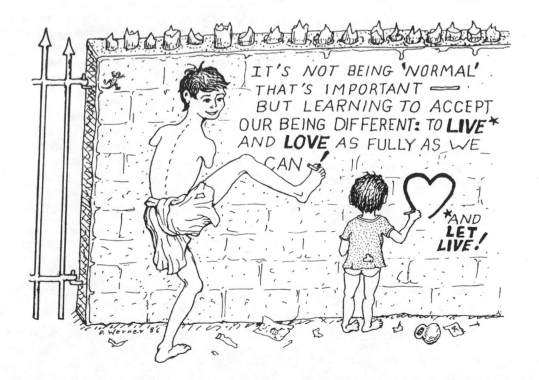

Thanks

Many persons have helped with the creation of this book and the innovative processes it describes. Following are some of the most important contributors.

First, heartfelt thanks go to the rehabilitation team of PROJIMO (Program of Rehabilitation Organized by Disabled Youth of Western Mexico) without whose creativity, hard work, and caring touch the substance for most of this book would not exist. Of the PROJIMO team, those whose contributions are portrayed on these pages include Conchita Lara, Mari Picos, Marcelo Acevedo, Armando Nevárez, Inez León, Cecilia Rodríguez, Rosa Salcido, Julio Peña, Martín Pérez, María de Jesús Leyva, Jaime Torres, Irma Llavió, Mario Carrasco Hernández, Miguel Zamora, and Marielos Rosales. Local children and youth who have helped to make equipment include Leopoldo Ribota, Martín Reyes Millán, Ernesto Navarro, Manuella Campista, Dionicio González, and Isidro González.

Also, hearty thanks go to the many disabled children, parents, and adults who participated in the problem-solving process.

Deep thanks go to Kennett and Jean Westmacott of *People Potential* in England for their emphasis on an empowering approach that puts the disabled person and family at the center of the problem-solving process. This innovative "partnership approach," introduced to the PROJIMO team, has provided much of the inspiration for this book. And for stretching our imagination for creative inventiveness, a strong vote of thanks goes to Reinder van Tijen of *Stichting Demotech*, *Design for Self-Reliance*.

Very special thanks for their essential contributions go to visiting experts in different areas of rehabilitation, therapy, and engineering who were involved in designing and creating personalized assistive equipment and in facilitating workshops—especially to Ann Hallum, John Fago, Ralf Hotchkiss, Oliver Bock, Michael Heinrich, Marybetts Sinclair, Jean Anne Zollars, and Kennett Westmacott.

For providing stories and photos of her creation of Appropriate Paper Technology aids for her daughter, Kim, warm thanks go to Sigi Lester.

Contributors to lively writings in the book include Oliver Bock, John Fago, and Gene Rodgers. Contributors of ideas and designs for specific innovative technologies include Monica Rook, Joep Verweij, and Annemick van Boeijen.

For introducing the author to innovative technologies in India, the author is grateful to San Yuenwah of UN-ESCAP, and to Lourdes Canziani of CORDE for information on new technologies in Brazil.

For specific outstanding photos in this book we thank John Fago, Renée Burgard, Ralf Hotchkiss, Ann Hallum, Kennett and Jean Westmacott, Sigi Lester, Lonny Shavelson, Mari Picos, and Shahidul Haque for SARPV-Bangladesh. For help with drawings we thank Efraín Zamora, Elizabeth Irwin, and Alicia (Tattie) Brelsford. (Most of the photos and line drawings in this book were done by David Werner.)

For help with scanning all photos and drawings and integrating them into the text we thank Efraín Zamora, whose tireless work was consistently outstanding. Thanks for assistance with scanning also go to Merlin Schlumberger, and to Liisa Turan for technical assistance with Quark Express.

For technical assistance with photo preparation, layout and design, formatting, computer troubleshooting, proofing, and a thousand odds and ends, I am deeply grateful to Jason Weston.

For their extremely important critical feedback on a draft of the book, I thank Ann Hallum, Kennett and Jean Westmacott, Mike Miles, Laura Krefting, Johan Borg, Ralf Hotchkiss, Pam Zinkin, and Sophie Levitt.

My deep appreciation goes to Renée Burgard for the final editing of the book and fine-tuning of the layout. Her artist's eye has done much to make this book more attractive.

For help with editing, proofreading and/or technical work, thanks go to Bruce Hobson, Trude Bock, Marianne Schlumberger, Tinker Spar, Jason Weston, Dorothy Weston, Edward J. Weston, Ted Weston, Tina Weston, and Lisa Wright.

Special thanks go to the Thrasher Research Fund, whose assignment to PROJIMO of a 3-year grant for the development of innovative technologies provided the initial motivation for this book.

For the primary financial assistance for developing *Nothing About Us Without Us* we are grateful to the Norwegian International Disability Alliance, and specifically to Harold Lundqvist and Pål Skogmo for their trust in the venture and their encouragement. For funding assistance for final publication of the book we are deeply thankful to the Mulago Foundation, to the Liliane Foundation Support Fund, and to Sti. Kinderpostzegels in the Netherlands.

Finally, as always, my deep appreciation goes to Gertrude (Trude) Bock, who has contributed her home and her heart not only to making this and my earlier books a success, but also to giving the hundreds of disabled children whom she has cared for new hope and greater opportunities.

David Werner

How to Use This Book

This is **an "idea book" about problem solving**—not a "cookbook" with precise instructions and measurements for making pre-designed aids and equipment. It is about **thinking problems through** rather than just following instructions. Nevertheless, you can use it as **a reference book** concerning different disabilities, assistive devices, and methods of problem solving.

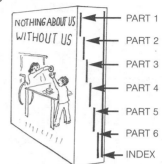

The book is divided into an **Introduction** and **6 Parts.** We suggest you **start by reading the main Introduction.** This gives an overview of the book's purpose and content. Each of the 6 Parts also has its own helpful introduction. Page-edges of these introductions are marked with short black lines. The book's index has page-edges marked with a long black line.

TO FIND WHAT YOU ARE LOOKING FOR IN THE BOOK, YOU CAN USE:

- The list of **CONTENTS** at the beginning of the book. This lists all the Parts and Chapters in the order that they appear in the book, and it gives page numbers.

- The **INDEX** at the end of the book (the pages with the whole outer edge black, starting on page 345). This lists in **alphabetical order** (a, b, c, d, and so on) all the topics or names that you may want to look up. **The Index is coded in this way:**

  - Names of persons who appear in the stories are listed in the Index alphabetically by their first name, like this: CARINA; EDGAR; MARI PICOS.

  - Names of assistive devices and technologies appear like this: **braces; communication boards; wheelchairs.**

  - Names of different disabilities or problems are listed like this: *blindness; speech problems; spinal-cord injury.*

  - All other entries are listed in ordinary letters, like this: Child-to-Child activities; India; land mines; women's rights.

If you cannot find what you are looking for, look under a similar name. For example, if you don't find *infantile paralysis*, look under *polio* or *paralysis*.

KEY PLAYERS. Most of the stories in this book come from PROJIMO, a community based rehabilitation program run by disabled villagers in Mexico. After the main Introduction to the book, there is a brief description of some of the **members of the PROJIMO team,** including MARI, CONCHITA, and MARCELO, whom you will meet often in the stories.

For further information on innovative technologies, or on groups to contact, see the two resource lists at the end of the book (just before the Index):

- **Resource List 1: Organizations and Programs,** page 341;
- **Resource List 2: Reading and Teaching Materials** page 343.

Please note: The first 4 Parts of this book focus on creating aids and equipment. **The last 2 Parts look at innovative approaches to the integration and participation of disabled persons** in the home, community, school, and work place.*

---

* Because this book is organized around individuals and their needs rather than by kinds of disability or assistive devices, to find information on a particular disability or device—such as *cerebral palsy*, or **special seats**—you may need to refer to several chapters or even Parts of the book. For this you will find the Index especially helpful.

CONTENTS

An Invitation to Readers
to Contribute Ideas to Another, Similar Book

We hope that this book is only the beginning of an ongoing, still very incomplete process of sharing helpful ideas. It tells personal stories of the search for solutions by folks who mostly live in one small corner of the world (western Mexico). And it focuses mainly on physical disabilities, because that is the area in which PROJIMO (the village program that gave life to this book) happens to have the most experience.

Likewise, the stories told here and the solutions found may not be the most instructive or appropriate (even locally). We work with what we have, within our limitations. However, **it is better to share blemished fruit than none at all.**

We imagine that many of you—the readers of this book—are disabled, or that you relate to or work with persons with a disability. Many of you have your own great stories of how you have searched for and discovered solutions. On reading this book, perhaps some of you will get ideas for more useful innovations than the ones we describe. (**We hope the book will inspire you to try out your own clever ideas—not just ours!**)

Among disabled persons around the world, their families, friends, and those who work with them, there is a wealth of exciting ideas, rich experiences, and innovative solutions (or partial solutions). **This book just touches the surface of what is possible.**

So, here is our invitation:

We hope that you, the readers of this book, will send us your own stories and experiences. Let us hear from you about innovations, gadgets, "appropriate technologies," and "easier ways of doing things"—discoveries that you would like to share with others. If possible, include drawings, photos, or both. (See page 340, on Suggestions for Effective Information-Sharing in Print.)

There are 3 ways in which we may be able to share your contributions:

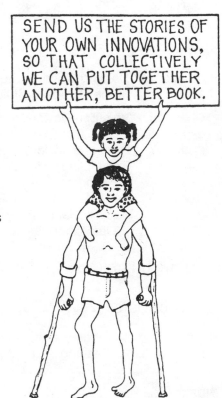

SEND US THE STORIES OF YOUR OWN INNOVATIONS, SO THAT COLLECTIVELY WE CAN PUT TOGETHER ANOTHER, BETTER BOOK.

- We can share them with the PROJIMO team of disabled village rehabilitation workers. Your findings may **trigger their imaginations** to experiment with new ideas, designs and possibilities, adapting them to their own local resources and reality.

- We hope to include some stories in our *Newsletter from the Sierra Madre,* which reaches health and disability workers in 130 countries. (Write to us at HealthWrights if you might like to subscribe.)

- If we get enough good ideas, we may put together another book similar to this one, but hopefully even more useful because it will be more of a world-wide, cooperative venture.

In describing your innovations, **please tell enough about the local situation and the people involved** to make the stories personal and heart-warming. Try to show that **technology should serve people,** rather than people serving technology.

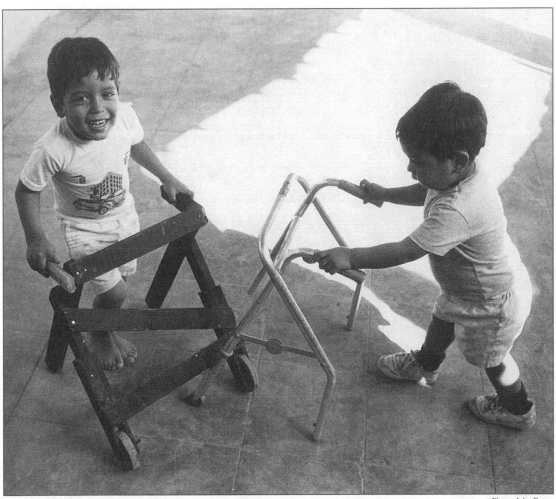

Photo: John Fago

The Old and the New—Each Has Its Place

The wooden walker, with its bigger wheels, rolls better on rough ground than the "modern" aluminum walker. The wooden front wheels act as brakes when the child puts his weight on them to step forward—a feature the aluminum walker lacks (see page 53). Also, because the wooden walker is heavier it gives more stability to the child with unsure balance.

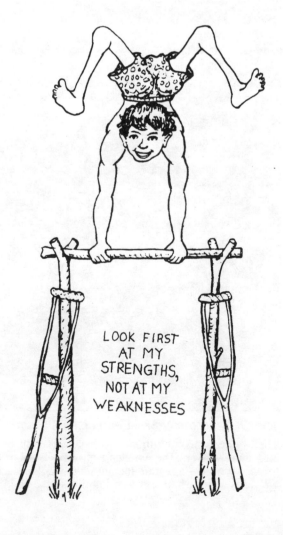

LOOK FIRST
AT MY
STRENGTHS,
NOT AT MY
WEAKNESSES

INTRODUCTION
Disabled Persons as Leaders in the Problem-Solving Process

This is a book of *true stories about people's creative search for solutions.* Written for disabled persons and their relatives, friends, and helpers, its purpose is *to share exciting, useful ideas,* and *to spark the reader's imagination:* to stimulate *a spirit of adventure!*

This book differs from most manuals on disability aids and equipment in 4 basic ways:

1. We make an effort to put the **person** and the **process** before the **product.** The 50 chapters cover a wide selection of disability aids that are relatively easy to make at home or in a village. But in presenting each innovation, emphasis is put less on the end-product (however important) than on the **cooperative process of discovery.**

In this approach, the *disabled person (and/or family members) often takes the lead, working as a partner and equal with service providers, technicians, or local crafts-persons.* With this sort of **partnership approach,** results tend to be more enabling than when assistive equipment is unilaterally prescribed or designed.

2. *Our goal is* **not replication,** *but rather* **adaptability** *and* **shared creativity.** *True,* most aids shown here can be easily replicated (copied exactly) at low cost at home or in a village workshop. However, placing strong emphasis on *replication* can be counter-productive . . . especially in the field of rehabilitation where *the needs, possibilities and dreams of each disabled person are different.* Too often, the routine construction of standardized designs contributes to a habit of trying to *adapt the disabled person to the assistive device,* rather than trying to *adapt the device to the disabled person.*

Therefore:

> Our objective is not to catalogue a set of aids and equipment to be copied, but to share an EMPOWERING PROBLEM-SOLVING APPROACH.

3. In most examples in this book, *we start by looking at an individual disabled person.* Placing that individual as central to the problem-solving process, we explore her or his unique combination of wishes and needs. Then we describe the cooperative, trial-and-error methods used in designing and testing possible solutions. The problem-solving is ongoing and open-ended. It may include anything from learning new skills or modifying the environment, to the invention or adaptation (or elimination) of an assistive device.

4. *Most of the rehabilitation workers and technicians responsible for the innovations in this book are themselves disabled.* Because they too have a disability, they are more inclined to work with a disabled "client" as a partner and equal in the problem-solving adventure. Also, being disabled, they often have insights (an insider's view) leading to new approaches that help enable the disabled individual with whom they work.

PROJIMO

Most of the innovations explored on these pages were created in PROJIMO: *Program of Rehabilitation Organized by Disabled Youth of Western Mexico.* This small community-oriented program is based in Ajoya, a village of 1000 inhabitants in the mountains of Western Mexico. The author of this book—himself disabled (see Chapter 11)—has worked as a facilitator and advisor to the program since it began in 1981. On the next page we give a brief account of how PROJIMO differs from similar community programs. For more information on the program we suggest you look at *Disabled Village Children,* a handbook which grew out of PROJIMO (see page 343). Or write to us at HealthWrights.

How PROJIMO Differs from Many CBR Programs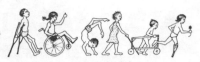

PROJIMO—the program in Mexico run by disabled villagers where most of the innovations in this book come from—differs from many Community Based Rehabilitation (CBR) programs in that:

- PROJIMO was started by, and is organized and run by disabled villagers.

- It grew out of and is linked to a villager-run primary health care program.

- The program includes a village-based rehabilitation center where disabled persons and family members can learn skills, take part in the creation of assistive equipment, and help and learn from each other.

- Services are provided, and assistive equipment is made by disabled persons who learn their skills mainly through apprenticeship, from one another and from volunteer rehabilitation professionals and skilled technicians. (These "experts" are asked to devote their short visits to teaching skills rather than providing services.)

- The quality and thought that goes into this work has developed beyond what you find in many community programs—because the PROJIMO workers have had years of challenging interchange with exceptional leaders in different fields of disability. Indeed, aids and equipment designed for and with disabled individuals sometimes meet their specific needs more effectively than those provided by large urban rehabilitation centers, and at a much lower cost.

PROJIMO's Need for Creative Problem Solving

Since its beginning, PROJIMO has been fairly innovative, not only technically but in its overall organization and structure. The disabled workers take pride in running their program on their own terms and in experimenting with participatory models of decision-making, management, and funding. In each of these areas they have had striking successes and failures. The program has evolved through a series of productive crises, the worst of which have threatened to destroy the program (see below). But each crisis somehow forces the team to re-evaluate its methods and to experiment with alternative approaches, which at times prove to be major steps forward.

PROJIMO began with the intention of serving physically disabled children. But soon children (and adults) with other disabilities, including developmental delay and multiple impairments, were brought for help. So the team has sought to expand its capabilities to meet these needs. But it is still most skilled and innovative with physical disability, an imbalance reflected in this book.

The Disabling Effect of Growing Poverty and Violence

Ironically, the biggest challenge to PROJIMO's survival has come about with the increase in spinal-cord injured teenagers and young adults. In the last decade, hundreds of these youths—most disabled by bullet wounds—have found their way to PROJIMO from all over Mexico. Their numbers reflect the mushrooming sub-culture of violence. As in much of the Third World, poverty, landlessness, and unemployment have grown with Mexico's structural adjustment to "free trade" and the inequities of the global economy. The widening gap between rich and poor leads to an increase in crime, alcoholism, drug trafficking, street-children, armed gangs, and wide-spread social unrest. The state reacts with ever harsher repression, corruption, police brutality, and institutionalized violence. All this has led to a substantial increase in disability, especially among young men.

NEW CHALLENGES FOR HARD TIMES. The youths arriving from this devastating *sub-culture of violence* are often both physically and psycho-socially disabled. Their habits with alcohol, drugs, and violence are deeply ingrained. PROJIMO has tried to set rules and has initiated peer counseling, but with mixed or delayed results. Meanwhile, the program's reputation has suffered; parents are reluctant to bring their young children. So PROJIMO has increasingly become a program catering to disabled teens and young adults (especially those with spinal-cord injury). In the long run this upsetting change may be for the good. Many children who used to come to PROJIMO now go to emerging programs—some started by PROJIMO's disabled "graduates"— conveniently located in several states of Mexico. But PROJIMO is still the only one of these programs that attends physically and psycho-socially disabled street youth.

From Violence to Caring

Not all of the disabled youths coming to PROJIMO with a history of drugs and violence turn out well. But some go through heart-warming transformations. Perhaps because of their own difficult childhood, their hearts often go out to those disabled children who are least pleasing and most vulnerable. The following true story illustrates this.

QUIQUE AND JOSÉ. Not long ago, a 7-year-old brain-injured boy named José was temporarily abandoned by his family at PROJIMO. Limited by extensive physical and mental handicap, José was fretful and unresponsive. He had no urine or bowel control. Repeated attempts to toilet train him failed. Whenever his bowels moved (too often!) he smeared his feces (shit) over his body, face and hair. Even PROJIMO's coordinators, Mari and Conchita, who are themselves disabled and usually very loving with disabled children, were at the end of their wits and patience with José.

Then an amazing thing happened: a friendship developed between José and Quique. Quique, a young man paralyzed from the neck down (quadriplegic), had an angry, belligerent temper. Repeatedly he was expelled from PROJIMO for drug dealing, drunkenness, and trouble-making. One day Quique was lying on his gurney under a mango tree when, unexpectedly, he and little José began to communicate. José could not speak, but some-how Quique caught his interest. When Quique talked to him—not as a misfit but as a friend— the boy began to grunt and eventually smile. With effort José rolled his wheelchair next to Quique and slipped his filthy little fingers into Quique's gaunt, paralyzed hand. From that moment the two were inseparable.

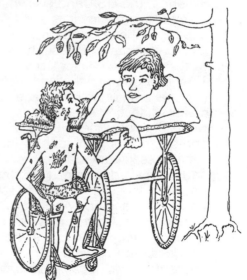

Quique assumed a protective responsibility for José. He demanded that the boy be bathed when he dirtied himself, and gently encouraged him to wash his own hands and feed himself. José began to show improvement in many ways, and smeared himself with his feces less often. Both he and Quique seemed happier.

Quique's strangely insightful, caring response to José was not unusual. Time and again, disabled youth who arrive socially scarred and violent have become among the most considerate care providers for those in greatest need.

Some of the most lovingly conceived innovations in this book were created by young disabled persons who emerged from the sub-culture of drug-trafficking and violence.

PROJIMO's Involvement With Innovative Participatory Technology

Toward the end of 1990, PROJIMO received a three year grant for Innovative Research from the Thrasher Research Fund in North America. Many of the innovations in this book were developed during this grant period, while some were developed before or after. In addition, to emphasize important points, a few innovations are included from other regions, ranging from India to Bangladesh and from Zimbabwe to Belize and Brazil.

Many of the innovations presented in this book have been developed by the PROJIMO team together with 3 sorts of participants:

1. **Disabled persons and family members** have been central to the problem solving process. Designs have been created to meet the expressed needs of disabled individuals and have been adapted, on their terms, to local social and environmental conditions, economic limitations, and locally available resources.

2. **Participants from community rehabilitation and disability programs in Mexico and Central America** have taken part in designing and building innovative aids during **short workshops** and **"educational exchanges."** Most of the participants were themselves disabled. Having a disability was considered a valued qualification, both for learners and facilitators. In this way, the methodology and "mystique" of the innovative approach has been widely shared.

3. **Volunteers from Europe, Latin America, the USA and elsewhere,** many of them innovators and experts in their respective fields, took part in most of these short workshops and mini-courses. They included prosthetists (leg makers), orthotists (brace makers), seating specialists, wheelchair designers, physical and occupational therapists, and instructors in early development and special education. Many (but not all) of these visiting specialists were also disabled. All came with an understanding that their role was *to teach rather than to provide services*, and *to work as partners and equals with local rehabilitation workers (mostly disabled villagers) and with disabled clients and their families.*

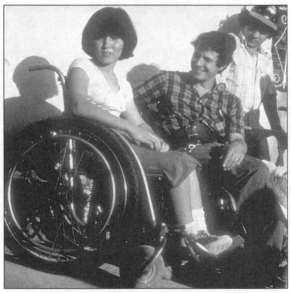

Ralf Hotchkiss, a wheelchair-riding engineer from California, with Concepción in a chair made in a wheelchair-making workshop at PROJIMO. Ralf has helped to design many great innovations together with disabled Third World wheelchair builders (see Chapter 30).

As a result of this unique combination of disabled community rehabilitation workers and disabled clients working together with visiting apprentices and outside specialists, many of the innovations described in this book have been created through a cooperative, equalizing process. As readers will notice, a lot of these aids and devices combine scientific sophistication and grassroots simplicity.

This sort of collective problem-solving process teaches us a lot. Above all, we learn to respect one another's contrasting insights and skills.

DISABLED PERSONS MAKE MAJOR BREAKTHROUGHS IN DESIGNS

A lot of professionals are unwilling to include disabled persons as partners in designing solutions to their needs, and often disabled persons are reluctant to assume such responsibility. Nevertheless:

> Many major breakthroughs in rehabilitation technology have been designed and created by disabled people themselves.

For blind people, of course, the most famous breakthrough was a brilliantly simple form of reading tiny raised dots with the finger-tips. This was invented by a blind French boy, Louis Braille. Rather than supporting his innovation, his teachers in the School for the Blind punished Louis and his classmates for experimenting with his new system. So they used it in secret! For those in positions of authority, it is often difficult when persons under their control take the lead. **In every sense the invention of Braille was revolutionary—and for blind people it was liberating.**

In recent years many of the most outstanding designs of communications aids, wheelchairs, and limbs have been developed by wheelchair riders, amputees, and other disabled persons. Dissatisfied with the equipment available to them, these persons invented something better.

THE BRAILLE ALPHABET

Louis Braille invented this dot alphabet at age 14. The dots are pressed into a thick paper from the opposite side with a pointed tool called a 'stylus'.

A major breakthrough in artificial limbs is the **flex foot,** which was invented by an amputee. When the person walks, the flexible foot-piece acts like a spring, simulating the push-off action of a normal foot. This makes walking easier, smoother, faster, and it takes less energy.

The lower leg and foot are made of a curved thin strip of **carbon fiber,** a strong, flexible space-age material.

The foot-piece bends more when the person steps on it, in effect loading the spring.

At the end of the step, the foot-piece gives a downward and forward push, propelling the person forward.

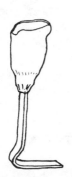

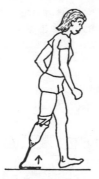

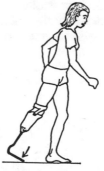

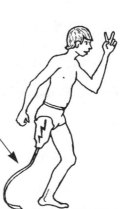

John Fago, a professional photographer who has an artificial leg, studied limb-making after visiting PROJIMO and then started making his own leg. Concerned more with function than appearance, he is designing a **flex leg** shaped like an upside-down question mark: ¿ — The entire leg acts like a spring, giving the user a powerful forward thrust. Also—with the help of a man who designs bamboo fishing poles—John is experimenting with making **a flex foot out of laminated bamboo,** instead of costly carbon fiber. His goal is to help poor communities to make flex-feet with local resources at low cost.

TECHNICAL AIDS AND EQUIPMENT ARE IMPORTANT

One reason for writing this book is that in many programs for disabled people in poor countries and communities, **too little attention is given to technical aids and assistive equipment.** The current trend is to down-play the technological side of rehabilitation. This comes both from disabled people's organizations and from planners of community based rehabilitation (CBR) programs:

- **Disabled activists and organizations** in the North are passionately concerned with disability rights. In their struggle to achieve a *Society for All*, they focus on social issues such as accessibility, equal opportunity for education, jobs, etc. They are less worried about technical aids. After all, most members of leading disabled people's organizations, especially in the North—and of Disabled Person's International, even in the South—belong to the middle class. They already have the essential personal aids they need. So their top priority is the struggle for their social rights. They have tended to project their own priorities onto the poor disabled people of the Third World, whose lack of assistive equipment (braces, wheelchairs, etc.) may be their biggest limitation.

- **The official World Health Organization (WHO) guidelines for CBR** have also (in the past more than at present) under-emphasized the importance of technical aids. Some CBR advocates assert that devoting attention to assistive equipment is a return to the "medical model" of rehabilitation, which they criticize (in large part, correctly) as being top-down, professional-dominated, costly, disempowering, and impractical. Technical information on assistive equipment in the WHO manual tends to be quite limited and superficial. Much stronger emphasis is placed on the social side of rehabilitation: schooling, skills training, job placement, community participation, etc.

It is true that social considerations are extremely important, and are still inadequately addressed in most urban "rehabilitation palaces." But **for millions of poor disabled persons, the lack of low-cost, appropriate mobility aids and assistive equipment is a major barrier to social integration—including schooling, jobs, and self-reliant living.**

For example, *wheelchair accessibility* is a big concern for those who have wheelchairs. But **95 percent of people who need a wheelchair don't have one.** Similarly, many who need leg braces or artificial limbs to subsist in difficult circumstances don't have them. Or they are given devices of such poor quality that they are of questionable benefit.

Appropriate aids can make a huge difference in terms of self-determination, social integration, and survival. But to create equipment that is appropriate, we need to work closely with the disabled persons concerned. We must consider the disabled person's unique combination of skills, wishes, impairments, opportunities, income, and motivation, as well as personal and environmental possibilities and constraints (within home and community). Designs may differ according to local resources, cost, accessibility, means of transportation to school or work, and the support system within the family and community.

ACHIEVING A *SOCIETY FOR ALL*: NEED FOR AN INTEGRATED APPROACH

To achieve a society in which disabled people can participate fully, 3 things are needed:

1. **Personal rehabilitation and assistive equipment** for improved function and mobility.

2. **Accessibility** in terms of the physical environment, transportation, etc.

3. **An accepting, welcoming attitude of the general population,** with readiness to provide equal opportunities. Supportive legislation can help open doorways to social rights.

Fulfilling only one or two of these requirements is not enough: all three must be achieved. The need for this integrated three-armed approach is pictured on the next page.

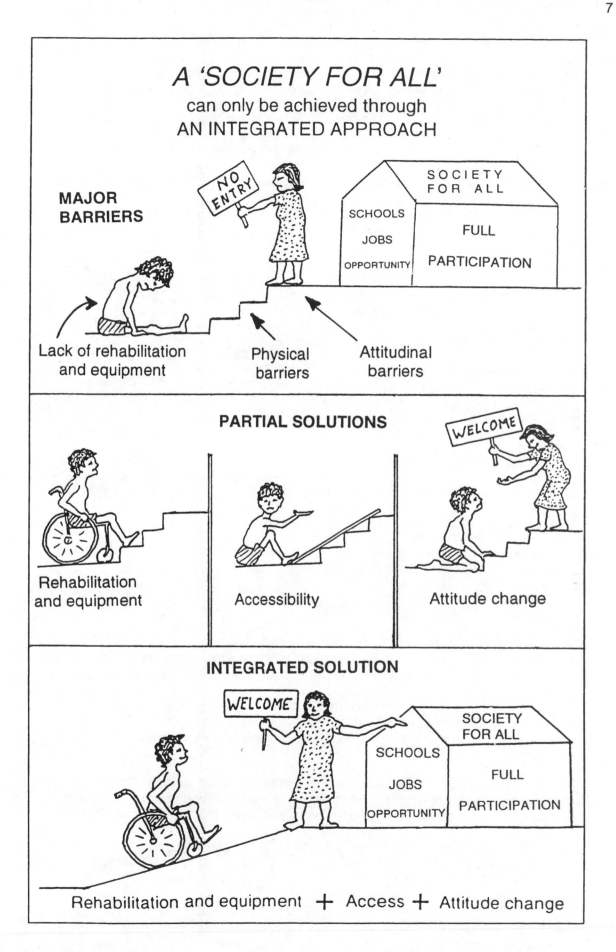

POVERTY AND DISABILITY: SURVIVAL COMES FIRST

Persons trained in the field of rehabilitation, as in other fields, tend to see people's needs in terms of their specialty. A rehabilitation worker, on seeing a disabled child in an urban slum, may think first of the child's disability-related needs. The worker may want to foster an "integrated approach," including assistive devices, access to schooling, and social involvement. But it is essential to remember that for that child and millions of other children, their basic health and survival needs come first.

 For many children, the biggest threat to their well-being is hunger

Most important for any child, whether disabled or not, is meeting her basic needs for food, shelter, and essential health care.

Too often, rehabilitation planners overlook or give too little attention to the economic limitations of the family. As a result, sometimes hundreds of dollars are spent on an orthopedic brace, hearing aid, or on special schooling—only to see the child die from untreated infection ... or from hunger.

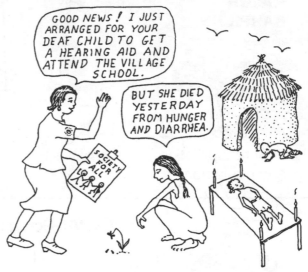

When including marginalized people in "development for all," it is essential to respond to their most urgent needs—as they see them.

Quite rightly, many community rehabilitation initiatives are putting more time and energy into helping disabled persons and their families find ways to produce food or add to their income. For example, some programs give a goat, rabbits, or chickens to a disabled child, and help her learn to care for and breed them.

Hard and Soft Technologies

Poverty and disability together put people, especially children, at double risk. Both must be dealt with. **People who are disadvantaged for whatever reasons need to *join in the struggle for equal rights and full participation in a fairer, more caring society.***

Therefore, when we think of "rehabilitation technology," it is important to consider not just the **hard technology of aids and equipment,** but also the **soft technology of ideas and action** that can help disabled persons to survive, meet their needs, and be more self-determined.

The last two Parts of this book look at innovative soft technologies. These include **activities and methods whereby disabled people can defend their rights, integrate into society, and learn skills to earn a living and keep the wolf from their door.**

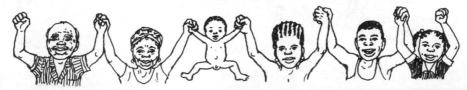

United action is needed to overcome the social disadvantages occurring with poverty and disability.

Adapting to Extreme Poverty in an African Squatter Settlement

One of the most innovative community based rehabilitation (CBR) programs that I (the author) have visited is in a huge shanty town called Matari Valley, in Nairobi, Kenya. This settlement was formed in colonial times by young women from rural areas who worked in the city as house girls and mistresses for white masters. When the girls got pregnant, they were thrown onto the streets and settled in Matari Valley. Today hundreds of thousands of single mothers survive there by brewing illegal liquor, selling their bodies, begging, and picking through garbage. A large number of children are disabled. Many mothers leave their disabled child shut up all day, sweltering in tar-paper shacks. The mothers do this, not by choice, but in their efforts to earn enough to feed their children at least one meal a day.

A CBR worker named Penina, who went to Matari Valley several years ago found that the first concern of mothers with disabled children was not "rehabilitation," assistive equipment, or schooling. **Their worries had to do with food, sickness, and survival.**

So Penina modified her rehabilitation plans. She put the survival and basic needs of the children first. She began by looking for ways to **help mothers earn a little income in their homes, so that they could spend more time with their children.** At times this meant giving mothers small loans to start selling lamp oil or charcoal. She helped groups of mothers form **child-care cooperatives,** so that they could take turns caring for one another's children while the rest sought outside work. She then helped mothers form sewing, chicken-raising and other **small work cooperatives** to produce an income and have **shared child-care where they work.**

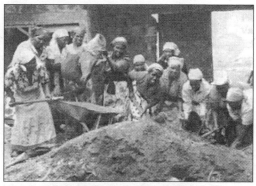

Mothers and grandmothers work together to build a cooperative bakery. Here they make mud bricks of earth mixed with straw.

Once the mothers were earning a bit more income, they could feed their children better and spend more time with them. So Penina began to introduce **early stimulation and developmental activities** into the child-care groups. From among those mothers who showed the most interest, love, and natural ability, she trained several to help as facilitators, teachers, and neighborhood rehabilitation assistants.

As day-to-day survival became less of a struggle, the mothers were able to devote more time to assisting their disabled children. Penina began to teach the mothers exercises and activities they could do in the home to help their children learn skills and become more independent. As much as was possible given the limited resources, she helped them to access the aids and services that they needed.

As the mothers began to see signs of improvements in their children, their confidence grew, both in themselves and in the potential of their children.

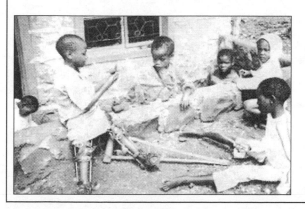

Eventually the mothers, with help from neighbors, built a modest community center (called *Maji Mazuri*) for meetings, rehabilitation, skills training, income generation, games, awareness-raising theater skits, and child-care. The women also built a cooperative bakery. **The initiative for disabled children became a spearhead for community development.**

Children at the Maji Mazuri Center

COMBINING THE BEST OF THE INDEPENDENT LIVING MOVEMENT AND CBR

In recent years, 2 major initiatives have evolved to help meet the needs, defend the rights, and promote the full integration of disabled people. These are the *Independent Living movement (IL)* and *Community Based Rehabilitation (CBR).* Active in many countries, both initiatives are a response to the discrimination, limited opportunities, inadequate services, and the need for self-determination that most disabled people experience in the world today.

The two movements have **different origins.** They also have **different strengths and weaknesses.** IL tends to be strong in areas where CBR is weakest, and CBR strongest in the areas where IL and disabled people's organizations sometimes are weak.

- INDEPENDENT LIVING: The IL movement was started from the bottom up by disabled people themselves. It began in the Western industrialized countries. Through organizations like Disabled People International (DPI), it has gradually made headway in the so-called developing countries. IL's biggest strength is **social action for equal opportunities, led by disabled activists.** Its biggest weakness is that it is largely a middle-class movement that often leaves out the poor. Also, living "independently" (or alone) is a very Western value. In societies with a strong sense of community, rooted in extended families, living "inter-dependently" (together) may be a more welcome goal.

- COMMUNITY BASED REHABILITATION: CBR, as an international initiative, was launched by idealistic rehabilitation experts working with the World Health Organization (WHO). Its biggest strength is that **it tries to reach all disabled people, especially those who are poorest and in greatest need.** It has an all-inclusive plan, including both government and private initiatives. But, too often, disabled persons still are treated as objects to be worked upon, rather than leaders, organizers and decision makers.

One of the biggest challenges for disability workers today is to find ways to **link the empowering self-determination of the Independent Living Movement with the broad outreach to poor people of Community Based Rehabilitation.**

A good place to begin is by encouraging disabled persons to take over more of the organizational and service-providing roles in CBR programs. Where possible, disabled people's organizations can lead or advise the programs (while making an active effort to include the poor and voiceless). *When disabled people learn to design and make assistive equipment, and to include the user in the process, success is more likely.*

Community Based Rehabilitation (CBR)	Disabled Person's Organizations Independent Living (DPI, etc.)
Major STRENGTHS:	Major STRENGTHS:
Rehab for all! Tries to reach all disabled people, with most concern for the poor. Comprehensive plan with social focus. Community education and involvement.	**Self-determination!** Disabled people take lead in defining their needs and demanding their rights. Goal is not to normalize disabled persons, but to stop society's unfairness.
Major WEAKNESSES:	Major WEAKNESSES:
Usually organized for—not by—disabled people. Structure often top-down. Tends to follow pre-determined recipes, rather than to seek liberating solutions.	Because members tend to be middle class, the poor are often left out, or their needs are misinterpreted to fit the priorities of Western disability activists.

TROUBLE-SHOOTING THE TIDE OF INAPPROPRIATE TECHNOLOGY

Some readers may wonder if this book is needed. Lots of manuals and pamphlets on assistive aids and equipment already exist. They range from high-power rehabilitation engineering to simple (sometimes overly simplified) collections of helpful low-cost gadgets. Some of these guide books have marvelous designs. But too often, more importance is given to the equipment itself than to the persons who may use it. Precise steps for construction are spelled out as if the final product were an end in itself.

There is a need for guides that put more emphasis on listening to disabled persons' wishes and suggestions, jointly evaluating their needs, experimenting to improve the design of assistive equipment, and adapting it accordingly.

The author and his co-workers have visited rehabilitation programs, both hospital-based and community-based, in many countries. **In program after program, we see well-made, attractive rehabilitation aids that simply do not meet users' needs.** (The same is true for exercises and therapy.) Often equipment is beautifully and skillfully produced following detailed instructions in guide books or training plans. But for some reason the end results do not provide the expected benefits or satisfaction.

> Not enough attention is paid to the specific needs, wishes, and ideas of the disabled person and family members.

At worst, assistive devices and exercises become dehumanizingly generic—ritualistic rather than functional. Around the world, two of the most poorly fitted disability aids are **parallel bars** and **special seating.** Here we will look briefly at parallel bars. We look at problems with special seating in Part 1.

Parallel Bars: Therapy or Torture?

Photographs or drawings of rustic parallel bars made of poles supported by forked sticks appear on fancy brochures of major CBR programs around the world. But on close inspection, as often as not, the bars are inappropriate for the child using them.

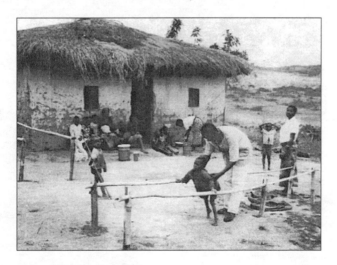

Here is an example from an international brochure showing a CBR program in Burundi, Africa.

What problems can you see with the parallel bars used for this child's rehabilitation?

Correct! **These bars are too high and far apart.** The child, who has weak legs, must bear most of his weight on his arms. This requires enormous strength. Only powerful athletes can support their full weight on out-stretched arms, as when they perform the iron cross on gymnastic rings. To make a child with flail legs try to do this on bars can turn therapy into torture.

PARALLEL BARS should be built or adjusted to the height and width best suited for the needs of the individual. Usually, placing the bars fairly close together (so the person's arms are next to her sides), at a height so her arms are almost straight when standing upright, is the easiest and most functional position.

Often this position creates difficulties.

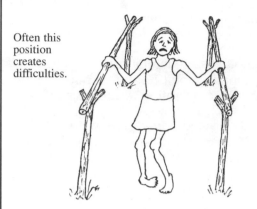

Often this position works better.

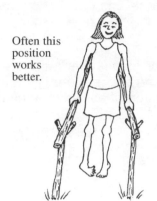
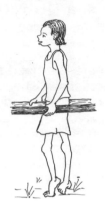

However, depending on muscle strength of the arms and hands, and other factors, some persons may find other positions or heights work better. For example:

A child who has strong legs but lacks balance may find it easier to walk with bars widely separated.

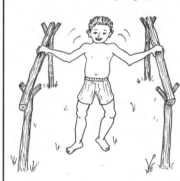

A child with weak upper arms may find it easier to rest his forearms on the bars. The bars will need to be elbow high.

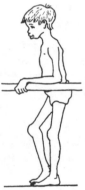

A child who tends to slump forward may find it easier to stand straight if the bars are high, so that he has to stand upright to rest his arms on them.

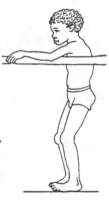

It is essential to pay attention to the concerns of the person who will use the equipment. Even a child who can not speak may have ways of communicating her preferences (through tears or smiles).

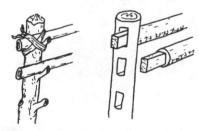

It helps if bars can adjust to different heights for different children (and to find out what height works best for an individual child). Above are 2 easy ways.

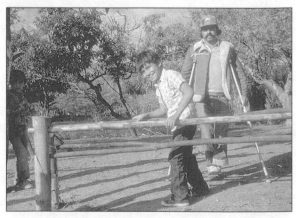

A child with cerebral palsy who has trouble controlling his arms experiments with multiple bars placed in different positions to find out what height and width work best for him.

Usually the best person to decide what works best is the disabled person herself.

The Need for Careful Evaluation of Instructional Materials

Unfortunately, photographs or drawings of assistive equipment are not always critically evaluated before they are included in training manuals. Likewise, many instructional materials—and training courses—do not put enough emphasis on thoughtful, innovative participatory problem-solving. There has been a tendency, especially in community based programs, to deliver overly simple cookbook-like formulas for solving the needs of disabled people. High-level decision makers often try to find answers to the problems of marginalized people through impersonal, standardized shortcuts (the technological quick fix) rather than through listening and responding to the wishes of those in need. In sum:

Today there is too much *doing things for people,* not enough *doing things with them ...* too much giving authoritative instructions and following of recipes, and too little creative, participatory problem-solving. Disadvantaged persons are reduced to objects, things to be worked upon, tinkered with, corrected, and normalized, rather than treated as unique individuals to be empowered on their own terms. Too often the disabled person—especially the child—is left out of the problem-solving process.

There is an urgent need for training materials and courses to place less emphasis on following standardized instructions, and more emphasis on an observant, problem-solving approach in which the disabled person and family members are included and listened to as equals.

Disabled Persons and Groups Take the Lead in Designing Better Solutions

To solve their problems, disabled people in some countries have begun to play a leading role. Especially in the North, but increasingly in the Third World, disabled people have organized and are demanding a say in decisions that affect their lives. Through the Independent Living Movement (IL), and increasingly through Disabled People International (DPI), they insist on social rights and equal opportunity in such things as accessibility, education, employment, and recreation. They demand a leading voice in programs and policy-making that affect them.

In many countries, organizations of persons with disabilities have adopted the slogan: "NOTHING ABOUT US WITHOUT US." But while disabled activists insist on self-determination concerning social issues that affect them, they have been slower to assume leadership in matters of rehabilitation and technical aids. Even in the North, most disabled persons still follow the dictates of rehabilitation professionals fairly

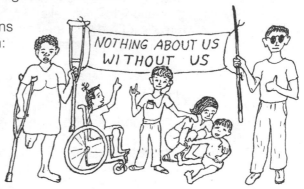

passively, without assuming much decision-making control. Disabled children, especially, have almost no voice in deciding what aids or equipment they are to use. This leads to errors in design that could be avoided. The author himself (David Werner) as a child was given orthopedic aids that did him more harm than good. Not until decades later did he at last obtain appliances that worked well for him ... thanks to a disabled village brace-maker at PROJIMO who included him as a partner in the problem-solving process (see Chapter 11).

ADAPTING SOLUTIONS TO THE LOCAL SITUATION AND INDIVIDUAL NEEDS

Throughout the Third World you see small children in adult-sized wheelchairs, and small thin adults in big, very wide, heavy chairs that they can barely move.

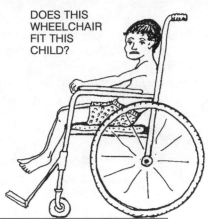

DOES THIS WHEELCHAIR FIT THIS CHILD?

A common shortcoming of large rehabilitation centers is that aids and equipment tend to be standardized and "generic" (a few basic models are intended to meet the needs of all). This is especially true when equipment is purchased in quantity from commercial (or foreign) producers. When standard commercial aids are prescribed, too often an attempt is made to adapt the person to the equipment rather than the equipment to the person.

> Disabled persons' needs differ, not only individually but also according to local customs, living conditions and environment.

A potential advantage of a small community-based rehabilitation center is that aids and equipment can be custom-made for each individual as the need arises, often at remarkably low cost. Such an approach allows greater flexibility in terms of personal preferences, as well as adaptation to local circumstances, resources, and environment.

Four Women with Spinal-Cord Injury: Their Different Mobility Needs

Consider for example, 4 young women, all about 20 years old, each with a spinal-cord injury of the mid back. These are *MIRA* from a village in Bangladesh; *RITA* from the mountains in Mexico; *LUZ* from a city in the Philippines; and *FARAH* from Egypt. Each, after loving support and encouragement from family and community, got over her initial depression and is eager to continue with life, earn a living, and take an active part in society. But to do so, each needs an effective means of mobility: a way to move around and go where she wants to, in spite of paralysis of the lower half of her body.

Let us suppose that each of these young women—Mira, Rita, Luz, and Farah—has had the luck to be given a costly imported wheelchair by an international donor called "Wheels of Fortune." At first, all four women were delighted with their shiny new imported wheelchairs. But within just a few months, all stopped using them.

Wheels of Fortune learned that this **low use-rate of donated equipment** was disturbingly common. So it sent a team of "social marketing" experts from the North (who did not speak the local languages) to analyze the problem. The experts concluded that "the recipients don't appreciate or care for things given to them free." Their solution was: "Require each recipient to pay at least part of the cost of all aids and equipment." With such *cost-sharing,* the experts insisted, "recipients will value more and take better care of the equipment they receive."

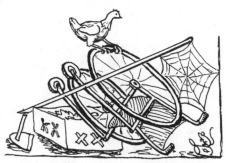

The four young women see the problem differently. If we were to ask them to analyze and state their concerns, we might find that each has good reasons for not using her chair. She would most likely insist that, **"If I had a chair that really helped me to move and do things more easily, I would gladly use and care for it!"**

Now let us imagine a different scenario. Let us suppose there are community rehabilitation workers who listen to each of the four young women and help them figure out the best local solution to their mobility needs. Together, they may be able to design more appropriate alternatives—liberating solutions that free the user to lead a fuller life in her home and community.

Here we present, briefly, the stories of these 4 young women. Though imaginary, their stories are based on reality. The solutions they find to their specific problems within their particular environments are based on actual innovations developed by concerned people in different parts of the world.

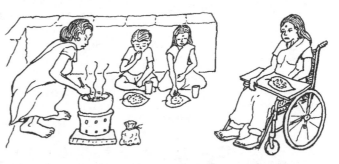

MIRA, **in rural Bangladesh,** became paraplegic (paralyzed from waist down) as a result of fighting between religious groups in her village. In the hospital, a social worker gave her a wheelchair from Wheels of Fortune. On the hospital floors, Mira learned to move about in her chair. But on returning to her village, she had problems. Traditionally, cooking was done at floor level on a cooking pot called a *chula.* Everyone ate sitting cross-legged on the floor. **In her wheelchair, Mira was separated from her kitchen work and from the family at mealtime.** For a while she sat in her chair without working; others served her food onto a board across the armrests. But Mira wanted to fit in better and to contribute more to family life. So she stopped using her wheelchair and began dragging herself around the dirt floor on her hands and backside. Maybe it was not the best solution, she thought. (It could cause severe and infected pressure sores. See Chapter 27.) But it was better than the isolation of sitting in her wheelchair.

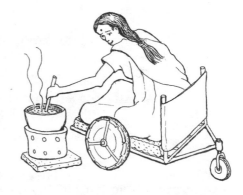

Solution: An answer to the needs of village women like Mira was found at the *Center for Rehabilitation of the Paralyzed* in Dhaka, Bangladesh. The Center is staffed and run mostly by spinal-cord injured persons who seek solutions to their own and other disabled persons' needs. They designed a "low-rider" wheelchair, or **trolley** to meet village women's need to cook and eat at ground level. First they created several working models. Then, in response to feedback and suggestions from different spinal-cord injured villagers, they adapted and modified the design. The trolley can even be used as a toilet (see page 194).

Because the chair is made completely of local materials and is fairly low-cost, it can be easily maintained at the village level. These low-riding trolleys have made it possible for women like Mira to return to their village homes and function effectively.

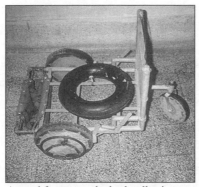

A metal-frame, wood-wheel trolley in Bangladesh. The rubber tube serves as a cushion and also as a toilet seat.

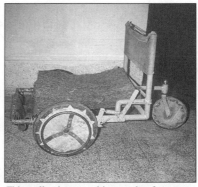

This trolley has a cushion made of coconut fiber coated with rubber. Firm but spongy, it helps prevent pressure sores (see p. 156).

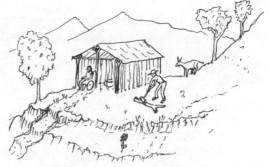

RITA lives in the mountains of Mexico in a small, pole-walled hut. She broke her lower back when she fell carrying water from a ravine. Like Mira, Rita's fancy wheelchair is of little use at home. She cannot ride it on the rough, narrow trails. Her hut has 2 small rooms for 8 people. The tiny kitchen has a big mud stove and no room to move around in a wheelchair. The kitchen counter, also made of mud, is at a height made for working standing up. And there is no space under it to position a wheel-chair. **There is simply no way for Rita to move or work effectively in her wheelchair.** Her stepmother sees Rita as useless and has begun to resent her presence.

Solution: If after her accident, Rita's rehabilitation workers had involved her in thinking through her therapy and assistive equipment, they might have found more useful alternatives. They would have realized how unsuited her environment is for a wheelchair (especially a clumsy, oversized one). Because her injury was low on her spine (L4), **it may make more sense to see if she can learn to walk with crutches— or at least figure out a way to stand up to work in the kitchen.** To do this, **leg braces** might help: possibly simple, lightweight ones made from plastic (see Part 2).

To prepare for standing and walking, Rita will need an **exercise program (1) to strengthen her arms and upper body,** and **(2) to maintain or increase the range of motion of her hips and knees.** If she can gradually stretch her hips and knee joints until they bend backwards a little, she may be able to stand and even walk (with crutches) without the need for long-leg braces. She can do this by "locking" her legs in a back-knee position, and by leaning her upper body backwards to stabilize her hips. She may even be able to work standing up, with her hands free (without her crutches).

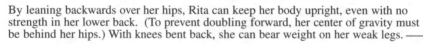

By leaning backwards over her hips, Rita can keep her body upright, even with no strength in her lower back. (To prevent doubling forward, her center of gravity must be behind her hips.) With knees bent back, she can bear weight on her weak legs. ➡

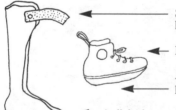

Simple below-the-knee **plastic braces** prevent foot-drop and help her avoid ankle-twisting on rough paths.

Rocker-bottom shoes allow a smoother gait (walking).

A flat area in the middle of the shoe soles permits greater stability for standing.

⬅ A slight downward angle of the foot pushes the knee back, adding stability.

With practice, Rita should be able to work standing in the kitchen. **A strap around her hips** may let her work more freely and securely.

With effort, she may even learn to walk with crutches on the steep trails. But she will need to develop **good balance, strong arms, and not get over-weight.**

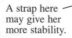

A strap here may give her more stability.

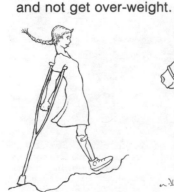

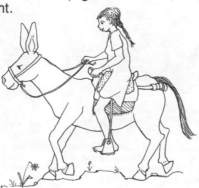

Perhaps the best solution for travel on the steep trails will be for Rita to learn to **ride the family donkey.**

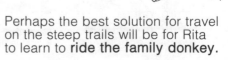

Luz lives in a crowded squatter town in the Philippines. Before her accident she worked as a *health visitor,* checking the weight of young children in their homes and giving nutritional advice to mothers. After her accident, she found that **her new imported wheelchair was too wide for narrow pathways or to fit through the very narrow doorways of many of the shacks.**

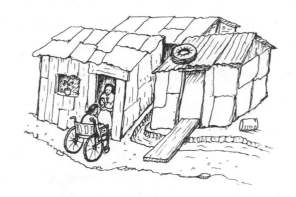

Solution: Fortunately, a program run by disabled persons called *House With No Stairs* (see page 342), has for years been experimenting with innovative designs of lightweight, low-cost wheelchairs. One of these has a horizontal folding mechanism (rather than a vertical "X"). This allows the user to easily make the chair narrower while riding it.*

So after they discussed Luz's needs with her, the workers took her measurements and went to work building her a **wheelchair with adjustable width.**

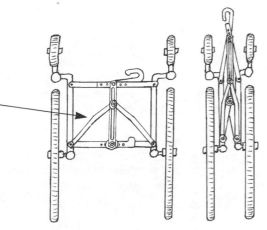

Folding mechanism as seen from underneath

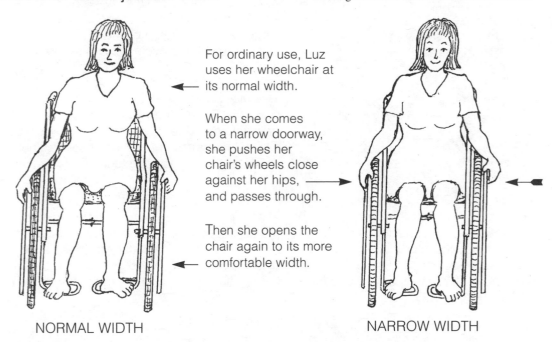

For ordinary use, Luz uses her wheelchair at its normal width.

When she comes to a narrow doorway, she pushes her chair's wheels close against her hips, and passes through.

Then she opens the chair again to its more comfortable width.

NORMAL WIDTH

NARROW WIDTH

Thanks to a wheelchair that was designed to help her overcome the barrier of narrow doorways, Luz was able to continue her work and earn a living helping other people.

---

* This innovation for pulling the wheels in close to the body in order to pass through narrow doorways has been further developed by Ralf Hotchkiss, a paraplegic wheelchair designer who has spent years teaching disabled groups to make and design locally appropriate wheelchairs. Among many others, Ralf has worked with the *House With No Stairs* wheelchair building team in the Philippines. For more discussion about this and Ralf's many wheelchair innovations, see Chapter 30.

FARAH lives in the Egyptian desert. Since her accident she has joined a women's cooperative where she can make clothing on a sewing machine, and sell it in local stores. But the cooperative is in another village, about 2 miles away on a sandy, rocky road. The narrow wheels of her imported wheelchair sink into the sand, making travel impossible.

Solution: Farah described her frustration with getting stuck in the sand and rocks to the local community based rehabilitation team. Together they tried to come up with a solution. They thought of putting extra wide bicycle tires on the wheelchair, so it would not sink in the sand. But they could not find tires that matched the wheels of her chair.

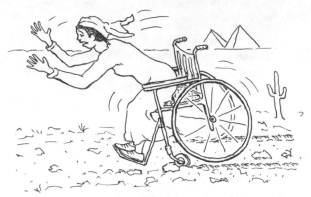

So they made a new, simple wheelchair using wide bicycle wheels. For the small front wheels they used thick disks made with several layers of plywood, covered with a wide strip of car tire. When Farah tried her new chair, the small front tires sunk somewhat less in the sand. But they got caught easily on small rocks. The wheelchair stopped so suddenly that sometimes Farah was almost thrown out of her chair.

Farah suggested bigger front wheels. But the CBR team pointed out that if the front castor wheels were larger, they would bump into the footrests on making a turn. What to do?

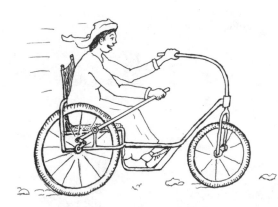

One of the CBR workers remembered a picture he had seen of a "tricycle wheelchair" with a single large front wheel, mounted in front of the footrests. So the team built a "trike" for Farah using extra wide bicycle tires on all 3 large wheels.*

The trike, powered by a hand lever, was a great success. Farah found it ran well on the sand and gravel roads. She could make it move so fast that it sailed through soft patches of sand without slowing down or getting stuck. She loved it!

In conclusion . . . The 4 young women—Mira, Rita, Luz, and Farah—all found different solutions to their different local and personal needs. This was possible because local rehabilitation workers listened to the women and involved them in planning and testing various innovations and adaptations. For 3 of the women, the solutions involved specially designed wheelchairs. But for Rita—who lived where wheelchair mobility was virtually impossible—it meant learning to stand and walk with braces, and riding the family donkey.

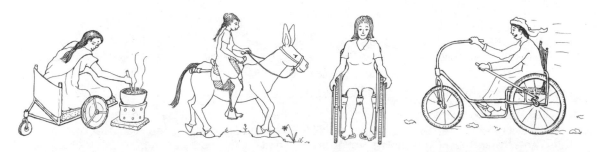

*There are many designs for tricycle wheelchairs, powered by one or two hands. See Chapter 31.

Examples from Real Life

While the stories of the four women with their different wheelchair needs are imaginary, they are based on experiences of real women. "Low-rider" wheelchairs or "trollies," such as the one adapted for Mira's needs, are produced for paraplegic women in Bangladesh by the *Center for Rehabilitation of the Paralyzed.*

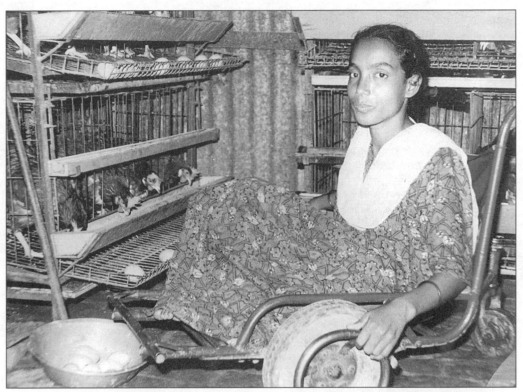

This woman in Bangladesh uses a trolley in her home business, raising chicken and selling eggs. Having an income of her own increases her independence and wins her community's respect. Photo by Shahidul Haque for *Social Assistance and Rehabilitation for the Physically Vulnerable* (SARPV).

Wheeled cots can also be adapted to local customs.

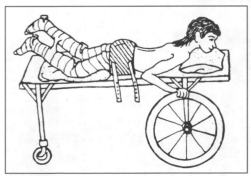

In most countries, trollies (wheeled cots or gurneys) are at a height so the person can eat and work at a table. This boy is on a gurney in order to remain active while his hip and knee contractures are straightened. (For more on gurneys and trollies, see Chapter 37.)

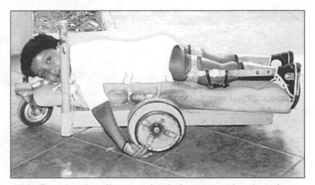

This floor-level trolley, or wheeled cot, was developed by the same program in Bangladesh that builds low-rider wheelchairs. It allows this boy to join his family for meals on the floor. (The boy needs to lie on his belly to heal pressure sores on his backside and to correct his hip contractures.)

About the PROJIMO Team

Many of the innovations described in this book were developed at PROJIMO, the village rehabilitation program in the mountains of western Mexico. As we explained in the Introduction, the program is staffed mostly by young disabled villagers. Because you will meet PROJIMO team members in various chapters, we thought you might like to know a bit about them. Most come from poor families and have lived through very difficult times. They first came to the program for their own rehabilitation, then decided to stay longer, learn new skills, and work together to help others. Many speak of their experience at PROJIMO as a kind of liberation or even a "return to life." Each has a fascinating story. Here we will say only a few words about some of the key members of the team.

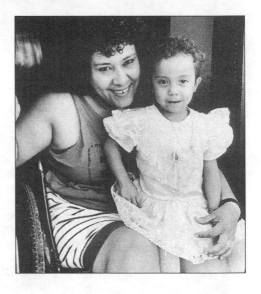

MARI AND ARMANDO. Mari Picos is one of the coordinators of PROJIMO. She was paralyzed from the waist down (paraplegic) in a car accident on her honeymoon. For two years she stayed in a dark room, unwilling to accept her disability or use a wheelchair. Twice she tried to kill herself. She was first taken to PROJIMO against her will. But in the course of her own rehabilitation, her heart went out to some of the disabled children. Eventually she became one of the leaders and organizers of the program. She became skilled at evaluating disability needs, peer counseling, brace-making, and at treating medical problems such as pressure sores, urinary infections, and epilepsy. She married Armando, now runs her own home, and they have a delightful daughter, Lluvia (meaning rain).

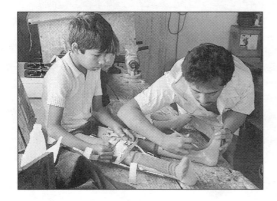

Armando Nevárez had polio affecting all four limbs. Doctors said he would never be able to walk. But they were wrong. PROJIMO helped him to get surgery and to begin to walk with leg braces and crutches. Armando became a skilled brace maker and now runs the wheelchair shop. He married Mari and usually treats her as an equal (which makes him exceptional in more ways than one).

CONCHITA AND MIGUEL. Conchita Lara became paraplegic from a fall when she was a teenager. For 4 years she was totally dependent on her family and very depressed. At PROJIMO, in her words, she "returned to life." Today, with Mari, she helps coordinate the program, makes artificial limbs, and does the program's accounting. She married Miguel Zamora, who is a driver and handyman for the program. They have two lovely children. Conchita's story is told in Chapter 42.

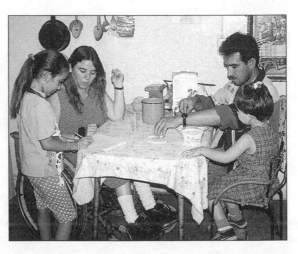

IRMA AND JAIME. Irma Llavió had polio as a baby. With all four limbs affected, she spent her childhood and adolescence crawling about on the floor, and she never left home. She was brought to PROJIMO by Martha Heredia, a leader in Mexico's budding independent living movement. For Irma, getting her own wheelchair and being with a group that treated her as an equal was liberating. She runs the kitchen, works in the toy shop, and helps her boyfriend, Jaime, in the wheelchair shop.

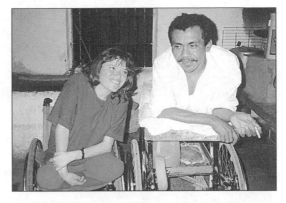

Jaime Torres, who is paraplegic and rides a wheeled cot because his hips are fused straight, has been working at PROJIMO for 6 years. For the first years he was chronically depressed, and sometimes he was drunk for days at a time. Then Irma arrived, and Jaime's spirit revived. He has become a master welder and wheelchair builder.

ROSA. Rosa Salcido, an older woman, is in some ways the heart of the program. One of the few non-disabled workers at PROJIMO, she is the personal attendant for most of the children and adults who are unable to care for themselves. Without children of her own, she has become a sort of universal mother, treating even the most difficult children with love and patience far beyond the call of duty. (See Chapter 32.)

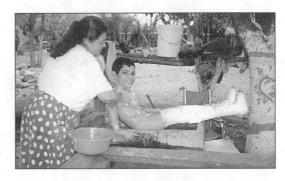

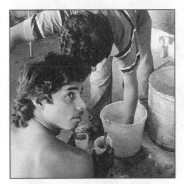

MARCELO. Marcelo Acevedo is one of the founders and leaders of PROJIMO. He had polio as a baby. Since his early childhood, the program has helped him with braces, crutches, and schooling, and trained him as a village health worker. He has become a very skilled, innovative brace and artificial limb maker, as well as a welder and wheelchair maker. Marcelo is one of the main trainers of others in these skills. I (the author) have Marcelo to thank for walking as well as I do today (see Chapter 11). Good-willed and gentle, Marcelo is often the peacemaker when conflicts arise. Marcelo (on the left) teaches Armando to make plaster molds for braces.

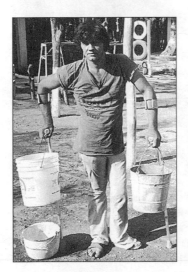

INEZ AND CECILIA. Inez Leon has one leg paralyzed by polio but is incredibly strong. Having grown up as a street child, in his teens he was brought to PROJIMO, and stayed. Trained in a hands-on way by Ann Hallum and other physical therapists, Inez has become a skilled therapy helper. After a long courtship he and Cecilia married and now have two little girls. Cecilia Rodriguez, who also had polio and uses a wheelchair, tutors disabled children and teaches them arts and crafts.

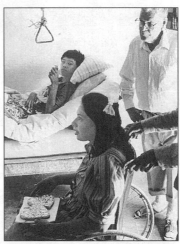

Cecilia with Osvaldo and Don Miguel.

MARIO. Mario Carrasco was born in a mountain village, but grew up on the streets of a coastal city. His involvement in drug trafficking led to the bullet wound that paralyzed him from the waist down. Angry and violent when he first arrived at PROJIMO, he became one of the most caring and capable workers there. (See Chapters 43 and 44.)

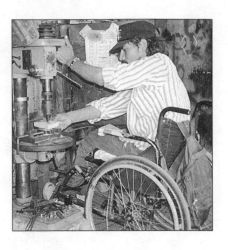

MARTÍN. Martín Pérez, like Mario, grew up on the city streets in the sub-culture of drugs and violence.

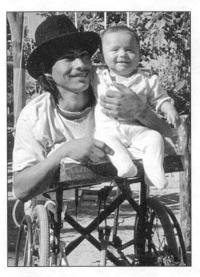

When he was 16 years old, Martín was shot by a gang rival and became paraplegic. At PROJIMO his fits of anger caused problems and sometimes brought Mari and Conchita to tears. But he became a very gifted wheelchair designer and builder. And he was very caring and helpful with the children who were most in need of attention and love. His work on creating a one-arm-drive wheelchair has been interrupted now by years in jail for trying to smuggle marijuana to his brother who was already in prison. (See Chapters 37 and 39.)

MARIELOS. If Rosa is the heart of the program, Marielos Rosales is the princess. Paralyzed in her lower body from a car accident, she was brought to PROJIMO for rehabilitation, then became involved in the toy-making shop, and now produces such beautiful play-things that she has more orders than she can fill. She also makes special seats, standing frames, and other wood and cardboard equipment for disabled children. When she does not have too much pain in her legs, she sings constantly and lifts everyone's spirits with her grace.

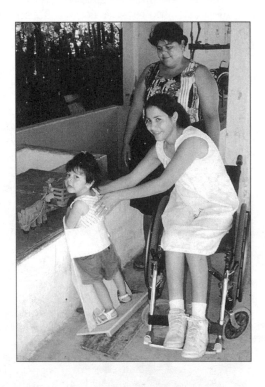

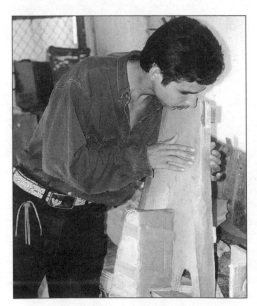

POLO. Polo Ribota was 13 years old when his father was killed. He has become and remains like a son to me (the author). Now in his early 20s, he lives in another village. But he often visits PROJIMO. He is always eager and willing to help build and design assistive equipment, frequently inviting the child who will use it to take part in its creation. (Polo is not disabled.)

Other PROJIMO team members, past and present, who appear occasionally in the stories and/or photos are *ROBERTO* Fajardo (one of the founders of PROJIMO, p. 90), *MARTÍN* Reyes Mercado (trainer of Child-to-Child activities, p. 286), *MARÍA DE JESÚS* Leyva (toy maker, p. 274), *JULIO* Peña (peer counselor, Chapter 28), *JAVIER* Valverde (brace maker and shoe maker, p. 307), *MANUELLA* Campista (toy maker, Chapter 49), *LEOPOLDO* Leyva (wheelchair builder, p. 259), *JUÁN* Morales (wood worker and brace maker, p. 31), *RAYMUNDO* Hernández (brace and wheelchair maker, p. 196), *DON MIGUEL* (handyman, p. 201), *RAFA* (toy maker, p. 279), *QUIQUE* (quadriplegic Spanish teacher, pp. 3 and 282), and *CHON* (a deaf village carpenter, see pp. 70 and 276).

Village children who have volunteered consistently with the program and have helped to make assistive equipment include *EFRAÍN* Zamora (who has since grown up and helped prepare this book, pp. 88, 126 and 292), *ERNESTO* Navarro (p. 67), *MARTÍN* Reyes Millán (213), *LLUVIA* Nevárez (Mari and Armando's daughter, p. 291), *DIONICIO* González (p. 330), and *BIANCA* (Cecilia and Inez's younger daughter, p. 285).

Skilled volunteers from North America and Europe who have helped to facilitate workshops at PROJIMO and cooperated with the village team in developing innovative aids and equipment include *ANN* Hallum (physical therapist, pp. 137, 181, and 292), *RALF* Hotchkiss (wheelchair designer, pp. 4, 148, 254, and much of Chapter 30), *KENNETT* Westmacott (director of *People Potential* in England, pp. 33, 72, and 206), *OLIVER* Bock (brace maker, pp. 82 and 88), *JEAN ANNE* Zollars (special seating expert, p. 42), *MICHAEL* Heinrich (engineer and cushion designer, p. 158), *BRUCE* Curtis (quadriplegic dancer and peer counselor), and *MONICA* Rook (occupational therapist, p. 45). Some of the many other volunteers who have made important contributions but are not specifically mentioned in the chapters are included in the Thanks page in the front of the book.

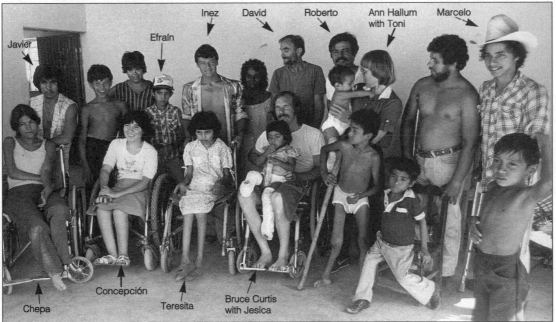

A group of some of the early participants of PROJIMO, about 1984.

Photo: John Fago

Note on the use of personal names in this book: Most names used for the disabled children and adults in the stories are their real names. However, to avoid confusion, we have occasionally used different names for persons with the same names. We apologize for any confusion.

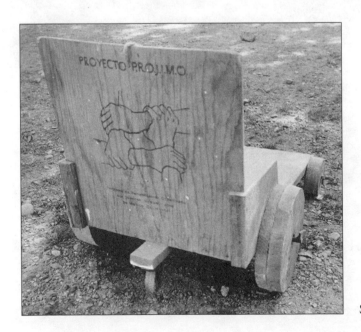

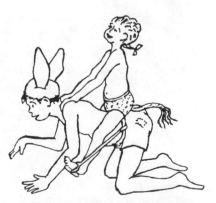

Special seating has many possibilities.

Part One

THE PURPOSE OF SPECIAL SEATING:
Freedom and Development, Not Confinement

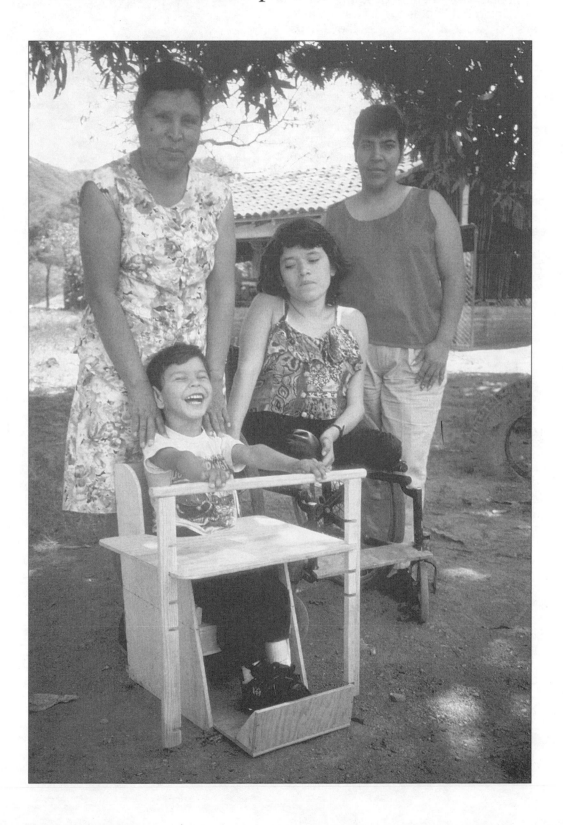

INTRODUCTION TO PART ONE

A Child is Not a Sack of Potatoes

Wheelchair riders often protest when people say they are "confined to a wheelchair" or "wheelchair bound." For them, **a good wheelchair is not confining but liberating.** It frees them to go where they want and to do what they choose. It permits them to accomplish more than they could do otherwise. It releases them, at least in part, from the handicapping effect of their disability.

The same is true—or should be—for special seating. It should not be confining, but liberating. The purpose of a special seat should not be to rigidly hold the child in a position that looks "good," but rather to help the child to learn to sit in a position that is beneficial. **A beneficial position is not necessarily one that looks normal. Rather, it is one that helps the child to stay healthy and to do what she wants or needs to do more easily and effectively.**

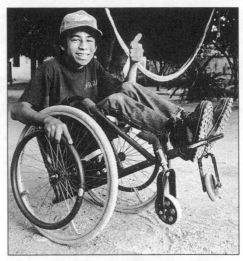

A good wheelchair is not confining, but liberating.

Usually the best special seat is one that provides the least amount of support needed to help the child do the most for herself.

For a child whose body stiffens like this,

don't do this,

when all that is needed is this.

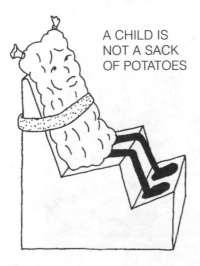

A CHILD IS NOT A SACK OF POTATOES

A child is not a sack of potatoes. Unfortunately, however, a lot of special seating is designed to hold children as if they were no more than sacks of potatoes.

Special seating, at its best, does not simply hold a child in a desirable position (although this may be a starting point for some children). It can sometimes help a child to improve balance, sit with less need of support, and learn new skills. In this chapter we will see examples of ways that seating can be designed for and with specific children to help them to gain better head control, discover the usefulness of their hands, observe their surroundings, dress themselves, and even use their leg muscles in preparation for walking.

SPECIAL SEATING: FIT OR MISFIT?

Special seating can be an important rehabilitation technology if it helps a disabled child to sit in a more self-controlled, more comfortable position, or if it enables her to do more things or learn new skills. However, in many programs **you will see special seats that do more harm than good.** The problem is not lack of concern. Often a lot of time, energy, and care have gone into making the seat. The crafts-person (perhaps a local carpenter) may be highly skilled. But two problems are common: First, **the design was selected from an overly simplified "how to do it" book, and the seat is not suited to the child's particular needs.** (This is especially true for children with cerebral palsy, whose combination of needs vary greatly.) Second, **the seat is too big for the child.** The following are photos of seats made for children with cerebral palsy. The photo on the left is from a brochure from Burundi (the same brochure with the photo of parallel bars we showed on page 11). The photo on the right is from a CBR program in Kenya which the author visited.

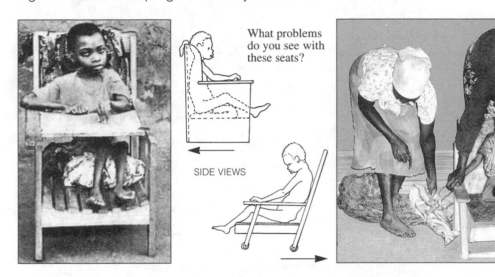

What problems do you see with these seats?

SIDE VIEWS

Note that both of **these seats are too big for these children.** In the first, the child's knees do not reach the front edge of the seat, so her unsupported feet stick out in front. The second seat could fit 2 such children, side by side. In these oversized seats, the children tend to slip forward. As their hips extend (get straighter), the spastic stiffening of their bodies increases. The result is a poor position, discomfort, and loss of control for eating or play. **Such misfitted seats can do more harm than good.** Using a standard child's chair, or simply sitting the child in the corner, is likely to work better.

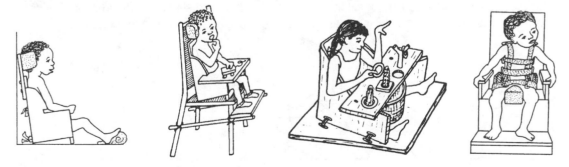

Above are a few examples of seating from the book, *Disabled Village Children*. Each seat works well for certain children ... but not for others! Especially for children with cerebral palsy, it is best to use a trial and error approach.

> **The best guide is what makes the child happy and helps her do things better.**

There are three main reasons why special seating is often inappropriate:

- There is a tendency to place **too much emphasis on construction of the equipment** and **not enough on making sure it meets the child's specific needs and fits her well.** Special seating, like all custom-made disability aids, should be approached through an experimental problem-solving process, by trial and error.

- A lot of instructional materials, especially those for community-level work, show pictures of a few special seats. But they **lack adequate instructions for measuring the child or for translating those measurements to the seating design.** (See Chapter 3.)

- In instructional materials, **designs are often misleading or inappropriate.** If a seat is built precisely as in a drawing, it may not be appropriate for the child shown (or, in some cases, for any child).

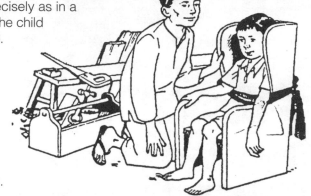

For example, here is a drawing from a brochure produced by a CBR training center in Asia. At first glance, the special seat appears well-fitted and appropriate. But look closer. Although it matches the child's size more closely than do the seats in earlier photos, the seat presents many problems for the child that is shown.

The problems are clearer when we look at the same seat from the side, as shown here:

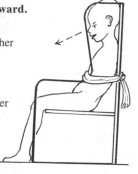

The sides of head-rest are too far forward. They block the child's vision to the sides.

The seat belt is too high. It causes, rather than prevents, slumping. Also, the belt provides no sideways stability because it passes around the sides of the chair.

The seat is too deep. The knees bent over its front edge force the child to slump with rounded back and extended hips: a tiring and harmful posture. It could increase spasticity.

The back of the chair pushes the child's head forward, lowering his line of vision. This makes it harder for him to watch activities around him, which can delay his development (see page 293).

Danger of falling. The chair tips back slightly but with no safety supports to prevent it from falling over backward. This is especially risky because the feet are on the ground. (There is no footrest.) A child with spasticity could easily push the seat over backwards.

If the child shown above has spasticity, the slouched position that the seat provides could trigger backward stiffening of the body, thus requiring the seat-belt to keep him in the seat. A few basic principles of seating and positioning of such children are shown below in simplified form. (Side supports and armrests, which may also be needed, are not shown in these drawings.)

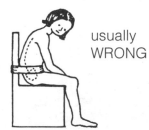

usually WRONG

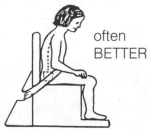

often BETTER

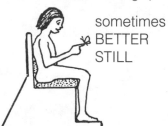

sometimes BETTER STILL

The seat belt is in a bad position for this child. Positioned at waist level, it may worsen rather than prevent the slouching posture.

To help pull the hips back and keep the back straighter, and to keep the hips bent enough to reduce spasticity, the belt must be low across her lap.

By raising the front of the seat or putting a dip at the back, spasticity can sometimes be reduced so that a restrictive belt is not needed.

To find out which of these—or other—options is likely to work best for an individual child, **experimentation is necessary, paying attention to the child's wishes and responses.**

A Great Variety of Seating Possibilities

When planning a special seat for a child, imagination is required to design and adapt a seat that:

- meets specific needs of the child (and whoever cares for her);
- fits into the local social and physical environment;
- is low cost, so the family or community can afford it;
- is simple and easy enough to make, so that the family can adapt or remake it as the child and her needs change.

A great variety of materials can be used: sticks, logs, wood, plywood, plastic, metal rod, cardboard boxes, paper, even mud.

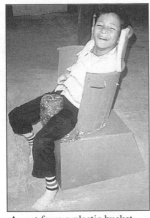

A seat from a plastic bucket.

Seats also range from simple to complex. The design depends on the child's particular needs and stage of development. Some seats serve mainly to keep spastic legs separated; others help a child sit in a more functional position. Some seats are designed to reduce muscle tone in a spastic child; others are designed to increase tone in a floppy (flaccid) child (see Chapter 4). Here is a sampling of different seating designs:

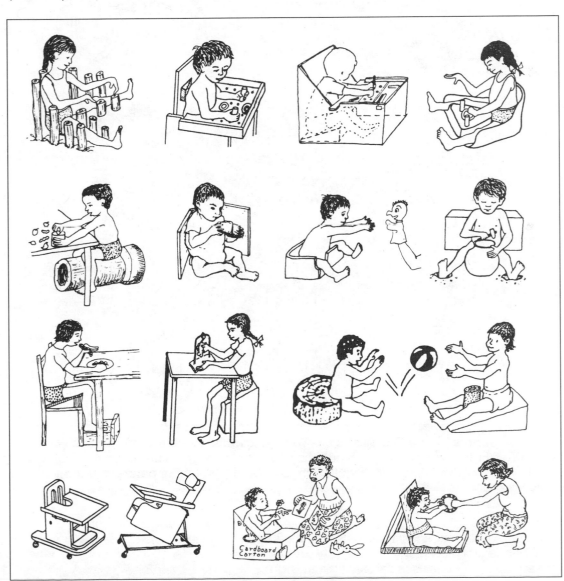

SPECIAL SEATING ON WHEELS

Wheels can be put onto special seats, for the benefit of both the child and her care-providers (mother, brothers and sisters, or others). The mobility (movement on wheels) achieved stimulates the child's development: exploration of her environment, enjoyment, physical coordination, self-reliance. And for the mother of an older, heavier child, being able to push her in a wheelchair, rather than have to always lift and carry her, makes moving her easier and protects her back.

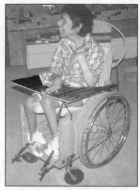

This wheeled wooden seat has rubber strips that pull this boy's legs forward to combat knee contractures.

Special seats can be built to fit into a standard wheelchair. Or wheels can be attached directly to the special seat. Here are **some examples of different forms of special seats on wheels:**

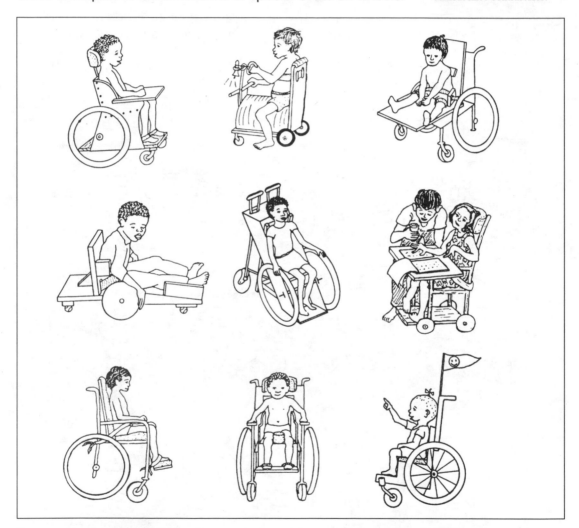

The 10 chapters in Part One illustrate several **innovative seating designs** (such as "positive," or forward-sloping, seating), the use of **unusual building materials** (paper and mud), and the involvement of **disabled children and parents as partners in the problem solving process.**

For more special seating ideas, including use of straps and wedges to improve positions or reduce spastic patterns, see the book, *Disabled Village Children.* Or see *Special Seating*, by Jean Anne Zollars (see page 344). Jean Anne helped develop the measuring device for special seating that is discussed in Chapter 3.

DESIGNING CHILD-FRIENDLY SEATS FOR THE NEEDS OF THE INDIVIDUAL CHILD

Every Child's Needs are Somewhat Different

Designing a special seat for a child's unique combination of needs can be a challenging adventure. It requires an experimental approach, with as much involvement of the child and parents as possible, to figure out what design to use and what supports and other features may benefit or appeal to the child.

No one—including a disabled child—likes to be in the same position for very long. For example, if our knees are bent for a few minutes, we want to straighten them. If they are straight for long, we want to bend them. The body tells us that such change in position is healthy and necessary. It keeps our joints flexible and working well. Therefore, it is wise that we listen to the child and that we **do not leave any child fastened in a seat (or standing frame or other assistive device) for too long.** Most children (but not all) will find a way of letting us know how long is long enough.

It is also wise to design the seat so that it **allows the child as much freedom and movement as possible,** while making sure it provides the minimum amount of positioning and support needed to help the child sit up well and function.

The Fish-and-Pond Seat—for Changing Positions and Fun. When possible, special seating should allow and encourage the child to change position. Children need to learn to sit with knees both straight and bent (and should be able to change position often). This *fish-IN-a-pond* seat for straight-leg sitting easily converts to a *fish-ON-a-pond* seat for bent-knee sitting. The seat was designed by the British simplified technology wizard, Don Caston, who adapted it to this child's needs on a visit to PROJIMO.

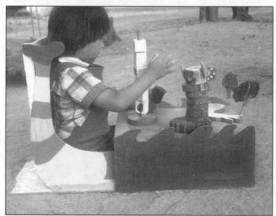

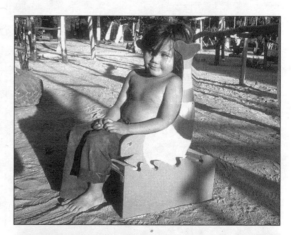

Making special seating and other assistive equipment attractive and child-friendly can make a big difference in how a child—and family—accept and make use of it.

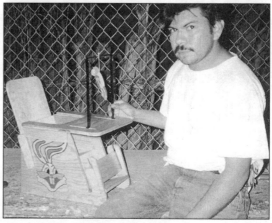

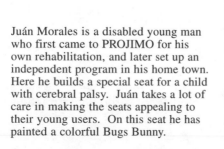

Juán Morales is a disabled young man who first came to PROJIMO for his own rehabilitation, and later set up an independent program in his home town. Here he builds a special seat for a child with cerebral palsy. Juán takes a lot of care in making the seats appealing to their young users. On this seat he has painted a colorful Bugs Bunny.

SPECIAL SEATING FOR SWINGS

Special seats can be built and adapted for a wide variety of circumstances, including playground equipment. For example, you can make a swing with an enclosed seat, so that a child who does not have enough hand or body control to sit in a standard seat can enjoy the fun and stimulation of swinging, like other children.

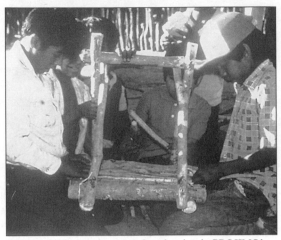

OMAR, a child with cerebral palsy, was brought by his mother to PROJIMO. His mother loved him a lot and wanted the best for him. But she overprotected him. When Mari suggested that Omar play in one of the enclosed swings in the Playground for All Children, at first both he and his mother were frightened.

Village children make an enclosed swing in PROJIMO's Playground for all Children (see pages 288-289).

But after just a few minutes in the swing, Omar was having a wonderful time. And his mother realized that her son could do more things than she had ever imagined. She said she would ask her husband to make a similar swing at home. Omar was delighted.

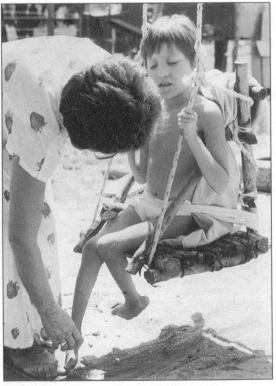

When Omar first sat in the swing he was tense and very unsure of himself. His mother was equally fearful.

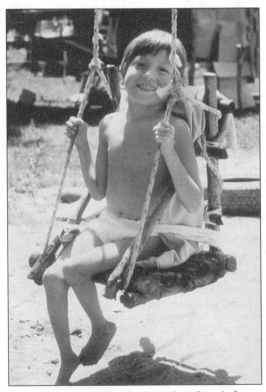

But after a few minutes in the swing, Omar's face beamed with delight. He was like a different boy. Both he and his mother discovered he could do more than either had thought possible.

For other designs of enclosed swings and specially adapted swing seats, see pages 57, 58 and 288. A swing seat made from an old tire for a girl with spasticity is described in Chapter 5.

A Seat for Carina to Dress Herself

CARINA is an alert young girl with cerebral palsy. She was 10 years old when she first visited PROJIMO. She and her mother had come to take part in a short training course on designing and making rehabilitation aids. The course—really an informal hands-on workshop where everyone learns from each other—was attended by a small group of participants, most of whom are disabled. They came from community rehabilitation programs in Mexico and Central America. A guest facilitator was Kennett Westmacott, an English furniture builder with long experience working with disabled persons and their families in developing simple, low-cost aids.

When it was Carina's turn to be seen, she was asked to join a small group of rehabilitation workers, some more experienced than others. In the shade of a mango tree, the session began with a friendly conversation. This was informal and relaxed, so that Carina would gain confidence with her peers and realize that they really wanted to get to know and understand her.

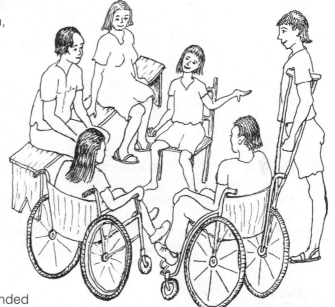

Understanding her speech was not easy for the group because Carina has difficulty with talking. When she is nervous, her body movements are less controlled and she finds it even harder to form words. But when Carina was surrounded by other disabled persons who showed real interest in her, she began to relax and her speech became easier to decipher. When she realized that she was the center of attention, and that people were doing their best to understand her in a non-judgmental way, she began to open up and enjoy the process.

Carina clearly had a mind of her own and wanted to become more independent. But her body simply would not do many of the things she wanted it to. For some time now, she explained, she had been able to feed herself. But it wasn't easy. Because much of the food she ate missed her mouth as it went in, sometimes she would let her mother help her. Now she wanted to manage on her own.

Carina had a walker (walking frame) that was made for her by disabled graduates from PROJIMO who had started a community-based program in the city where she lives. But she was still learning to use it. It was frustrating. The harder she tried, the more difficult it seemed to become. Her mother explained that Carina sometimes went through periods of fairly rapid improvement, but then seemed to go through times when little noticeable improvement took place. That was when Carina and she got discouraged. Carina's twisted smile and the gestures she made while her mother talked showed that she agreed. When one of the senior rehabilitation workers explained that this was how most disabled children develop—in apparent spurts and plateaus—both Carina and her mother seemed relieved.

Someone asked, "Carina, of things you like to do, what would you most like to do better?"

Carina tensed with excitement and chewed out the words, "Put ... on ... my ... clothes."

"And what else would you like to do?" someone else asked her.

She repeated, more forcefully: "PUT ... ON ... MY ... CLOTHES!"

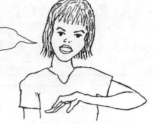

Her mother explained that for months Carina had been trying to dress herself. Sometimes she would struggle to do so for a long time before finally, sometimes tearfully, accepting assistance.

One thing was clear. Carina had told the group what was, at present, her most urgent felt need. It was her bid for budding independence and self-reliance. Her body, for all its unruliness, was her own.

"Is there anything we can do for her or make for her that can help her to dress by herself?" asked Kennett. It was anybody's guess. People said they needed to know more about precisely what Carina could and could not do, and where the problems were.

"Sometimes I can *take off* my clothes all by myself!" said Carina proudly.

It was time for Carina to demonstrate what she could and could not do. She was asked to start with what she could do successfully: get undressed. Carina was eager to show off her skill. She managed, with considerable difficulty, to remove her blouse. Then she did her best—unsuccessfully—to put it back on. Finally, and against her protest, her mother helped her.

Observation and identifying problems. By watching Carina, and with explanations from her mother, the group tried to evaluate Carina's skills and problems with dressing. They saw that **her cerebral palsy was of mixed types.** She had some **spasticity** (involuntary tightening of certain muscles), some **athetosis** (repeated forceful uncontrolled movements) and **occasional low muscle tone** (moments when her body became floppy and would sag forward). Unable to stand without support, Carina tried to undress and dress while sitting.

Even when seated, Carina had trouble staying upright and controlling her arm movements.

When trying to pull on her blouse, her body would suddenly sag or stiffen, throwing her off balance, usually backward.

In a high-back chair, her body arched backwards and made dressing impossible.

On a stool (or sitting on the ground), she would fall over, either backwards or forwards.

Ideas for possible solutions. After observing what Carina was able to do, what she was unable to do, and the nature of her difficulties, the group—including Carina and her mother—conducted a brain-storming session.   All ideas were welcome, including constructive criticism.

Someone suggested that Carina wear **loose-fitting clothes** which she could pull on easily over her head, and that she avoid tight-fitting garments with difficult buttons or zippers. Carina's mother said she already did this—except, of course, when Carina wanted to look more elegant. Carina grinned her emphatic agreement.

Someone else had the idea that Carina **sit near a firm post or pole** that she could **hold onto with one hand,** while pulling on her clothes with the other.

Another idea was some kind of a seat **that would give the support or protection she needed to keep from falling over,** but which would allow the **space and freedom** she needed to pull a blouse or dress down around her body.

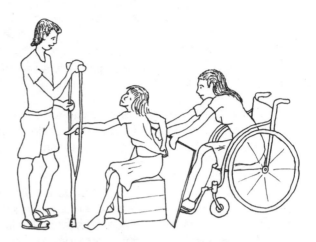

Experimentation. The best way to find out if these ideas worked was by experimenting. Carina sat on boxes of different heights, while participants firmly held a pole for her to hold onto. They tried **holding the pole upright, sideways, and at different heights to find out what she felt worked best.** Also, they tried using a wide board for a **back-rest,** holding it at different heights, angles, and positions. Carina loved all the attention and tried her best to put on her blouse in all the suggested ways.

Why does Carina fall over backwards? Carina had somewhat more control with the combination of a tilting backrest and a pole to hold on to. But still, she had to work hard to sit upright. "Her body keeps trying to fall over backwards!" observed her mother.

On analyzing the difficulty, the group realized that **Carina had trouble sitting upright partly because of the stiffness of her hips.** (The combination of spasticity and contractures prevented her hips from bending enough for her to sit upright.)

NORMAL SITTING POSITION

To sit upright, the hips bend at a right angle.

The back-bone and the thigh-bone are at 90 degrees.

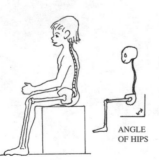

ANGLE OF HIPS

HIP TILT CAUSES INSTABILITY

The difficulty with sitting causes more tension and spasticity, thrusting the child backwards.

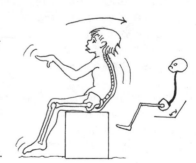

STIFF HIPS— BACKWARD HIP TILT

Because the hip-bone (pelvis) tips back, the child sits with the back bent. She must work hard to keep from falling backward.

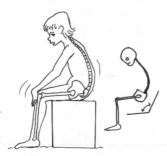

TILTING THE SEAT FORWARD FOR MORE STABILITY

The seat tilt lets the thigh-bones slope down toward her knees.

Now the back-bone can go straight up. The child can sit straighter and is more stable.

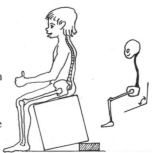

Tilting Carina's seat forward. The workshop participants experimented to see if Carina could sit straighter and more securely when sitting with the seat tilted forward. To everyone's delight—especially Carina's—it made a big difference. Her back rose straight from her hips, and she found it was easier to sit without having to use her hands to keep her balance.

Carina tried sitting on the seat at several different angles of tilt. In each position she tried twisting her body, moving her arms and hands about, and trying to take off or put on a piece of clothing. A small amount of tilt appeared to help most. A lot of tilt seemed to make her spasticity worse, and again she had trouble with falling over backwards. At last she and her helpers decided that she sat straightest and had most control when the seat was only sloping a little.

Again they tried having Carina try to dress, using a post to hold onto and a sloping back-rest, but this time with the seat tilting forward. Finally, Carina and the group agreed on a combination of features that worked best.

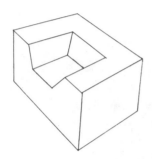

Designing and building a seat. Next came the design for a trial seat. Everyone had ideas. In the end, a plan was drawn for **a sunken seat built within a large plywood cube.** The top of the cube formed a narrow U-shaped shelf on which Carina could place her clothes within easy reach. The shelf also provided an area where Carina could reach out when she began to fall.

The sides and back of the seat tilted outward, to allow Carina room to pull down her dress. They gave support only when she began to fall. The seat itself tilted forward a little, allowing her to sit straighter.

There was a long debate as to what to use as a hand-grip while dressing. Carina's mother wanted something movable—and removable. Suddenly Carina gave an eager cry and pointed at her walker. Why not? The walker was about the right height. They tried it and it worked.

With a little practice, Carina learned to shift from the walker to her seat, and then to position the walker in front of her for hand support.

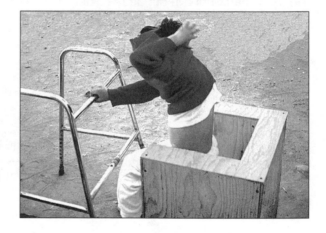

Testing and evaluation. From the first, Carina was able to dress with more control. A couple of times she even managed to put on her blouse without her mother's help. As Carina practiced with her new seat, her confidence grew. With less fear of falling, she was less tense. This reduced her spasticity, so she was able to work at getting her blouse over her head without suddenly stiffening and falling backward. When she first succeeded in putting on her blouse alone, Carina was in seventh heaven.

In a few months, Carina's new cube seat proved so successful, *she no longer needed it.*

"Positive seating." It was very clear that **Carina sat straighter, with more control, when the seat tilted forward.** The remarkable benefits of forward tilting seats—or *"positive seating"*—for certain children are further explored in Chapter 4.

Seats with Changing Positions to Meet Jazmín's Different Needs

CHAPTER 2

Need for Seating that Adjusts to Help a Child Gain Greater Body Control

Especially for the child whose body is floppy and has little head control, it is important that seating be designed so as to help the child gain more trunk (body) and head control. Before designing the seat, it is a good idea to check how much head control and trunk control the child has, by holding him in a sitting position. It is often best for the mother or family member to do this, and it is essential that she understand the principles involved.

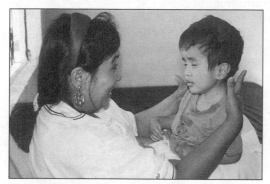

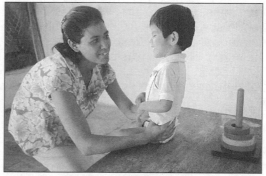

To check head control, sit the child on your lap or on a firm object. With your hands, provide just enough shoulder or trunk support to keep the child sitting upright. With your fingertips, position the head straight up. Then gently lessen the head support to see if the child can hold (or partly hold) his head up, even for a moment. Catch the child's head softly with your fingertips when it begins to fall.

To check trunk (body) control, sit the child firmly and hold his body just under his arms. Gradually move your hands lower on his body to find out how low the support can be for him to keep in an upright position. If he can keep his balance and remain sitting upright when you hold him low at the hips, he is developing fairly good trunk control. This boy's mother was surprised at how much trunk control her son had.

These two activities, used here for evaluation, can also be used to improve a child's head control, trunk control, and balance. Do them several times a day. As a general rule:

> **Use the least amount of support needed to help the child do the most she can for herself.**

For special seating, this same principle applies. It is often helpful if the seating is adjustable, allowing the child to sit in positions for stimulation as well as for relaxation.

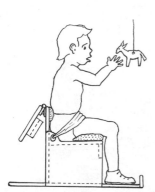

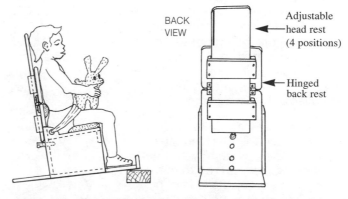

BACK VIEW

Adjustable head rest (4 positions)

Hinged back rest

In this position the seat encourages the child to use her muscles and to develop control and balance.

When the child begins to get tired, the seat can be easily placed or adjusted to another position in which the child can rest and relax.

For Jazmín—A Seat That Changes Position

JAZMÍN was 3 years old when her mother first brought her to PROJIMO. Her brain had been damaged at birth. She still had almost no head control. When her mother tried to sit her up, head fell forward and her body flopped to one side. She had spent most of her life lying in a crib. At PROJIMO, Mari (one of the coordinators of the program) showed Jazmín's mother several activities that she could do to help Jazmín gain more head control. These included the "fingertips at the base of the skull" activity shown on page 37.

After working with Jazmín's mother to evaluate her daughter's abilities and needs, Mario (a carpenter who is paraplegic) and Mari designed and made a special seat for her. It was basically a plywood box with the seat, the back, and width measured to her size.

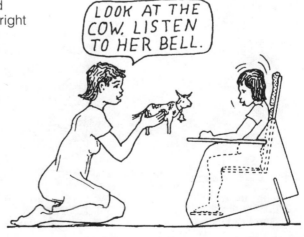

Jazmín's large head tended to fall forward even when she was tilted somewhat back. So Mario made a headrest that angled backward from the seat back. That way, Jazmín could rest her head against the headrest without her head falling forward. But although this let her rest comfortably, it did little to help her gain head control. For this reason a piece of plywood was prepared, with slits of different lengths, so that it could lift the back of the seat to different heights. A soft chest band helped to keep her from slumping forward.

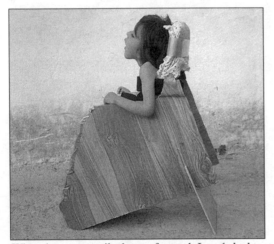

When the seat was tilted more forward, Jazmín had to make more effort to keep her head from falling forward.

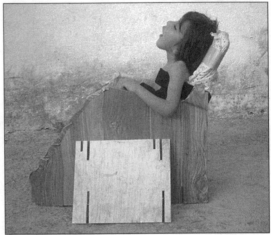

When the seat was positioned so it tilted far back, Jazmín could rest without her head falling forward.

Because the angle of the seat could be adjusted securely in 5 different positions, her mother could experiment, seeking the angle at which Jazmín was barely able to keep her head upright. Over time, this would help her develop head control. As her control improved with the combination of special seating and fingertip exercises, her mother could leave Jazmín sitting longer in the upright position before letting her rest in the back-slanting position. And, little by little, she could tilt the seat further forward, encouraging yet further improvement in head control.

Mari also encouraged Jazmín's mother to talk with her daughter when she did any activity with her. Jazmín's mother learned to move bright colored objects in front of her face, encouraging her to follow them with her eyes and to try to lift her head.

LOOK AT THE COW. LISTEN TO HER BELL.

A problem with Jazmín's seat was that her body still tended to flop over to the right, with her head hanging over the side of the seat.

To help Jazmín sit straighter, the team made wedges of layered cardboard and positioned them to hold her hips in place and to center her body. But still, her body and head flopped far over to the right side. ———→

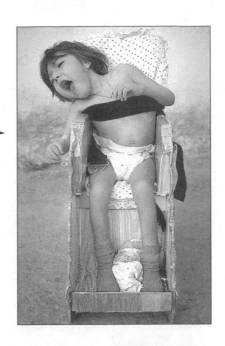

By experimenting with her hands, Mari found that when Jazmín's head was supported gently on the right side, this kept her upper body from flopping over to the right. She thought a head support on the right side would help. But it should be easily removable. Removing it at times might help Jazmín become less dependent on it, and it might encourage her to keep her body and head upright. Eventually, the side-support might not be needed.

Armando made a simple, easily removable, side-of-the-head support by heating a piece of sheet plastic over a flame and bending it as shown below.

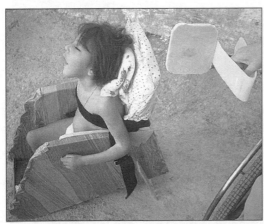

For comfort, a foam pad was attached to the part of the headrest that would support her head.

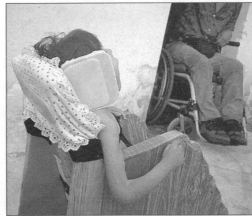

The U in the plastic could be slipped firmly onto the head-rest, over the cushion.

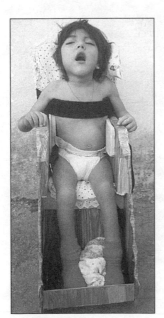

With the right side of her head supported in this way, Jazmín could sit much straighter. The thin plastic support was rather flexible, so that when Jazmín pushed her head against it, it would bend a bit. This permitted some head motion. Yet when she stopped pushing, the support would gently move her head to a straighter position.

With the help of head-control exercises and a special seat designed to meet her needs, together with more stimulation by her mother, brothers, and sister, Jazmín began to gain better head control. Once she could hold her head up, she took more notice of action and movements around her.

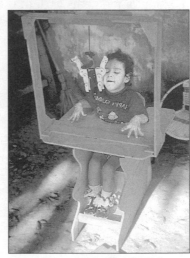

The table on this special seat has an overhead bar with toys hanging from it. The bar frame slides back and forth, adjusting to the child's reach.

Adjustable-position seating designs similar to the one made for Jazmín have been modified and adapted by PROJIMO to meet the needs of many different children. Here is an example of a seat for a baby named *FÁTIMA*, who had floppy cerebral palsy and developmental delay.

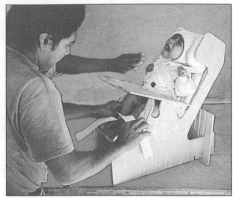

When the seat is positioned tilting back, the baby is secure and can relax. She feels more confident about reaching out and using her hands in this safe, back-tilted position.

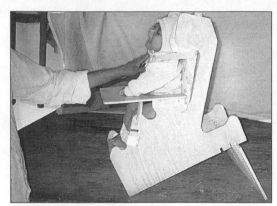

When the seat is tilted forward more, the baby must use her neck and back muscles to stay upright. As her head and trunk control increase, she can be tilted farther forward and stay there longer.

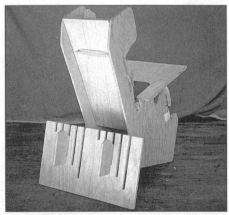

The adjustable back-board of the seat has a series of vertical slots in it. These allow the seat to be positioned at many different angles.

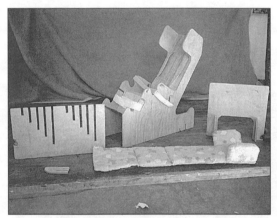

This photo shows the seat with its detachable components: the back-board, the table, and the pad to cushion the baby's bottom, back, and head.

Many of the seats built at PROJIMO include an adjustable overhead bar from which colorful toys, rattles, and bells can be hung. These attract the child's attention and stimulate her to lift her head, reach out, and start to develop hand-eye coordination.

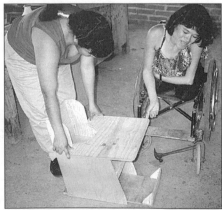

The mother of Tinín, a child with cerebral palsy, helps Irma build a special wooden seat for him.

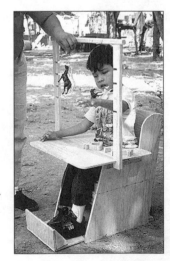

Irma and Tinín's mother attached a bar that can be adjusted over the table. Toys hung from the bar encourage the boy to lift his head and to use his hands. (For more on Tinín see pages 54-55.)

CHAPTER 3

Measuring and Fitting Devices
for Children who Need a Special Seat or Standing Aid

The Need for Careful Measurement and Fitting of Special Seating to Meet each Child's Needs

If special seating is to help a child sit well, gain better head and body control, or move and do things more easily, **it is essential that the design be appropriate for the child's needs, and that it fit the child correctly.**

In many parts of the world, one sees disabled children sitting in specially-made seats or wheelchairs that simply do not fit them. Often the seat is far too big. ⟶ *Before building a seat for a child, it is important to* **take correct measurements.** *Equally important is to* **carefully evaluate the child's individual needs, interests, limitations, abilities and possibilities, as well as her likes, dislikes, and fears.**

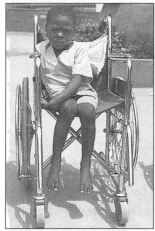

Apart from other difficulties, the over-sized wheelchair of this paraplegic child in Angola increases her spinal deformity.

The most important test of a special seat is: Does the child like it?

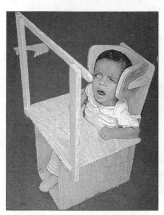

Although this seat was especially made for her, this child howled every time she was put into it, and she never learned to accept it.

Even a child who is mentally delayed or cannot express her wishes with words may have strong feelings about how she is treated or seated. I (the author) have seen occasions where a beautifully built, accurately fitted seat is painstakingly made for a child. Yet the child screams every time she is put in the seat, and despite repeated attempts and coaxing, she never learns to accept it. (For an example, see page 66.) Sometimes the child may have good reasons (see the special seat made for a child with hydrocephalus, page 293). Such a seat can perhaps be modified or rebuilt so that it is more acceptable. But *clearly, it is preferable to make a seat that from the first comes close to meeting the child's needs.*

One of the best ways to find out what type and size of seating may best meet a child's needs and preferences is to **experiment with a variety of different pre-existing seats.**

For this reason, PROJIMO likes to keep on hand a collection of special seats of different types and sizes. Often a seat that does not quite fit a child can be provisionally adjusted by putting a block over the footrest or a thick pad against the backrest. If the angle (tilt) of the seat needs to be changed, try putting one or two books under the front or back of the seat, according to the child's particular needs. **Such experimentation, by trial and error, is important before actually designing and building a seat for an individual child.**

MEASURING A CHILD FOR A SPECIAL SEAT

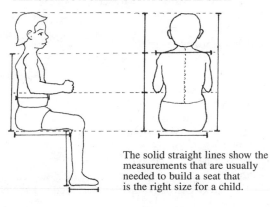

The solid straight lines show the measurements that are usually needed to build a seat that is the right size for a child.

An "Evaluation Seat"—for Fitting, Measuring, and Testing to find the Best Positions for a Child

Building an appropriate seat for a child who has a lot of spasticity or deformities often involves much more than simply taking accurate measurements of the child. Trials with different seating possibilities can be very helpful. But a pre-existing seat that both fits the child and has the combination of features and positions the child needs is often not available.

PROJIMO has experimented with the design and construction of a completely adjustable "fitting-and-measuring seat," in which a child of any size can be tested in a range of positions.

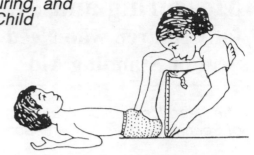

A good way to take the basic measurements for making a seat is to lie the child on his back with hips and knees bent at right angles. But such measurements are only a small part of the evaluation and testing needed for good seating.

Such a seat needs to have independent adjustments—for width, depth, height, and for the angle of the seat, the foot-rest, the back, and the headrest (when needed). It must also have adjustable, removable supports for positioning and alignment of the hips, back, shoulders, and head. And it should have a removable table with adjustable height, angle, hand holds, and other features.

Fortunately, a physical therapist, Jean Anne Zollars, was making visits to PROJIMO to help teach short courses on special seating. She helped to design and build the early experimental special seats.

The first experimental measuring seats designed and built at PROJIMO could be modified for children of many sizes and needs. But they were too complicated, too big, and too difficult to adjust.

Eventually, the team made simpler designs that were easier to adjust. These include the adjustable seat-with-wheels shown on the next page.

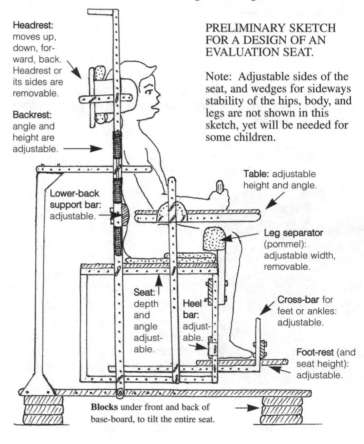

Headrest: moves up, down, forward, back. Headrest or its sides are removable.

Backrest: angle and height are adjustable.

Lower-back support bar: adjustable.

Seat: depth and angle adjustable.

Heel bar: adjustable.

PRELIMINARY SKETCH FOR A DESIGN OF AN EVALUATION SEAT.

Note: Adjustable sides of the seat, and wedges for sideways stability of the hips, body, and legs are not shown in this sketch, yet will be needed for some children.

Table: adjustable height and angle.

Leg separator (pommel): adjustable width, removable.

Cross-bar for feet or ankles: adjustable.

Foot-rest (and seat height): adjustable.

Blocks under front and back of base-board, to tilt the entire seat.

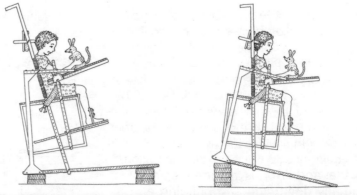

These drawings show how the early, experimental measuring seat could be adjusted to test a child with the seat tilted both back and forward (see p. 47).

A wheeled, adjustable measuring seat

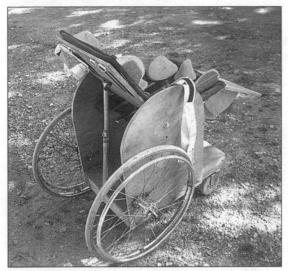

This model of a measuring seat has wheels, and can be used for measuring and fitting a child for a wheelchair.

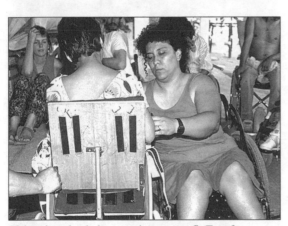

Using the wheeled measuring seat to fit Tere for a wheelchair, Mari tries the backrest at different angles.

Adjustable wedges

To provide special support for persons who need it, wedges of different sizes and shapes can be made. For the adjustable wheelchair shown here, the team molded wedges made of sawdust mixed with white glue. Wedges can also be made of paper maché or layers of corrugated cardboard (see page 73).

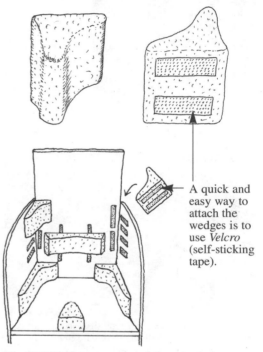

A quick and easy way to attach the wedges is to use *Velcro* (self-sticking tape).

The PROJIMO team equipped the wheeled seat with a variety of adjustable wedges and a removable knee separator (pommel).

PARTICIPANTS FROM OTHER LANDS IMPROVE THE DESIGN

Some of these measuring seat designs were developed during a series of short courses at PROJIMO by participants from community rehabilitation programs in different Latin American countries. One participant in the course was Monica Rook, an occupational therapist from Holland who was helping to facilitate a CBR program in Belize. After returning to Belize, Monica and her team designed a simpler, easier-to-build measuring seat, details of which are shown on the following page. →

It is exciting when course participants improve on innovations in their own programs and countries.

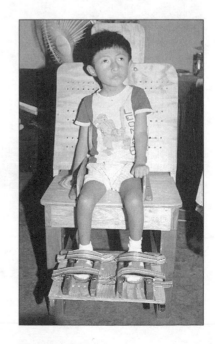

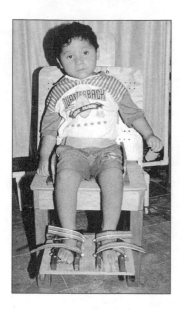

The adjustable chair from Belize is made of wood. Wooden support pieces of various sizes and shapes are attached to the seat and back of the chair. These can be positioned, adjusted, or removed depending on the child's needs. The supports—which can be used to stabilize the feet, hips, trunk, shoulders, and head—are attached by bolts. These fit through rows of small holes drilled in the footrest, seat board, and back board. The seat belt and foot straps are also adjustable.

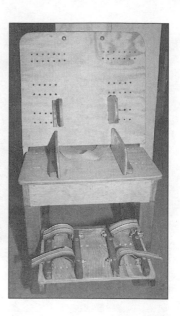

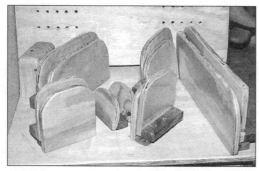

Supports and wedges of various sizes and shapes can be placed in all sorts of angles and positions.

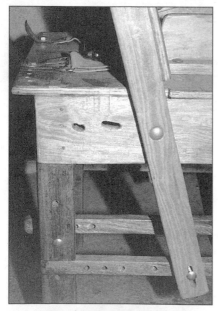

The angle of the seat back and the depth of the seat are adjustable, with bolts that pass through holes in the side boards and the bottom rungs of the chair.

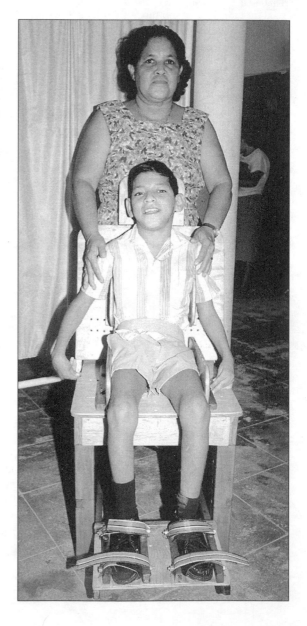

An Adjustable Frame for Fitting and Measuring a Child for a Standing Frame

Using a similar technology with adjustable pieces of wood, Monica Rook and her team of community rehabilitation workers in Belize also invented a device for fitting and measuring children who need a custom-made standing frame.

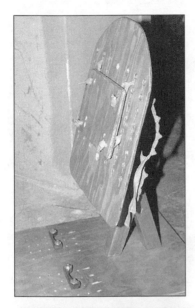

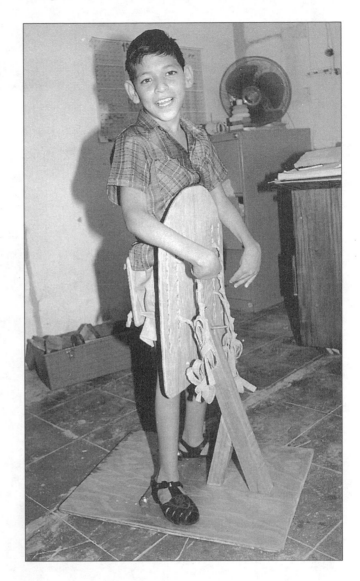

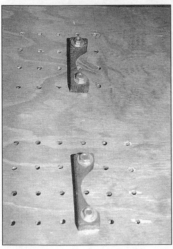

The feet are held in position by wooden heel-stops which can be adjusted with bolts that pass through the floor board. The standing board is hinged, and the angle (tilt) can be easily adjusted.

An adjustable standing frame can also be useful for holding a child in different positions, for different activities.

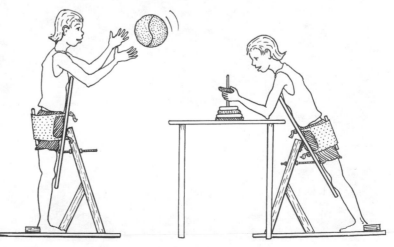

Use of Sand-Bags to Help a Child Sit

"Special seating" can sometimes be quite simple. Here the mother of *CRUZ,* who has cerebral palsy, helps her son sit upright by placing sand-bags across his folded legs and behind his hips. Later, PROJIMO created a cardboard seat for Cruz (see Chapter 8).

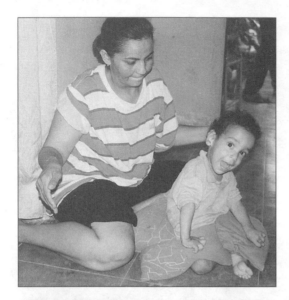
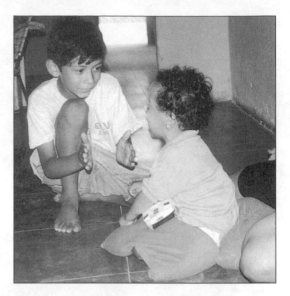

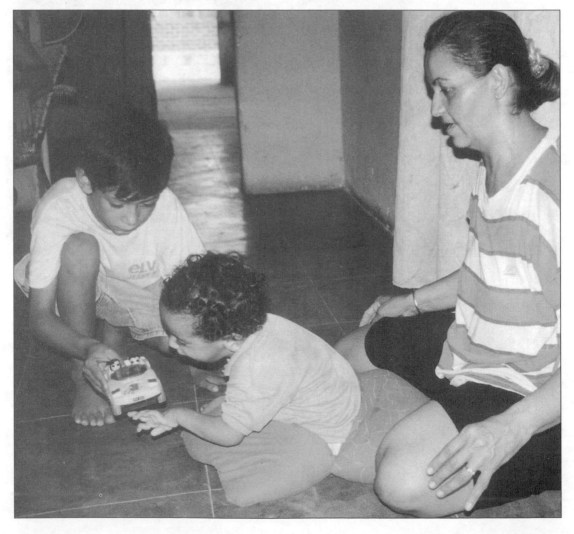

Positive Seating to Help Toño See, and Edgar Learn to Walk

CHAPTER **4**

TOÑO was 4 years old when his concerned parents brought him to PROJIMO from a neighboring village. His brain had been damaged shortly after he was born, apparently by meningitis. He was multiply disabled and very small for his age.

In the first meeting with Mari and other members of the village rehabilitation team, Toño's worried father explained, "I'm not even sure he can see. We try to sit him up so he can look at things around him. But he just droops his head and stares at his lap. He doesn't show interest in anything."

Observation and examination. Watching Toño, the team observed that his overall development was quite delayed. He responded very little to people and things around him. He did not reach for or play with toys.

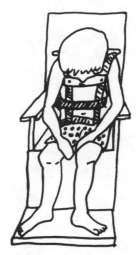

Mari tested Toño's vision by moving a small light in front of his eyes. Occasionally, his eyes followed the light, but sometimes they did not. "I think he sees," said Toño's mother. "He's just not used to looking at things."

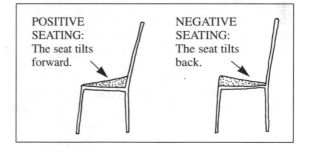

Toño could sit by himself, but his whole body was floppy and he had little head control. The team tried sitting him in a special seat that was his size. An H-shaped strap held his body upright. But even then, his head drooped far forward. To keep his head from falling forward, they had to tilt the seat so far back that his head faced upward rather than outward. Only when he cried did his drooping head come up for a moment.

"That gives me an idea," said Mari. "Let's try *positive seating.* It might help him sit more upright." She explained that *positive seating* means that the seat tilts forward (see Chapter 1, page 35). This differs from *negative seating,* the common position where the seat slants slightly back.

POSITIVE SEATING: The seat tilts forward.	NEGATIVE SEATING: The seat tilts back.

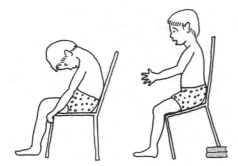

Experimentation. Mari asked Toño's father to sit the boy in a simple child's chair. He drooped over at once. Then Mari asked his father to put a book under the back of the special seat in which Toño sat, to tilt it a bit forward. The boy's head still drooped. But, when another book tilted the seat farther forward, an amazing thing happened. Toño's body gradually straightened and he lifted his head.

When Toño's father walked across the room in front of his son, the boy turned his head, following with his eyes. "He sees me!" exclaimed his father in delight. "That's the first time he has ever watched anybody move in front of him! My boy can see!"

Why Positive (Forward Tilting) Seating Helps Some Children

Positive seating (sloping the seat forward) does not help all, or even most, children with cerebral palsy or developmental delay. But it does help some children with stiff, backward-tilting hips, or those with low muscle tone who have trouble sitting upright. It is especially useful for children who can sit briefly without support, but who tend to droop forward with sagging head. Often it helps them to sit straighter and raise their head.

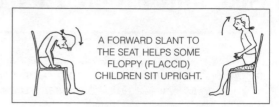

A FORWARD SLANT TO THE SEAT HELPS SOME FLOPPY (FLACCID) CHILDREN SIT UPRIGHT.

NOTE: Some therapists dislike the term "positive seating." This is because both positive (forward sloping) and negative (backward sloping) seating can be either helpful or harmful, depending on the particular needs of each child.

The concept of positive seating is still new to many rehabilitation workers and therapists. **It is often helpful for children who, for 2 different reasons, have difficulty sitting upright.**

1. As mentioned in Chapter 1, some children with spastic cerebral palsy have **stiffness of the hips** (pelvis) that prevents them from sitting with their back at right angles to their thighs. When they sit on a level (horizontal) seat, they tend to fall over backwards. Or they sit slouched with their back in a C-shaped curve.

When the child sits on *a forward-tilting seat,* or wedge, this allows her back to rise straight up from the hips. (The pelvis is rotated to an upright position.) On this forward-slanting seat, the child is more stable, less tense (which reduces spasticity), and often has better head, body, and hand control.

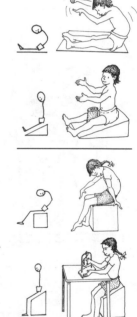

2. Some children have **low muscle tone**, as in the floppy (flaccid) type of cerebral palsy, and in some mixed types. On a level seat, they tend to slump forward and have difficulty raising their heads.

For such children, *a forward-tilting seat* (positive seating) often does wonders. The forward slant causes the child to push with her legs to keep from sliding forward. This use of the leg muscles increases overall muscle tone, which (in some cases) allows the child to lift her head and hold a more upright posture.

CAUTION: Each child is different. Results with positive seating vary from excellent to counterproductive. Be sure that—if muscle tone is increased—it gives the child greater control, rather than triggering a stiff, spastic reaction (as it does in some children).

POSITIVE SEATING AS PREPARATION FOR WALKING

Positive seating sometimes stimulates a child to use her leg muscles (to avoid slipping off the sloping seat). This helps to strengthen the thigh muscles that straighten the legs. Use of these muscles is essential for standing and walking. Thus positive seating helps some children prepare for walking at a later time. This was the case with Edgar.

Ways that Positive Seating can Speed the Development of Certain Children

- It helps a child with back-tilted hips to sit upright. This increases stability and relaxes spasticity so that the child is more able to use her hands and do things.

- It can help the floppy child to sit upright, increasing body and head control.

- By enabling the child to lift her head, it enables her to watch the world around her. This stimulates vision and involves her in family activities. It can speed her physical, mental, and social development.

- By encouraging use of the leg muscles, it helps prepare the child to walk.

EDGAR was 7 years old when his mother and older brother brought him to PROJIMO from a distant village. Like Toño, Edgar is developmentally delayed and has a type of cerebral palsy which is primarily floppy (flaccid), with poor balance. Also like Toño, Edgar would sit with his head drooping forward, totally uninvolved with the world around him. He spent a lot of time staring down at his upturned hand. His mother had tried hard to interest him in toys and other things, but he made no effort to take hold of them. The only thing he did with his hands was to sometimes pick at his clothing, or pull his hair. His mother was discouraged.

The PROJIMO team carefully evaluated Edgar's needs. They helped his mother and brother do playful activities with him, and gradually Edgar began to take more interest in things. They designed a special seat for him with a table and a removable frame from which were hung brightly colored toys, bells, and rattles. These encouraged him to lift his head, look at them, and begin to touch and handle them. (The design for this seat is shown on page 32.)

But with all these stimulating objects and activities, Edgar showed only a little improvement. He still spent most of his time with his head hanging forward. When he did lift his head, it seemed to be with great effort, and in a moment his head would droop again.

A try with positive seating. It was around this time that the team learned about positive (forward-tilted) seating, and decided to try it with Edgar. They repeated the experiment they had used with Toño, but this time they sat the child on a box instead of a chair.

With the box tilted forward, Edgar sat up straighter. He also seemed more alert. He looked at things around him like someone who had just awakened from a dream.

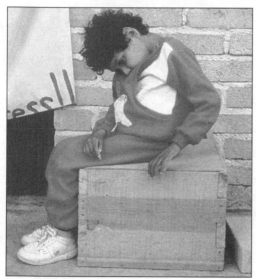 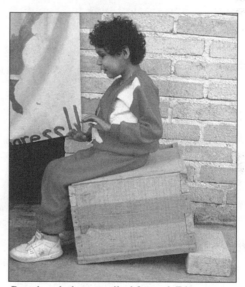

With the box flat on the ground, Edgar sat in his typical slumped position.

But when the box was tilted forward, Edgar gradually straightened up and lifted his head.

After only about a minute, however, Edgar looked tired, and he slowly began to droop again. Although at first he seemed to enjoy sitting on the sloping box, now he began to fret. When his mother removed the brick from under the back edge of the box, Edgar looked relieved. But he continued to droop like a wilted flower.

After a few minutes, the team tilted the box forward again. As before, Edgar straightened up and became more alert. But in a moment he again grew tired and slumped over. Mari explained to Edgar's mother that, to sit upright, Edgar had to use muscles he seldom used in his thighs, back, and neck. So he tired quickly. For Edgar it would take time to gain the strength he needed to stay upright for long. He would need a schedule, with short periods of forward-tilted seating alternating with rest periods with the seat tilted back. As the boy's strength increased, the length of time he could sit upright on a forward-tilted seat would also increase. In time he might learn to sit upright, even on a non-sloping seat.

Designing Edgar a wheelchair with adjustable seat tilt

The team realized that getting Edgar used to sitting upright in a forward-tilted seat would require frequently shifting him back and forth, from a seat that tilted forward to one that was level (or that tilted somewhat backward).

However, Edgar's mother worked all day in a small restaurant. Sometimes she took Edgar with her. More often she left him at home alone for most of the day. The child was getting too heavy to carry long distances.

It would be too much to expect Edgar's mother to carry him to the restaurant and then to spend all day moving him in and out of a seat with a forward slant. Things needed to be made as easy as possible for his busy mother.

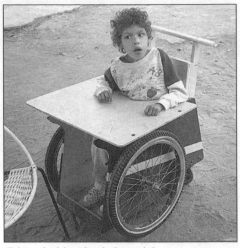

Edgar, in his wheeled special seat.

So the team decided to try to design *a combination of wheelchair and special seat,* so that Edgar's mother could push him to and from the restaurant. The wheeled seat needed to be easily adjustable, so his mother could quickly change the tilt of the seat-board from a forward to a backward tilt . . . if possible with the child still sitting in it.

The following design was the result:

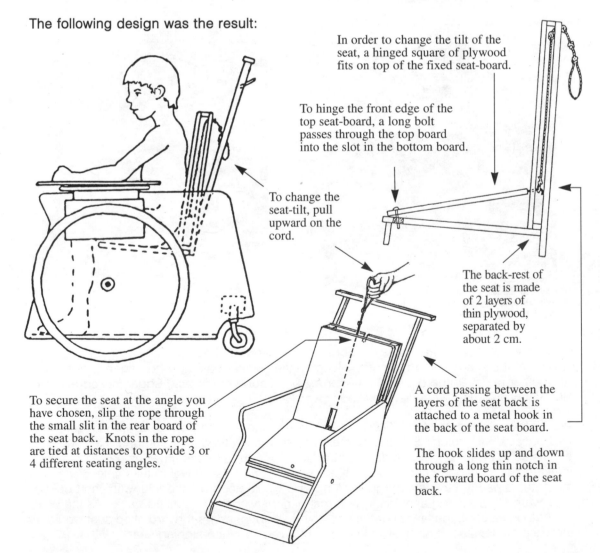

In order to change the tilt of the seat, a hinged square of plywood fits on top of the fixed seat-board.

To hinge the front edge of the top seat-board, a long bolt passes through the top board into the slot in the bottom board.

To change the seat-tilt, pull upward on the cord.

The back-rest of the seat is made of 2 layers of thin plywood, separated by about 2 cm.

A cord passing between the layers of the seat back is attached to a metal hook in the back of the seat board.

The hook slides up and down through a long thin notch in the forward board of the seat back.

To secure the seat at the angle you have chosen, slip the rope through the small slit in the rear board of the seat back. Knots in the rope are tied at distances to provide 3 or 4 different seating angles.

Additional features of the wheelchair with adjustable positive seating

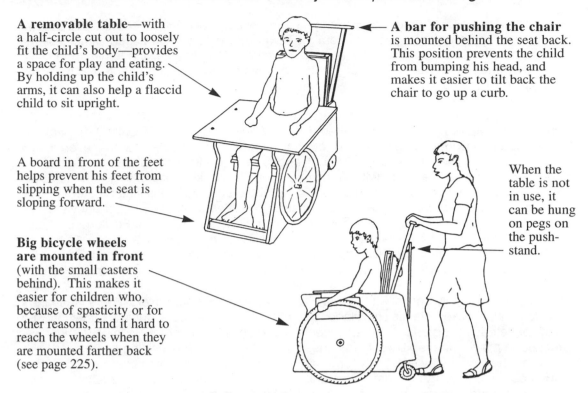

A removable table—with a half-circle cut out to loosely fit the child's body—provides a space for play and eating. By holding up the child's arms, it can also help a flaccid child to sit upright.

A board in front of the feet helps prevent his feet from slipping when the seat is sloping forward.

Big bicycle wheels are mounted in front (with the small casters behind). This makes it easier for children who, because of spasticity or for other reasons, find it hard to reach the wheels when they are mounted farther back (see page 225).

A bar for pushing the chair is mounted behind the seat back. This position prevents the child from bumping his head, and makes it easier to tilt back the chair to go up a curb.

When the table is not in use, it can be hung on pegs on the push-stand.

Designing this chair, the team observed that changing the slope of the seat changed the height of the child relative to the table. Therefore the table height had to be adjustable. They created a simple design that allows **adjustment of both the table height and angle.**

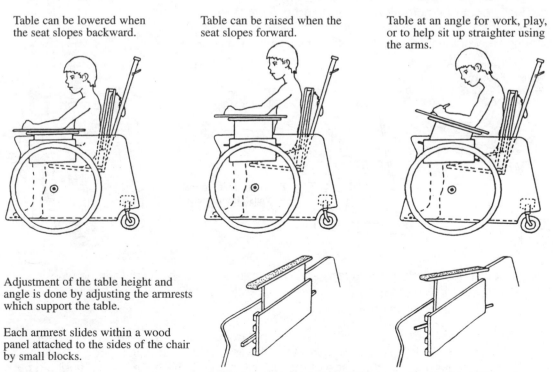

Table can be lowered when the seat slopes backward.

Table can be raised when the seat slopes forward.

Table at an angle for work, play, or to help sit up straighter using the arms.

Adjustment of the table height and angle is done by adjusting the armrests which support the table.

Each armrest slides within a wood panel attached to the sides of the chair by small blocks.

A thin rod of hard wood slipped between the blocks at different heights and angles determines the position of the armrests and table.

The many adjustable features of this chair allow the family and child to experiment with different combinations of adjustments, to find out what works best for the individual child.

OUTCOME WITH EDGAR — AND HIS FURTHER PROGRESS

As with many children, in evaluating Edgar's progress it is difficult to separate the benefits brought by the physical equipment from the human support and increased stimulation that accompanied it. Certainly all the attention, movement, handling, talking to him, and encouragement that Edgar received during his days at PROJIMO contributed to his sense of self-worth and readiness to hold his head higher.

Equally important was the renewed interest on the part of Edgar's mother and the enthusiasm of his 12 year older brother, Adolfo. Adolfo helped the PROJIMO carpenter, Mario, to build Edgar's wheelchair. Through this involvement, Adolfo became even more eager to try it out with his younger brother, and to help him to use it effectively. In the course of a few days at PROJIMO, Adolfo learned a lot of skills for working with the boy. With words, objects, and stimulating noises, he would encourage his little brother to raise his head and look around, adding to the effect of the tilted seat. Also important were Edgar's rides all around the village. Back in their own village, now that Edgar had wheels, both his mother and brother were much more inclined to take him out and include him in their activities. His new seat seemed most effective in getting Edgar to raise his head when he was bumping over rough terrain, and when the scenery was constantly changing.

Edgar and his family continued to visit PROJIMO periodically for several years. Members of the team also visited his distant village whenever they had an opportunity. Edgar showed slow but steady progress, physically, mentally and socially. Much of his improvement was related to his growing ability to hold himself upright. At first, when sitting in a forward-tilted position, he would stay erect only for a minute or two before slumping over again. But with practice, he sat upright longer. Eventually, he began to spend more time sitting up and looking around him, even when he was not in his forward-tilting seat.

Preparation for walking. The forward-tilted seat also stimulated Edgar to use his leg muscles. The boy gradually became more able to stand and even to take a few steps with assistance. To help him get used to bearing his weight, they made a standing frame for him. ➡

Holes for straps.

A knee separator can be added.

Holes for feet (straps may also be needed).

The standing board held Edgar's legs and hips in a straighter position than he was accustomed to. Initially they had been very stiff, with beginnings of contractures (inability to straighten completely).

As with the positive seating, at first Edgar was put in the standing frame for very brief periods (2 or 3 minutes). As he got used to it, the time was lengthened. Edgar's mother and Adolfo also learned to do "range of motion" exercises to help the child straighten out and make his stiff joints more limber.

Edgar showed overall improvement for about two years. Then, sadly—after the death of his father—he had **a severe setback involving self-abuse.** This is discussed in Chapter 8.

Two Very Different Walkers for Edgar

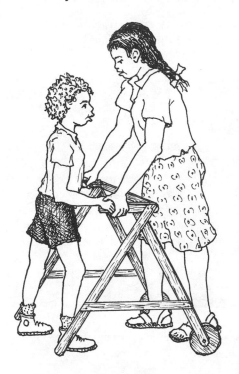

For Edgar, standing with his **standing frame** made it easier to hold up his head. This probably helped for the same reasons as did tilting his seat forward. The voluntary use of his leg muscles triggered an increase in muscle tone throughout his body.

After Edgar had used the standing frame for a few months, the team thought he might be ready to try a walker. PROJIMO's carpenter, Mario, experimented with different styles and heights. Then he built a simple **wooden walker** for Edgar. Adolfo and a couple of the village children helped Mario.

◄— Here, a school girl who assists in making simple equipment at PROJIMO helped Edgar learn to walk. As you see, Edgar (for short but increasing amounts of time) was able to hold up his head.

This walker's wooden wheels allow it to roll forward without having to lift it (which Edgar could not do because of weakness and poor balance). Also, the wheels' large size (compared to many walkers) works well on uneven ground.

The walker has automatic brakes similar in effect to those of some very costly commercial walkers. The braking action was discovered by accident. The wooden wheels turn loosely on a bolt between 2 wooden struts. When the child pushes the walker forward between steps, the wheels roll easily. But when the child puts his weight on the walker to take steps, the wheels press against the side struts, acting as a brake. This braking effect makes walking easier for the unsteady child with poor balance.

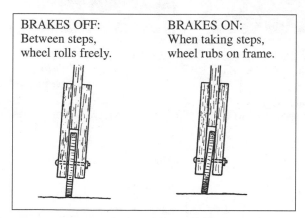

BRAKES OFF:
Between steps, wheel rolls freely.

BRAKES ON:
When taking steps, wheel rubs on frame.

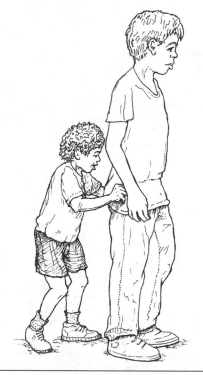

Although the walker worked when someone helped Edgar hold onto it, for a long time he made little effort to hold or walk with it by himself. What Edgar seemed to enjoy most was hanging onto the back of Adolfo's shirt and walking behind him. Fortunately, Adolfo enjoyed this too. **So his big brother became Edgar's custom-made "human walker."** —►

Rehabilitation equipment can be important. But for child development, **the warmth, stimulation, and adventures with persons the child feels close to are essential.**

Merry-Go-Round as Therapy for Tinín

Positive seating does not work for all children with floppy cerebral palsy. Tinín is a child for whom other approaches worked better. When his mother brought him to PROJIMO at age 5, he had great difficulty sitting upright, as can be seen in these photos.

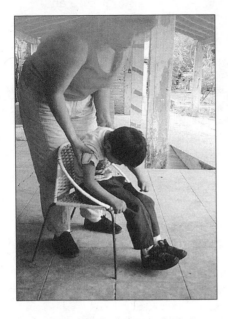

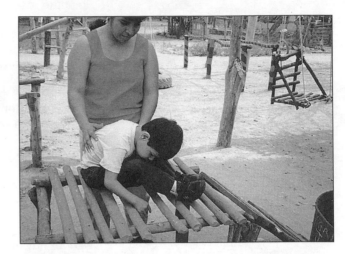

The PROJIMO team experimented with positive (forward-tilting) seating, but Tinín slumped forward so far that he would fall off the seat, unless held. In Tinín's case, negative seating (with the seat sloping backwards) seemed to help more than positive seating.

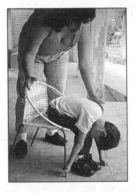

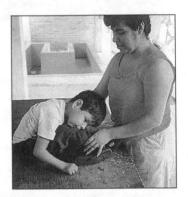

While the team tried everything they could think of to help Tinín sit upright, his mother had the idea of putting him in the merry-go-round in PROJIMO's "Playground for All Children." Actually, the idea was Tinín's. Of the 10 or so words he spoke, one was "car." Since he first saw the merry-go-round, which has a small car on it with a pretend steering wheel, he kept pointing to it, saying "Car!" Clearly he wanted to sit in it. So his mother followed his wishes.

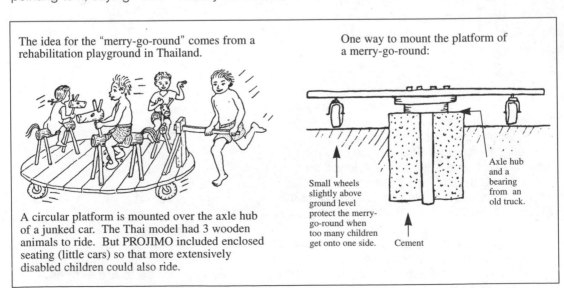

The idea for the "merry-go-round" comes from a rehabilitation playground in Thailand.

One way to mount the platform of a merry-go-round:

A circular platform is mounted over the axle hub of a junked car. The Thai model had 3 wooden animals to ride. But PROJIMO included enclosed seating (little cars) so that more extensively disabled children could also ride.

Small wheels slightly above ground level protect the merry-go-round when too many children get onto one side.

Cement

Axle hub and a bearing from an old truck.

Sitting in the small "car" Tinín tried hard to sit upright; but even with his excitement and desire, he was only partly successful. Yet when his mother—sitting across from him—started to turn the merry-go-round with her foot, Tinín began to straighten up.

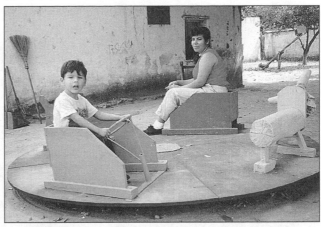

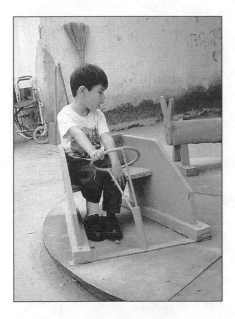

The faster the merry-go-round went, the more Tinín straightened up. He hung onto the steering wheel for dear life. Therapy was never more fun!

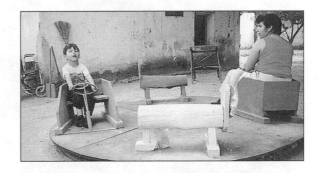

Considering how his holding onto the steering wheel seemed to help Tinín to sit upright, the team began to experiment with special seating. They designed a simple backward-slanting wood seat. Above its plywood table, they added a removable cross-bar, held by upright bars with notches that snugly grip the edge of the table. The series of notches allows the bar to be set at different heights and slipped forwards or backwards, to whatever positions appear best.

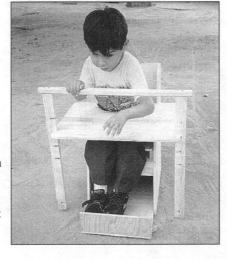

With the cross-bar in its lower positions, Tinín can hold onto it to sit up straighter.

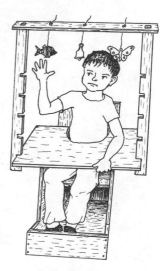

With the cross-bar in its highest position, things that interest Tinín can be hung from it.

By following Tinín's interests and by taking an experimental approach, his caretakers found equipment and activities that helped him to gain more control of his body, and to sit in a way that enabled him to learn new skills and take part more fully in life around him.

The Special Seat as a Tool for Stimulation

The special seat—combined with an overhead bar with toys hanging from it, and lots of interaction between the parents and the child—can do a lot to help a child gain better head and hand control, and to become more involved in the world that surrounds him.

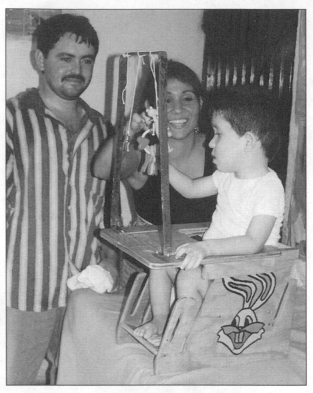

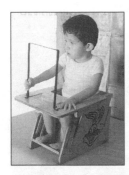
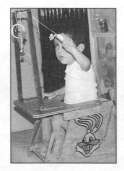

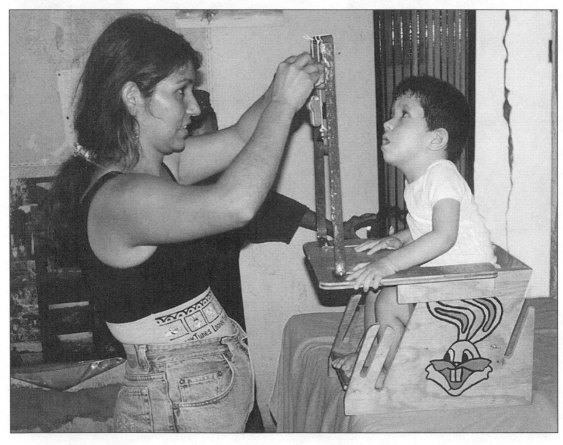

CHAPTER 5

A Tire Seat to Reduce Celia's Spasticity

CELIA, who has cerebral palsy and developmental delay, was brought to PROJIMO in a specially adapted buggy, or stroller, prescribed by a rehabilitation specialist. But there were problems with how she sat. Although a chest band held her more or less upright, she frequently went into a spastic pattern. Her head and shoulders pressed backward, her arms extended widely, and her legs stiffened in an asymmetrical position. ———————→

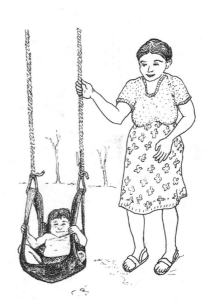

The PROJIMO team and Celia's mother experimented with different seating, trying to find a position that would reduce Celia's spasticity and give her more control of her body, especially of her head, arms and hands.

An innovation: The most effective seating arrangement proved to be a tire swing. It can be made like this. ——→

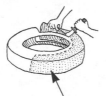 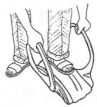

Cut away this part of the tire.

Then turn the tire inside out.

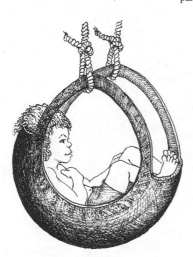

The double curve of the tire gently bent the child's head, shoulders, and hips forward. And it held her legs in a bent, relaxed position. ←———

In the tire swing, Celia had much more head and hand control and little sign of spasticity.

She was even able to reach forward and hold the tire rim. ——→

PROJIMO encouraged the family to make a tire swing in their home, and to improvise other seating arrangements that would provide a similar function.

Problems: Shortcomings of the tire swing are: (1) It is suspended in one location and cannot be easily moved. (2) The tire works well for Celia, but for many children, a spastic pattern can be better reduced by flexing the hips to a 90-degree angle, which the tire swing does not do. (3) The tire holds the child in a semi-reclining position. But, for maximum function, it often helps to sit more upright.

Usefulness for other disabled children: The design for the tire swing can be found in the book *Disabled Village Children.* This kind of tire swing has been used in many countries, both in children's playgrounds and for rehabilitation of children with physical and mental delay. However, its potential as a device for special seating, especially for children with spastic cerebral palsy, still needs to be more fully recognized and implemented.

OLD TIRES *have a hundred uses in*
A PLAYGROUND FOR ALL CHILDREN

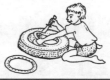

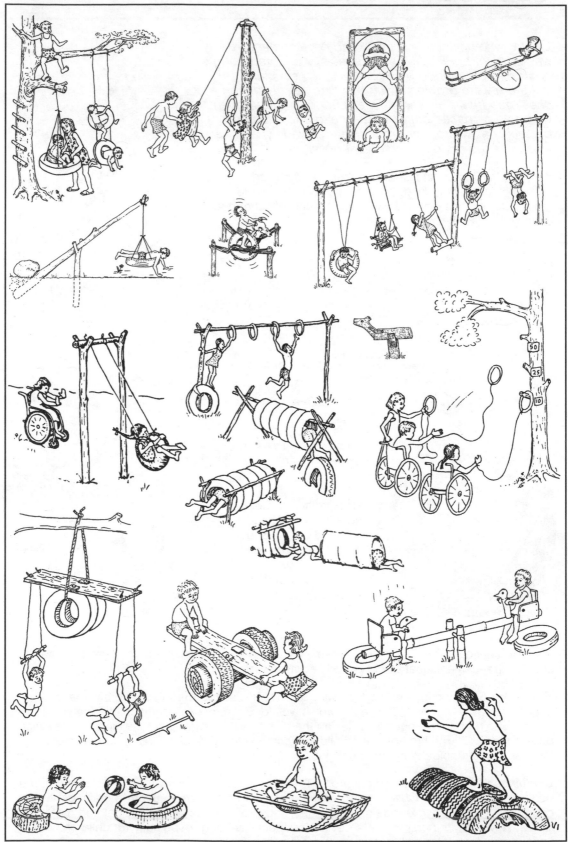

A Mudguard for Dalia

CHAPTER **6**

DALIA is a lovely 5-year-old who is developmentally delayed. Her mother brought her to PROJIMO to see if anything could be done to help her "learn to walk and talk."

On observing Dalia's responses to people and things around her, the PROJIMO team felt the child had a lot more potential than she had realized. She seemed quite alert—but her attention span was short. She would play with a toy for a moment, then drop it. She was beginning to speak a few words, but she had trouble pronouncing them.

Physically, Dalia had difficulty with hand control and with balance. She had a lot of spasticity, mostly in her lower body. She could not stand, even with assistance.

Dalia's mother explained that, as a single working mother, she often had little choice but to leave her daughter alone at home for long periods. For her safety, she locked Dalia in a small room. "I'd like to take her out with me and do more fun things with her, like visit friends who have children," she said. "But she can't walk and she's getting heavy."

Mari—a wheelchair rider herself—thought a wheelchair might help. She had Dalia try a variety of children's chairs at PROJIMO, to see if any suited her. One small second-hand wheelchair fit her well. Dalia loved it! She made a great effort to roll it by pushing on its wheels. Time and again, her mother said, "Use the hand rims!" But Dalia kept pushing the wheels. (They were easier to grip.) When at last she rolled the chair forward, everyone cheered. *Here was a disability aid that held the child's attention, that helped to improve her hand control, that could stimulate interaction outside the home, and that gave her greater independence—all in a form she enjoyed and might well persist with.*

Dalia's mother foresees a danger. Dalia's mother recognized the benefits of the wheelchair. But she was worried. "I won't dare take her outside in it!" She explained that they lived in a slum on the edge of the city. The dirt alleys were full of garbage and "doo-doo."

"You see, Dalia always puts her fingers in her mouth. Now that she's discovered she can move in her wheelchair, she'll always have her hands on its wheels! Filth from the street is sure to end up in her mouth and make her sick. Her health is already delicate."

For this reason, Dalia's mother preferred to use a stroller from PROJIMO. It was rather like a baby buggy and, in it, Dalia would lie back passively, unable to reach the small wheels. Mari, a

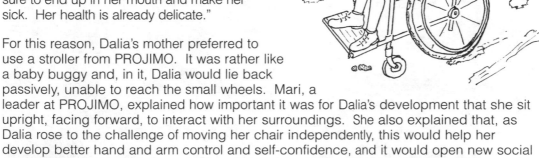

leader at PROJIMO, explained how important it was for Dalia's development that she sit upright, facing forward, to interact with her surroundings. She also explained that, as Dalia rose to the challenge of moving her chair independently, this would help her develop better hand and arm control and self-confidence, and it would open new social (and developmental) horizons for her. This might, in turn, help her improve her speech.

But Dalia's mother still worried about the filth from the street. "I guess I just won't be able to take her outside in the wheelchair," she sighed, "unless there's some way to keep her hands off the wheels when we pass through filthy areas."

Looking for a solution: The challenge for the PROJIMO team was to design some sort of "mud guard" to keep the child's hands from reaching the wheels of the wheelchair when passing through mud and filth. The mud guard needed to be simple, low cost, and lightweight. It also needed to be easy and quick to put on and remove.

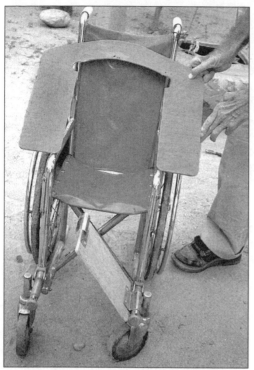

The author holds the U-shaped mudguard in front of Dalia's wheelchair.

An innovative solution: A simple U-shaped armrest was cut from plywood.

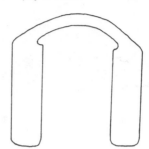

The two arm supports were wide enough to prevent the child from reaching around them to grasp the wheels.

The back bridge of the "U" was curved to fit around the curved fabric back of the wheelchair. By folding the wheelchair slightly, the armrest could be instantly placed or removed. No clamps or ties were needed.

The entire arm-rest took only half an hour to make (the time to cut out the design with a saber saw, to round the corners and edges, and to sand them). The only cost was that of a 50 cm square sheet of 1/4 inch plywood.

The ease with which the mudguard can be put in place and removed makes it more likely that Dalia's mother will take it off when inside the house. It is important that the mudguard be removed when it is not needed, so that Dalia can increase her hand-skills and learn to move about independently in her wheelchair.

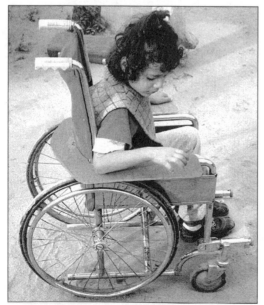

Armrests keep Dalia from reaching the wheels.

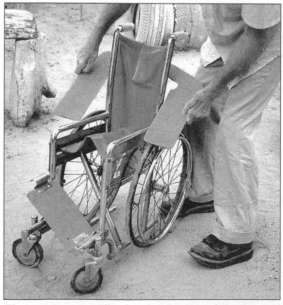

The armrests are easily placed and removed.

CHAPTER 7

Listening to Rufina
Listen to her Body

Learning from a Young Girl with Athetosis How to "Listen to Her Body," to Help Her with Control for Sitting and Moving

RUFINA is a bright little girl with athetoid cerebral palsy. She was brought to PROJIMO from Más Válidos, a community rehabilitation program in the state capital. (Más Válidos was started in 1985 by two disabled youths who had gone to PROJIMO for their own rehabilitation, and then stayed for a year to apprentice as rehabilitation workers.) Rufina was accompanied by two social workers, but no family members. Her parents are poor migrant farm workers who dared not request time off, for fear of losing their seasonal jobs.

When Mari asked Rufina how old she was, the child shook her head. But she looked about 7 or so. Rufina is shy, yet she has a ready smile and a stubborn will. Although she understands language well, her difficulty with mouth and tongue control make her speech hard to understand. She does her best to communicate using sounds, signs, and gestures.

The girl's physical ability is quite limited due to spasticity combined with athetosis (uncontrolled movements which keep her body and limbs twisting and writhing). She came to PROJIMO in a bright red wheelchair that had been donated by a charitable organization. In her adult-sized chair, her body's continuous strong thrusts into extension (arching backwards) made it a never-ending battle for her to stay in the chair and not pitch off of it.

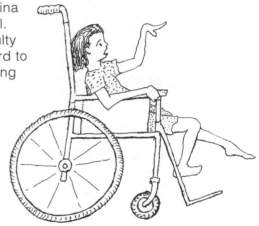

Rufina in her giant wheelchair.

Rufina has strong hands and can grip things fairly well. However, she had been delayed in developing manual skills, because her hands were constantly kept busy trying to make her uncooperative body stay inside her wheelchair. Because of this, she was unable to feed herself, or to use her hands for play or other activities, making her almost completely dependent on others for all of her needs.

A SERIES OF TRIALS AND ERRORS

The PROJIMO team observed Rufina's difficulties in her huge wheelchair. Their first suggestion was to seat the girl in a child's wheelchair of the correct size for her body.

Another idea was to fit her wheelchair with an insert so she could sit with her hips at a 90-degree angle. They tried each of these adaptations, together with various hip, belly, and chest bands. Also, they put a raised pad on the front half of the seat to try to keep her from scooting forward when her body stiffened.

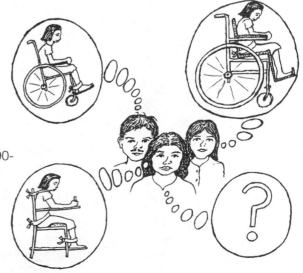

Altogether, the team tried over a dozen different kinds of seating, strapping, and angles of tilt.

Nothing seemed to help.

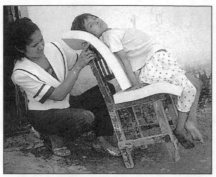

Fitting a regular chair with cushions did not work. Rufina's body arched up stiffly.

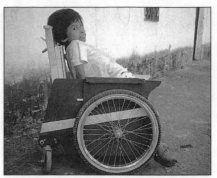

This chair, with positive seating, did not work either.

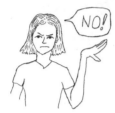

With each of these trials, they asked Rufina whether she thought the adaptation helped her to sit better or made her more comfortable. Each time she emphatically said NO. She made it clear that she felt better and more in control in her big red wheelchair. At first the team thought she was just afraid to try something new … or that she was emotionally attached to her handsome (if inappropriate) first wheelchair.

But, on observing the girl carefully, the team realized that all the adaptations they had tried only seemed to make her body movements worse. The hip and body straps triggered such forceful thrusting that they were counter-productive. Her body used up so much energy pushing against the restraints that she streamed sweat and quickly became exhausted.

With each new trial, Rufina insisted that she preferred her own wheelchair. The team knows how important it is to listen to a child and to respond to her wishes. And, reluctantly, they had to agree that none of their improvisations helped. Inadequate as the huge wheelchair was, they had found no better alternative. They were almost ready to give up and let Rufina continue her struggle to keep upright in her beloved chair. But that was a shame, since it did not let her use her hands for other activities.

Then the team had one last idea. They saw that one problem with the giant wheelchair was that Rufina's right knee hooked over the front edge of the seat, pulling her forward.

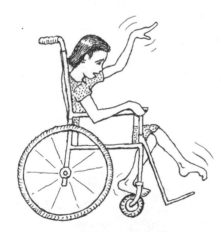

This caused her to push herself backwards, and to start to slip out of the chair, a process that she was constantly having ⟵ to fight.

So they tried one last experiment: **a long, padded board, placed on the seat,** to extend her legs straight forward. ⟶

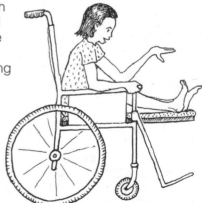

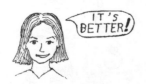

"So how do you like it now?" Mari asked her, expecting the same negative response. But this time Rufina smiled and said: "It's better!"

Indeed, she was able to sit up straighter and seemed to have more control of her body and hands.

This time, when they experimented with a fairly loose body-band, her body appeared not to fight it as much. And Rufina agreed that it helped.

Rufina takes the lead. Excited by her new ability to sit upright for moments without struggling, Rufina took the problem-solving initiative. Now that her hands were freer, she could experiment to improve her stability. Leaning forward, she grasped her left foot and, with a lot of effort (but insisting that no one assist her), she doubled her left knee. The uncooperative leg kept trying to straighten, but the sponge padding on the seat-board helped to keep the bent leg in place. Then she caught her right foot, bent the knee, and tucked the foot under her left knee. This cross-legged position gave her better body and hand control than ever.

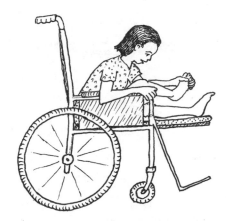

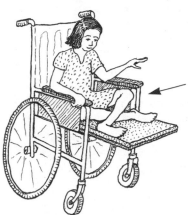

But one thing bothered her. When she crossed her legs, her knees pressed against the metal wheel-guards, under the arm rests.

"Would you like us to remove the wheel-guards so that you can sit cross-legged more easily in your chair?" Mari asked her. Rufina nodded energetically. Within an hour, the panels under her armrests were removed, leaving more space for her knees. Now, Rufina could sit cross-legged more easily.

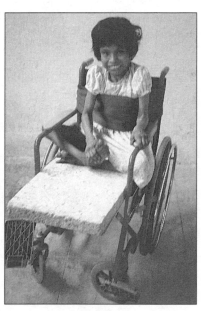

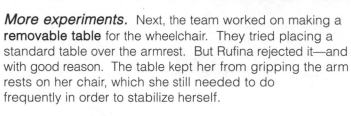

More experiments. Next, the team worked on making a **removable table** for the wheelchair. They tried placing a standard table over the armrest. But Rufina rejected it—and with good reason. The table kept her from gripping the arm rests on her chair, which she still needed to do frequently in order to stabilize herself.

So the team designed a narrower table that fit snugly between the arm rests. To the team's delight, Rufina was able to eat fairly well from a plate on the table, and even to pick up a glass of water and drink it without much spilling.

Everyone was thrilled with the results, especially Rufina. The PROJIMO team was pleased, not only with her new comfort and ability, but with the key role the child herself had played in the problem solving process. **Not only had the girl's participation led to better seating and improved function, it had also given her a new sense of self-confidence, equality, and personal worth.**

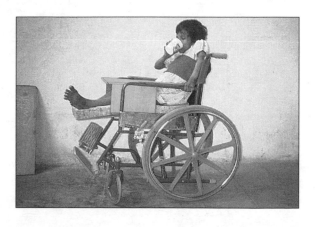

Another Suggestion to Help Children Like Rufina to Sit Better

Before this book went to press, the author asked a number of persons with different disability-related skills to read the draft and make suggestions. No one took on this task with more care and concern than Ann Hallum, an instructor of physical therapy who has made several teaching visits to PROJIMO. (Ann is one of those rare teachers who treats her students as equals, and challenges them to think problems through, rather than to just follow instructions.) She caught mistakes in the book, helped make points clearer, and had many good suggestions.

On reading about Rufina, Ann suggested a measure that she has found helps some children with athetosis (sudden, forceful uncontrolled movements of the body and limbs) to sit in a more stable position. Her suggestion is as follows:

USE OF A THIGH BAND FOR CHILDREN WITH ATHETOSIS

Ann explained that, instead of using a "pelvic band" (hip strap) to stabilize the hips, it sometimes works better to put the band across the thighs, close to the body. The "thigh band" often helps to prevent the sudden stiffening of the body that tends to make the child arch up, throwing her out of her chair. It pulls her backside down so that she sits squarely against her butt bones, which can help stabilize her in an upright, sitting position.

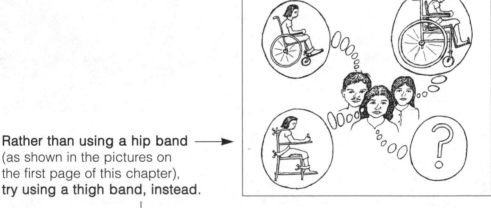

Rather than using a hip band (as shown in the pictures on the first page of this chapter), **try using a thigh band, instead.**

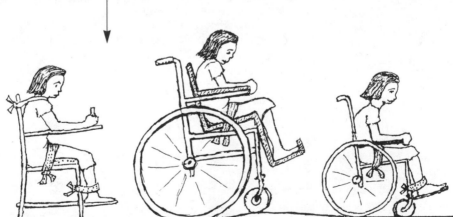

NOTE: For another example of changes (improvements and corrections) to earlier drafts of this book, see the two different versions of the exercise sheet for persons with an amputation of a leg, on pages 181 and 182.

Paper-Based Aids

Seating and Standing Aids for Cruz and Kim, and a Helmet for Edgar

APPROPRIATE PAPER-BASED TECHNOLOGY

Most of the special seats described in this book have been made, at a fairly low cost, with wood or plywood. But for many families, even local wood is too expensive or difficult to obtain. For this reason, in Zimbabwe, Africa many years ago, an elderly man named Bevill Packer began to make special seating and other assistive devices out of waste paper and cardboard. In this Appropriate Paper-Based Technology (APT), layers of paper and/or cardboard are glued together with a paste made from flour and water. Paste can be made from maize flour or even with left-over "sadza," a wheat-flour baby food widely used in Africa. Well-made paper-based seating aids and other devices can be unbelievably strong. ⟶

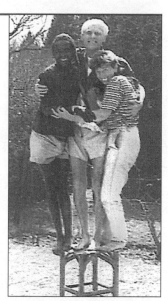

This stool, made only of paper and cardboard, can support 3 people. The photo is from the APT manual mentioned on page 73.

Apart from being **low-cost** (in terms of materials), paper-based technology has other advantages. It is:

- **Easy and fun to make.** Children love to help make this equipment. (However, care with technique is needed for the results to be strong and durable.)

- **Adaptable to personal needs.** Seat-backs and supports can be molded to meet individual needs. Adjustments can easily be made, hollows scooped out, or lumps or wedges added where needed, for greater comfort, protection, or support.

- **Gentle to the touch.** The finished seat or device has a surface that is somewhat flexible, especially when made of corrugated cardboard (from "thick wall" cardboard boxes). This provides a softer, giving, personal touch and is gentler where it comes in contact with knees, butt bones, and other bony areas. It tends to be more comfortable and protective (against pressure sores) than wood, plastic, or metal.

During the last few years, the art of Paper-Based Technology has spread over much of Africa, and is now being discovered in other continents, including the Americas and Europe.

For years, PROJIMO and Project Piaxtla in Mexico have made limited use of paper-based technology for things such as paper-maché puppets, learning aids, and wheelchair cushions. (A cardboard cushion to prevent pressure sores is shown on page 157.) PROJIMO has only recently begun to experiment with using APT for special seating, standing boards, and other assistive devices. The aids in this chapter are among PROJIMO's first experiments.

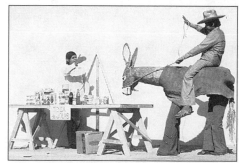

This donkey, with a head of paper maché, was made by Piaxtla health workers and used in a farm worker theater skit to awaken villagers to their constitutional land rights.

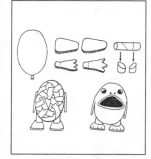

To make a paper-maché frog, strips of newspaper several layers thick are pasted over a balloon.

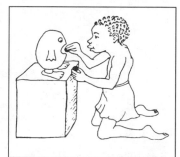

A child with developmental delay plays at feeding a frog by putting small stones into its mouth.

CRUZ is a 2 year old boy with cerebral palsy that is in part floppy (low muscle tone) and in part spastic (uncontrolled tightening of muscles). His mother devotes a lot of time to helping him develop his body, mind, and spirit to their best potential. Cruz's brothers and sisters play with him, talk to him, and help him with activities.

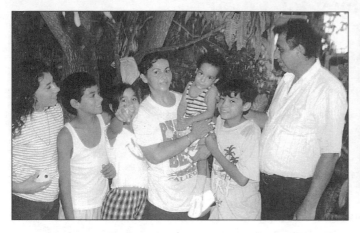

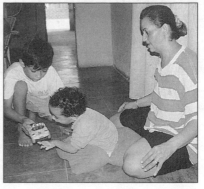

Cruz learns to sit, with the help of sandbags on his legs and behind his hips (see page 46).

Thanks to this loving family effort, Cruz has gained fairly good head control and, with effort, he manages to open his hands to wave hello and goodbye. He also tries very hard to speak. His words are difficult to understand, but his family has learned to interpret them, and they encourage him to speak as much as possible. The boy thrives on all the hugging, handling, and encouragement he receives.

A wooden seat the child hated.
Cruz's mother brought him to PROJIMO from a nearby village. She understood his condition so well that the rehabilitation workers learned as many practical developmental activities from her as they were able to teach her. It was agreed that Cruz might benefit from a special seat. Juan designed and built a handsome plywood seat for him with a removable backrest.

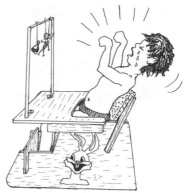

But for some reason, Cruz hated his wooden seat. Usually a cheerful child, no sooner was he placed in the seat than he began to scream and wail. His mother was sure he would get used to it, but after two months he still refused to accept it.

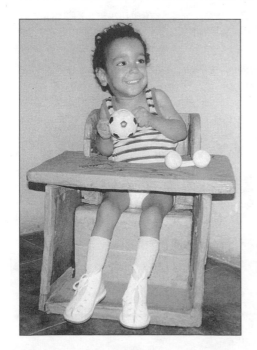

A cardboard seat that he liked.
PROJIMO had been experimenting with paper-based technology. So they tried sitting Cruz in a still-unfinished seat made of laminated cardboard (layers of cardboard from old cartons, glued together). To everyone's surprise, Cruz was all laughs and smiles. His mother was amazed at the difference.

We are not sure why Cruz, who had such a strong dislike for the plywood seat, took such an instant liking to the cardboard one. The positioning and support provided by each was much the same. We suspect that the cardboard seat—with its thick, rounded, relatively soft, yielding structures—was somehow friendlier and more similar to human touch. By contrast, the plywood seat, even with its cushioned lining, was more rigid and unyielding. Despite the smiling rabbits painted on its sides, the wooden seat was not as child-friendly.

A Cardboard Seat Built for Cruz

The seat was designed with many special features. A removable post, or pommel, was placed between the boy's thighs to keep him from slipping forward. A table-top fits around his waist to help stabilize his lower body. A removable, U-shaped hip support fit into the seat to stabilize his hips. It held him slightly forward from the seat-back so that when he wanted to, he could sit up without leaning against the seat-back. (This idea came from watching Cruz's mother place sand bags around his hips to help him sit upright.)

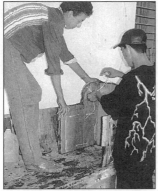

All of the seat parts, including the table top, the pommel, and the U-shaped hip support, were made by **pasting together (laminating) layers of corrugated cardboard** cut from old cartons.

To make the seat, large sheets of cardboard were bent to form the sides and back. After gluing, they were sewn with string to hold them as the paste dried.

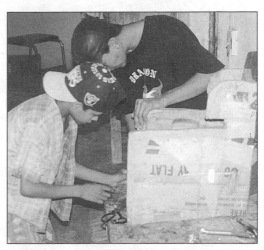

Village children helped to build the cardboard seat.

On his first try, Cruz sat fairly well in the seat. But there were problems that required some modifications:

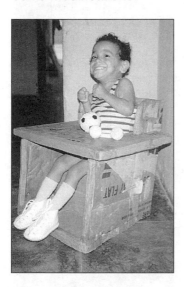

1. When Cruz was excited, his legs stiffened and his tense body pushed backward. ←

So **a removable ankle bar** was added to keep his feet on the foot-rest. The bar was made of cardboard, reinforced by a flat metal rod, bent to help position his feet. A **removable foot separator** of layered cardboard was added to help him position his feet well. ———→

2. Although the U-shaped hip-support at times seemed to help Cruz sit upright, often he would slump or push back against the seat back.

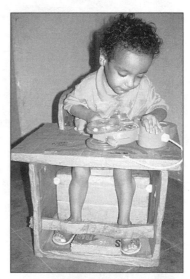

So a 2-piece **low-back support** was made of layered cardboard. It could be easily removed as he gained better hip and back control.

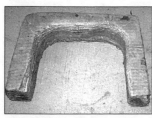

U-shaped hip support made of laminated cardboard.

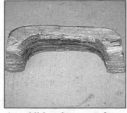

An additional support for higher stabilization of hips.

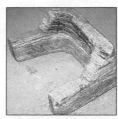

The 2 hip supports can be used together or singly.

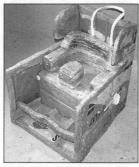

Both hip supports plus groin pommel stabilize hips well.

Addition of an adjustable tilt to the seat. On experimenting with the angle of the seat, it was found that sometimes Cruz sat more upright when the seat tilted forward. (See discussion of positive seating in Chapter 4, page 48.) So a mechanism to change the seat angle was added.

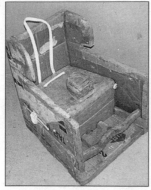

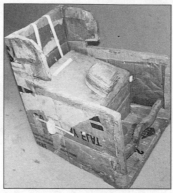

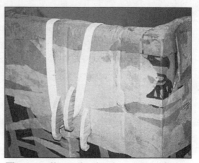

A thin cloth strap was attached to the back edge of the seat-board.

By pulling the strap the seat could be positioned at different angles.

Three small wooden hooks were made, with posts that fit tightly into holes drilled into the back side of the cardboard seat-back.

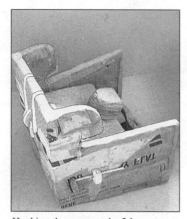

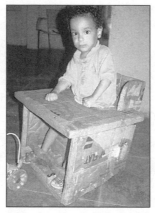

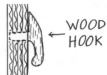

Hooking the strap on the 2 lowest hooks gives the seat a steep tilt.

When Cruz sits on the forward sloping seat, he sits more erect, with more trunk control.

By hooking the cloth strap on one or more of these hooks, the seat could be adjusted to 7 different angles.

WOOD HOOK

The forward tip of the seat seemed to help Cruz sit in a more upright position. The tilt caused him to push downward with his legs to keep from slipping forward. This increased the muscle tone in his back. But since the foot-bar kept his knees bent, he avoided spastic arching backwards.

All of these adaptations and additions were simple and fun to make because the cardboard frame and attachments were so easy to cut, drill, and modify. Almost the only tool needed was a knife. Removable pieces molded from cardboard could be firmly attached by pressing them (or the pegs attached to them) through grooves or holes cut into the frame. The thickness and texture of the cardboard frame provided a firm grip for the inserted posts and attachments.

The different pieces and attachments to Cruz's seat are almost all removable and many are easily adjustable. The final version of the seat with its removable parts is shown here.

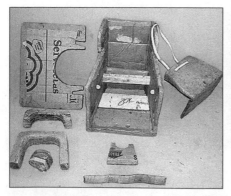

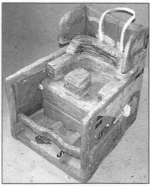

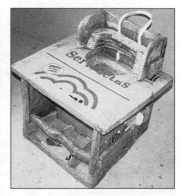

An instruction sheet for making cardboard seats is on page 72.

A Cardboard Standing-Frame for Cruz

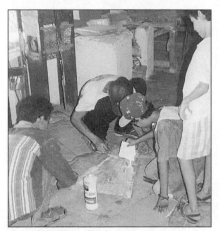

Village children paste together sheets of cardboard to make a standing-frame.

Cruz's mother, brothers, and sister often held him upright, and Cruz did his best to stand. At first his legs stiffened in a tip-toe position. But, if he was held quietly for a while, the spastic muscles would gradually relax and his feet would flatten on the ground. Cruz's mother had bought him new, high-top shoes, which seemed to help him position his feet better.

The PROJIMO team felt Cruz might be ready for a standing-frame. Again, they decided to use mainly corrugated cardboard. The cardboard was reinforced with wooden struts, and had a wooden base-board.

In a preliminary trial of the standing frame, Cruz stood fairly well on it. His feet rested flat on the base-board and were held apart by the foot-holes in the vertical frame. The boy seemed delighted with being able to stand by himself.

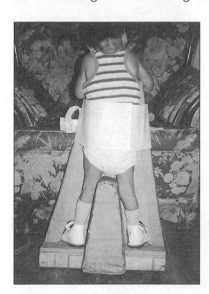

However, his knees angled inwardly as he stood. ⟶ He needed something that would hold his legs straight and apart. So a **leg-separator** was made by re-shaping and gluing together 2 cardboard boxes to form a long, thin ⟵ triangle.

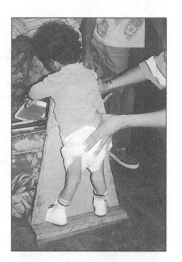

A big advantage of a standing-frame made of cardboard is its smooth, soft surface, and its capacity to bend or sink in slightly, under pressure. The cardboard, therefore, provides more gentle support for bony areas such as Cruz's knees.

In conclusion: PROJIMO's early trials with cardboard assistive devices show great promise. The PROJIMO team still needs to improve its technique, to create smoother and cleaner products. But the results are working remarkably well. Cardboard provides a number of advantages over other materials: especially its low cost, and the ease with which the structures can be modified and adapted to meet individual changing needs.

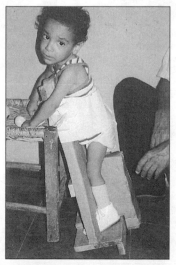

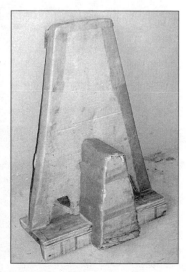

A Cardboard Head-Protector for Edgar

Children with epilepsy (fits), who suddenly lose consciousness and fall, often need a padded helmet or head protector to prevent head injuries.

EDGAR, whose brain was damaged at birth, had been brought repeatedly to PROJIMO from a distant village by his mother (see Chapter 4). His condition had steadily improved. But after his father was murdered, he developed a serious problem, perhaps related to family stress. His mother lost her restaurant job. She worked long hours away from home, selling odds and ends to keep her children fed. She had little time for her disabled son. Sometimes Edgar's brothers and sisters played with him after school. But for many hours a day, Edgar—who could neither walk independently nor talk—sat in a corner or lay on a mat, unattended.

Bored and lonely, the boy had developed harmful, self-stimulating behaviors. He rocked back and forth, stared at his hands, hit his face with his fists, and banged his head on the floor. His mother said he hit himself to make himself cry, to get attention. The team suggested that she give him more attention when he was not hitting himself, to reinforce his positive rather than his harmful behavior. But they realized she was depressed, overworked, and needed help. So they found neighbors and a village health worker to take turns caring for Edgar, to provide him with human contact, and to stimulate him with rewarding activities.

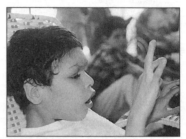

From banging his head on the floor, his brows and forehead were chronically swollen.

But patterns do not change overnight. Edgar needed some kind of head protection. But the family's visit to PROJIMO was brief. In 2 hours, the bus would leave for their distant village. So Mari and her helpers decided to quickly improvise a simple cardboard head-protector.

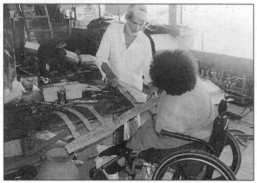

1. After measuring Edgar's head, Chon (who is deaf) helped Mari cut a long strip of cardboard, with several "arms," to form a head-band with criss-cross straps.

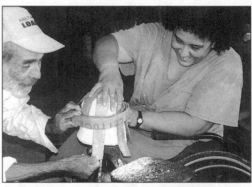

2. To make the helmet fit, Mari and Chon used an old plaster leg-mold which they rounded and filed to the size of the boy's head.

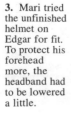 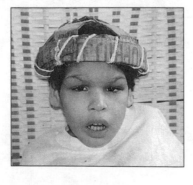

3. Mari tried the unfinished helmet on Edgar for fit. To protect his forehead more, the headband had to be lowered a little.

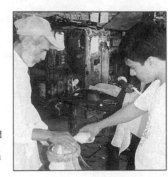

4. After making a few adjustments, Chon and a young helper glued the cardboard helmet together. To hold it in place, they sewed the layers of cardboard together with string.

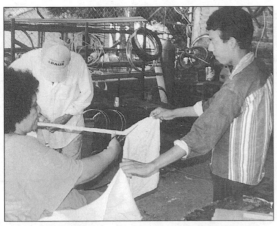

5. Martín helped Mari cut strips of a soft towel to be used as padding for the helmet.

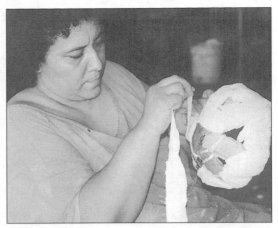

6. Mari wrapped the cardboard head protector with the strips of soft towel.

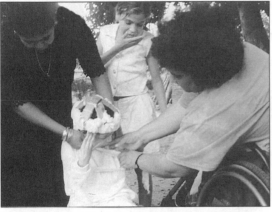

7. Mari attached a chin strap of soft cloth to the head protector. Here she and Edgar's mother tie it gently in place.

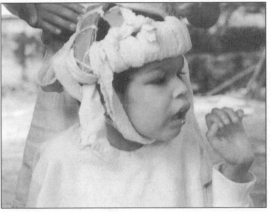

8. The new head protector was finished in two hours. The final steps were hurried, and the glue was still moist. But Edgar's mother said she would cover it more neatly with cloth padding at home.

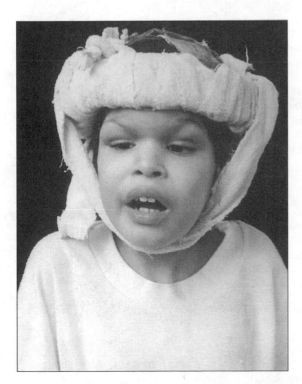

We hope that the cardboard helmet will help protect Edgar and prevent further damage caused by his hitting his head.

Far more important, however, is the need for community support, loving attention, warm physical contact, and playful, stimulating activities. Fortunately, the community health worker in the village, who used to work at PROJIMO, is very capable and conscientious. He has agreed to find a warm-hearted local woman who works well with children, and who has the time to care for Edgar for 3 or 4 hours a day. The health worker will provide training and advice to Edgar's care-provider, so that Edgar gets the rehabilitation and the developmental stimulation he needs.

Suggestions for Making an APT Specially Designed Seat
(adapted from a sheet prepared by Kennett and Jean Westmacott)

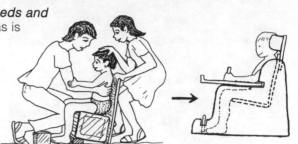

1. *Plan the seat according to the child's needs and possibilities.* With the child's help (as much as is possible), experiment to find a helpful sitting position. Try different placement, angles, and amounts of support. (To do this, use chairs, hands, boxes, sandbags, and wedges as needed.) Look for a position the child likes, that provides good posture and encourages more self-control and use of head, body, and hands. **Sketch a seat design accordingly.**

2. *Measure the child.* With the child in a sitting position, take measurements for the height, depth, and width of the seat, and the height of the seat-back (see page 42).

(see page 42)

3. *Make several laminated (layered) cardboard flats.* For the sides, back, seat, armrests, and lapboard of the special chair, cut corrugated cardboard sections from old cartons. Paste together 4 to 10 layers with the corrugation alternating (each layer criss-crossing the one below).

4. *Pressure-dry.* Put a flat board, with heavy weights on it, on the cardboard until it drys completely and is hard. (This may take several days.)

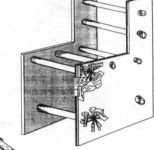

5. *Make cardboard tubes (for girders and struts).* Rub paste onto large sheets of thin, dense (not corrugated) cardboard and roll it around a straight bamboo or broomstick. Pull off and **let dry.** Make 8 or more tubes, depending on your design.

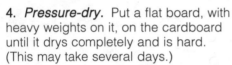

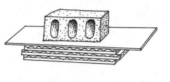

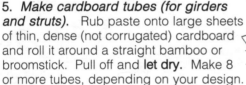

(If thin, solid cardboard is not available, cross-struts can be made by cutting bars from a laminated section of corrugated cardboard.)

6. *Cut holes* in the chair-sides that will fit tightly around the cross tubes. (For best alignment, place the two chair-sides together and cut the holes in both sides at once.)

7. *Assemble and check.* Cut the sides, seat and back flats to the correct size. Assemble, and make necessary adjustments. (If possible, try sitting the child in the chair before gluing.) Let tubes stick out a little. Slice tube ends lengthwise, bend strips over, and paste them firmly to chair-sides with many thin layers of strong paper strips. (Or rub tube-ends with a stone to flatten them. Torn edges stick better than cut ones.)

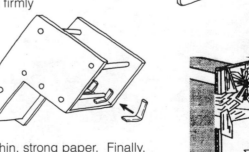

8. Turn chair over and *paste "angle irons"* of dense cardboard bent at a right angle between seat and sides.

9. *Paste over all other edges* with layers of thin, strong paper. Finally, **cover the whole chair with a finishing layer of strong paper.** (Cement bags, wall-paper, or pages from old magazines work well.) Using paper with colorful pictures makes it more fun! Decorate as sparks your fancy!

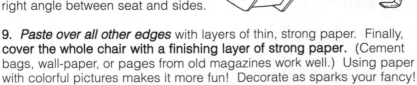

10. When totally dry and hard—it may take a week or more—*varnish to seal.* A plastic (polyurethane) varnish provides good, safe protection.

How PROJIMO's Cardboard Aids Differ from the APT Developed in Zimbabwe

The methods used at PROJIMO for cardboard special seats and other assistive devices have been adapted from those developed in Zimbabwe by Bevill Packer and described in his fine book *Appropriate Paper-Based Technology (APT): A Manual.* (For the full reference, see Resource List 2, page 344.) The Zimbabwe methodology, summarized on the facing page, has been modified somewhat to meet the situation in rural Mexico in the following ways.

TYPES OF PAPER. The Zimbabwe APT seats use 4 main kinds of paper, in different ways:

1. **Corrugated cardboard** such as that used in cardboard cartons. Laminated sections of this thick, light cardboard are often used for the sides and backs of special seats.

2. **Extra-strong paper** such as that used for cement bags. Strips of this are used for edging, and for joining pieces of the frame together. Pasted in place, it makes strong angle joints.

3. **Thin (solid) cardboard** such as that used for shoe boxes. This, and other strong, thick paper is mainly used to make structural supports, often in the form of tubes (see facing page).

4. **Ordinary newsprint, wrapping paper, and the like.** These are usually used by tearing the paper along its grain into thin strips. In a criss-cross pattern these are pasted into layers, either upon a flat surface, or over a form of the desired shape (paper-maché technology).

In Mexican villages, only the first two kinds of paper are readily available: **corrugated cardboard cartons,** and the **strong brown paper** from old cement bags, building-plaster bags, and corn flour (*Maseca*) sacks. Therefore, at PROJIMO, paper-based devices are made almost entirely of corrugated cardboard and surfaced with strong brown paper. Because of the air spaces within corrugated cardboard, walls of assistive devices must be extra thick.

For support struts such as those that hold up the horizontal seat of a Zimbabwe APT chair, you can use round tubes of thin cardboard. PROJIMO uses rectangular "beams" made by laminating corrugated cardboard. These must be extra thick to have enough strength.

PASTE. Zimbabwe APT recommends making a thin paste with flour and water, as follows:

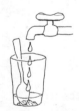

Mix one soup-spoon of refined (white) wheat flour in ½ cup of cool water.

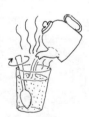

To this mix, add ½ liter (½ quart) of boiling water. Then boil for several minutes, stirring well.

The Zimbabwe manual emphasizes that for gluing strips of paper or thin cardboard, a *very thin paste* be used, so that it penetrates the paper's surface. (Use of thick paste may later attract termites!) However, when making flat boards by pasting together layers of corrugated cardboard, it is essential to work fast and use very little paste. You must "Race the stretch!" says the manual. If the cardboard gets too wet (from too much paste or from working too slowly) the inner, wavy (corrugated) layers tend to come loose or lose their shape. Drying time is also longer. *To end up with strong, flat, smooth boards, the laminated cardboard must be pressed on a flat surface under a weighted plank until completely dry.*

To glue together small cardboard structures, PROJIMO sometimes uses carpenter's *white glue* instead of flour-and-water paste. It dries faster and may be stronger but costs more.

CARDBOARD PLUS OTHER MATERIALS. While the Zimbabwe APT Manual encourages using only *paper products* as building materials, PROJIMO has experimented with combining paper with other low-cost and scrap materials. For example, the special seat for Cruz has a few wood hooks and pegs. Its narrow foot-bar consists of a scrap piece of metal bar (for strength) covered with layers of corrugated cardboard (for padding). Cruz's walker combines the use of cardboard and wood. Each material has advantages.

PAPER-BASED TECHNOLOGY IS NOT JUST FOR POOR COUNTRIES:
Examples from England

Paper-based technology (APT) is not only appropriate for poor countries. Its adaptability and versatility make it useful anywhere. In England, Ken and Jean Westmacott run a workshop called *People Potential* where they train families of disabled children to design and create home-made assistive devices. The examples below were made by Sigi Lester for her daughter KIM who has Rett Syndrome, a profound mental and physical disability. Sigi became so skilled at making aids for her daughter that she now runs her own courses on APT, teaching parents of disabled children. All her equipment is beautifully decorated.

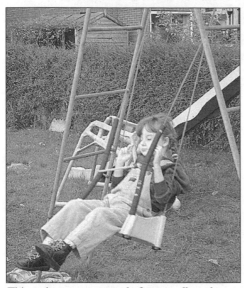

This swing seat was made from cardboard layers. A low back-rest helps Kim gain better body control. Molded hollows under her butt keep her from sliding forward and help her to sit straighter. Sigi covered the seat with a non-slip material to prevent Kim from slipping forward, and thus improve her posture.

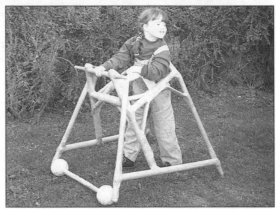

Kim's mother made this walker from rolled tubes of thin, pasted cardboard. The A-frame gives just enough trunk support so Kim can begin to take steps. Wheels made with hard plastic-balls (toilet floats) strengthened with layers of pasted paper, roll well on soft ground.

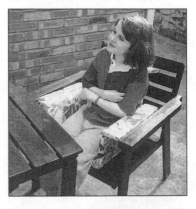

This APT chair-insert with armrests enables Kim to use the same furniture as the rest of the family, yet gives her the extra support that she needs.

An anti-slip surface ensures good posture and safety.

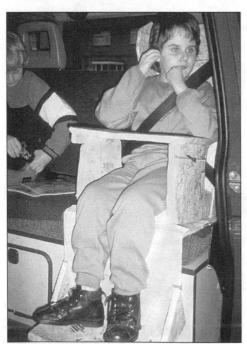

Kim loves her APT car-seat because it is covered with colorful old maps. The seat swings toward the van door for easy access.

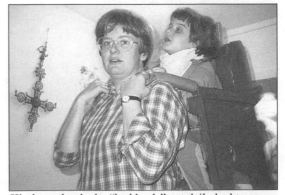

Kim's mother had a "bad back," yet daily had to carry Kim up and down many stairs. She made this APT carrying-seat molded to fit against her own hips and back. She got the idea from the way Sherpas in Nepal carry people (see p. 143). The seat is decorated with golden stars and a moon on a dark blue background.

Mud Seats and Other Aids for Nadu, in India

The "Spastics Society of Tamilnadu," in India has a large, well-equipped center in the city of Madras. It also has an outreach program to rural areas, where most people are quite poor. Families there have few resources to build aids and equipment for their disabled children. They make their houses of mud with palm-leaf roofs. There is almost no furniture: people cook, sit, and sleep on the earth floor.

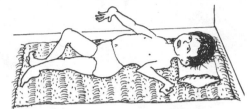

NADU is a little girl in a remote village. She has cerebral palsy, and the rehabilitation workers visited her family's home. Her family fed, dressed, and cared for her lovingly. But Nadu had spent the first five years of her life lying on the floor. Because she could not sit or stand by herself, her parents did not know what else to do.

Nadu also had difficulty with speech. Mentally, she seemed a little slow. Part of her developmental delay probably came from lying on the floor all day, looking up at the ceiling.

The visitors tried sitting Nadu in corners and against walls, but her spastic body and uncontrolled movements soon left her sprawled again on the floor. She needed special seating. However, building materials were scarce, and screws and nails were unavailable.

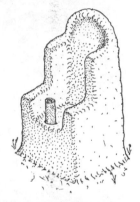

"Here, our main building material is mud," explained Nadu's father.

Mud! With suggestions from the visitors, the family made a special seat and other aids out of mud. **The mud seat** had a pommel made from a thin log (padded with an old cloth) to keep Nadu from slipping forward.

Later, they built her **a standing frame made from mud.**

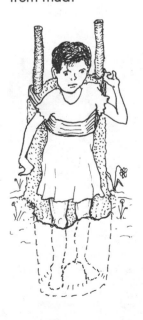

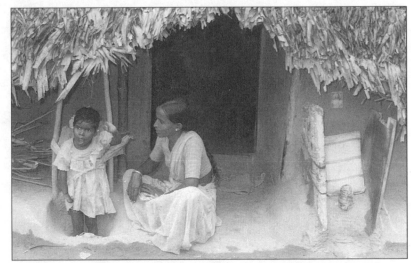

Nadu and her mother at their home. On the left, Nadu stands on her **mud standing frame** with her feet in a hole in the ground. To experiment with positions that help her stand best, the position and angle of her feet can be adjusted easily (with a trowel). To the right of the door is a **special seat made of mud.** One side and the back of the seat are both made from scraps of foam-plastic packing crates.

The rain storm. Sadly, a few months after Nadu's aids were built, a rain storm turned them into a pool of mud. But the loss was temporary. Soon, her family built new and better mud aids. These included a ground-level seat for sitting with her legs extended.

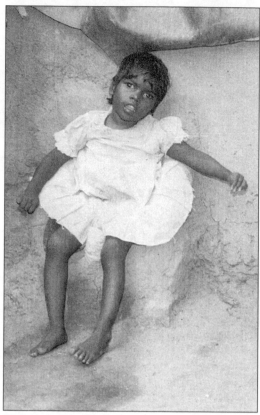

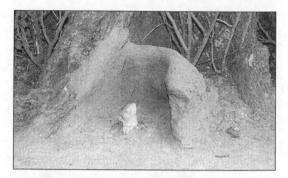

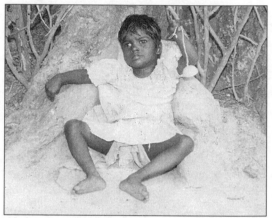

Nadu's chair-level seat lets her sit with bent knees.

Nadu's ground-level mud seat, seen in the two photos above, used a flared tree-root as an arm rest. It had a padded post between her legs.

One advantage to aids made of mud is that they must be rebuilt after each rain storm. This provides an opportunity to periodically re-adapt them to meet the child's changing needs.

A sloping mud platform was also built by the family for Nadu to lie on. Her head and arms extended over the front edge. This helped her gain better head control, and encouraged her to use her hands to play with objects in front of her.

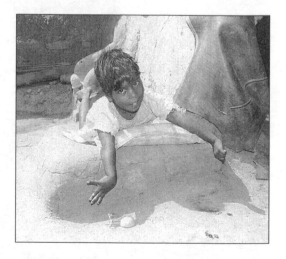

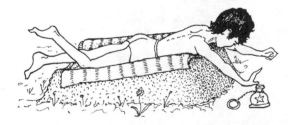

The mud-made equipment for Nadu, while rustic, allowed the girl to sit and stand upright, and to participate more in the world around her. It also gave her family new enthusiasm for working and playing with her. Nadu soon began to speak better, to laugh more, and to take more interest in things around her.

A Wheelchair Seat Helps Dora Overcome Chronic Depression

CHAPTER **10**

DORA is a school teacher from Guadalajara, in her mid-30s. Until she was about 25 years old, she was energetic and full of life. Then she began to develop muscle weakness and spasticity, first in her legs, then in her whole body. Diagnosed as **multiple sclerosis,** *it was at first only a nuisance; then it became disabling. For a while, she used a wheelchair. But a huge pressure sore formed on her left buttock. After that, she had to remain in bed. Her health worsened until she was very thin and pale. Doctors said her condition was too delicate to risk surgery to close the sore. Despite medical attention, counseling, and a supportive family, her condition continued to worsen. At last—on an off chance—her mother took her to PROJIMO, 300 miles away.*

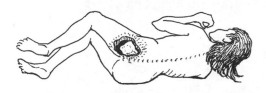

When Dora arrived, the PROJIMO team welcomed her and did their best to respond to her needs. By then, her physical condition was life-threatening. The huge pressure sore had destroyed all the skin and flesh of one buttock, leaving the entire butt-bone (ischial tuberosity) exposed.

Long-term infection and oozing from the sore had left Dora severely anemic and protein deficient. But, her state of mind was even more critical than her physical condition. Dora was deeply and chronically depressed. She had spent most of the last 4 years, day and night, lying in a bed in her parents' home. Her doctors had forbidden her to sit in a wheelchair, or even to sit up in bed, because of the enormous pressure sore on her buttock.

First Steps

On talking with Dora and her mother, Mari realized that, in order to improve her condition, one of the first tasks was to help her to overcome her depression.

"I don't want to go on living if I have to spend the rest of my life cooped up and lying in bed." Dora said. "But the doctors say I have no choice. They tell me I have to get stronger before they can operate on my buttock. But I just keep getting weaker!"

Dora looked at Mari with tears in her eyes. "If I could only move about like you do in a wheelchair! Then I could go outside, visit friends, do lots of things!"

"Have courage!" said Mari. "Together we'll do our best to figure something out."

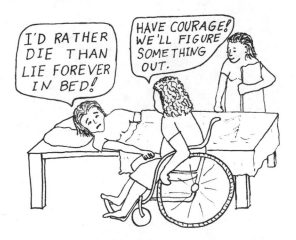

Mari and the PROJIMO team met with Dora and her mother to look for solutions. To improve her physical health, she would need an iron-, energy-, and protein-rich diet. But she was so unhappy that she ate almost nothing. Everyone agreed that, for Dora to improve physically, it was important for her to improve her feelings about herself and her life. She needed a renewal of hope—and a sense that life was worth living.

Dora's first wish was to get out of bed and move about: in other words, **mobility.** But how was this possible with the giant lesion on her buttock? "Her sore will never heal with her lying on it. She's too weak for surgery, and she's so unhappy that her overall health keeps deteriorating," said Mari. "What to do?"

The Gurney That Didn't Help

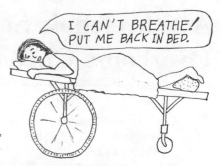

One idea the team had was to arrange for Dora to lie face-down on a wheeled cot, or *gurney* (trolley). They have used gurneys for many spinal-cord injured persons with pressure sores. Lying face-down takes the pressure off the sores. Also, actively moving about on a gurney can lift people's spirits, improve circulation, and speed healing. (See Chapters 37 and 38.)

Dora was eager to try. But, lying on her stomach proved uncomfortable because of her spasticity and contractures. Also, as severely anemic as she was, she had trouble breathing. Struggling for air and soaked in sweat, she begged sadly, "Put me back in bed."

After this failed attempt, Dora was more discouraged than ever. Her mother was ready to take her back to Guadalajara. Another meeting was held. Dora kept repeating her wish: "If only I could move about in a wheelchair!"

An Unusual Wheelchair Seat

Impossible as it seemed, the team set about designing a wheelchair for Dora that would put **no pressure on the buttock with the sore.** Mario—who has had severe pressure sores himself (see page 157) —built a plywood seat to fit inside a standard PROJIMO-built Whirlwind wheelchair. The plywood frame helped to hold her legs and feet in a good position.

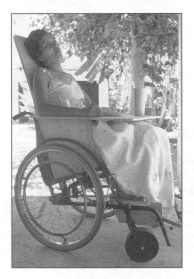

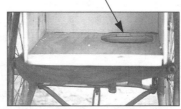

A large hole was cut in the plywood seat to fit directly under Dora's destroyed buttock, so that air could freely circulate to the bandaged sore.

Mario made a **special cushion** out of layers of cardboard (see page 157). He also put a hole in the cushion under the left buttock.

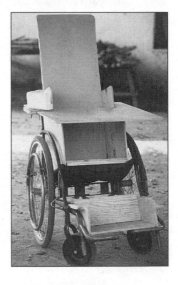

The **sides of the seat extended far enough forward** so that padding could be placed to help Dora sit upright, even with all her weight on one buttock only.

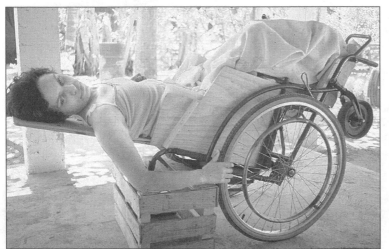

The **high seat-back** holds up Dora's head when the chair is tilted back. This way, **her chair can be tilted far back at frequent intervals.** This is essential to prevent new pressure sores on the healthy hip, which supports her full weight when seated.

"It works!" Dora tried the new seat and was enthusiastic. It took some time to arrange padding next to her thighs and flanks so that she could sit fairly straight and comfortably. To protect the healthy buttock, the chair had to be tilted back for a while every 10 or 15 minutes.

With the basic chair completed, Dora and the team began to look for ways to help her to function better. They equipped the seat with a removable table so that she could read and write, do manual activities, and feed herself.

However, feeding herself and drinking from a glass was a problem. The combination of spasticity, weakness, and the tremor of her arm made it hard to lift food or drink to her mouth without missing her mouth or spilling it.

An Elbow Stabilizer to Facilitate Eating and Drinking

Inez (who assists people with physical and occupational therapy) helped Dora to experiment with different devices and positions to make eating and drinking easier. Dora found that when Inez held her elbow firmly on the back corner of the table, she had more control. So the next job was to figure out a simple way to stabilize her elbow without someone having to hold it in place.

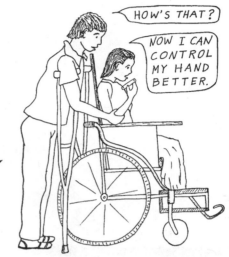

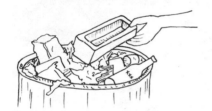

In the garbage bin, Inez found a small, broken, foam-plastic packing box, with an inside width of about 3 inches (10 cm). With a pocket knife, he fashioned the box to fit around Dora's elbow. He attached it with Velcro (self-sticking but removable tape) to the back corner of Dora's wheelchair table.

By inserting her elbow in the foam-plastic box attached to her table, Dora found she could eat more easily and even drink without much spilling. She was delighted. It was the first time in 4 years that she had been able to eat and drink without assistance.

Not Her Sore, but rather Her Spirit was Healed

Dora and her mother stayed at PROJIMO for several weeks. By the time she left she was eating better, gaining weight, and looking healthier. She felt much more positive about her own existence. The pressure sore had not even begun to heal, and probably never would without extensive surgery. However, if Dora's health continues to improve, surgery at some time may be possible.

But something more important than healing the sore was the healing of her spirit. Her mother said that she was again beginning to see some of the old spark and joy of life that had made Dora such a good teacher. First things first.

NOTE: For innovative ideas on prevention and treatment of pressure sores, see Chapters 27, 28 and 38. For overall basic information on pressure sores, see the book, *Disabled Village Children*, by David Werner.

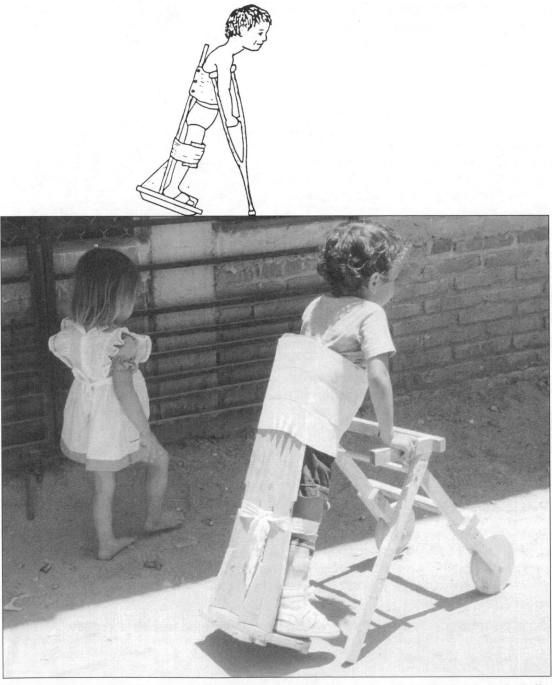

Joel, who has spina bifida, learns to walk using a wooden walker and a "parapodium" (standing frame for walking) made at PROJIMO.

Part Two

CREATIVE SOLUTIONS FOR WALKING AND FOR LEG AND FOOT PROBLEMS

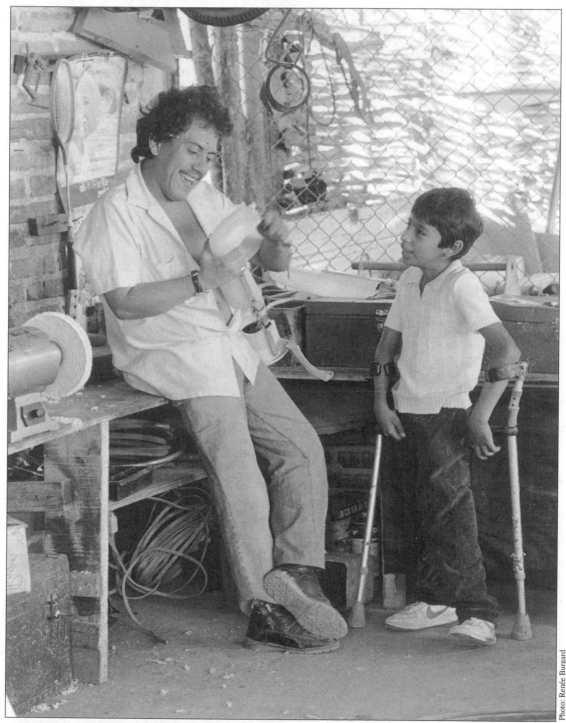

Photo: Renée Burgard

INTRODUCTION TO PART TWO
New Approaches to Meeting Common Problems

PART 2 looks at methods, aids, and equipment related to walking, and at ways to correct or cope with various problems in the legs and feet. The first several chapters in Part 2 (Chapters 11 to 14) look at leg braces (calipers). Chapters 18 and 19 concern artificial legs.

Use of Plastics. The introduction of plastic as a basic material for making leg braces and other orthopedic appliances has been a big step forward. For many children who have had to wear heavy, uncomfortable, metal braces, the chance to use light-weight, comfortable, snug-fitting plastic braces can be liberating.

BRACES FROM JUNK PLASTIC.
Professionally made plastic braces are often so costly that many people who need them cannot afford them. Fortunately, in various countries and communities, people have found ways to make plastic braces and other appliances at low cost—using everything from plastic cups and buckets to PVC water pipe and plastic sewage pipe.

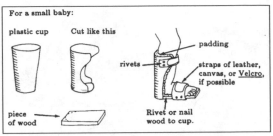

Part 2 of this book looks at the use of plastics—from simple throw-away containers to modern oven-molded polypropylene.

The chapters in Part 2 will give a range of examples of these innovative uses of plastic to create low-cost braces and artificial legs. Two chapters explore ways that empty plastic bottles or plastic pipes can be used as "foot-tubes" to help correct in-turned feet.

"MODERN" BRACES. In addition to innovations with old plastic containers, PROJIMO uses "modern" plastic brace-making technology, simplifying it for use in a village workshop. Sheets of polypropylene plastic are oven-heated and draped over plaster leg casts to create individually designed braces.

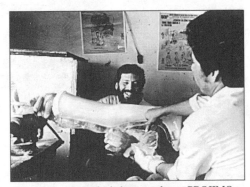

Artificial Limbs. People in India have made one of the biggest breakthroughs in appropriate, low-cost artificial limbs: the Jaipur foot. But, because this is well-known and pro-duced in many countries, Chapter 19 looks more closely at the Mukti limb, a leg made from a section of plastic drain-pipe.

Raymundo, a paraplegic brace-maker at PROJIMO, drapes a hot sheet of polypropylene plastic over the mold of a boy's leg, and trims off the excess. Oliver Bock (with beard), a visiting orthotist (professional brace maker), helps and teaches Raymundo.

Skeleton for Teaching. To better understand how a leg or foot can best be braced, or to plan effective therapy, it helps to have some understanding of how the bones, muscles, tendons, and ligaments work together. To demystify the anatomy of the lower limb, Chapter 20 introduces the design and use of a simple plywood skeleton used for teaching.

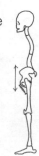

Participatory Problem Solving. As in the rest of this book, most of the chapters in Part 2 will focus on how the technologies described have been designed and adapted to meet the particular needs of a person with a disability.

Leg Braces for David:
The Need to Solve Problems as Equals

CHAPTER 11

Making Sure Aids and Procedures Do More Good Than Harm

When I (David Werner) was a young boy, I gradually developed a strange, waddling gait (way of walking). Often I fell down and twisted my ankles. At school, some of the other children, to tease me, imitated the way I walked. They said I looked and moved like a duck. Soon I was nicknamed "Rickets," and for years everyone called me that, even some teachers … even my friends. I hated the nickname and the teasing. But, in some ways, they may have helped me to become a better person. I came to feel a kind of empathy for other kids who were belittled or made fun of. All my life I have been a defender of the underdog.

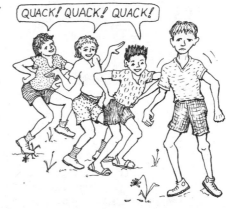

When I was about 10 years old my parents, who were increasingly concerned about the problem with my feet, took me to a foot doctor. In those days, no one knew that my strange gait and frequent falls were early signs of **progressive muscular atrophy** *(a hereditary condition which was diagnosed years later as Charcot-Marie-Tooth Syndrome).*

Torture by arch-supports. The doctor examined my feet. Finding them weak and floppy, he prescribed arch-supports. An "orthotist" (brace maker) across town would make them.

When the arch-supports were ready, the orthotist put them on my feet. "Do they hurt?" he asked. "No," I said. So I was sent home with instructions to wear them every day.

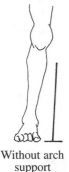

Without arch
support

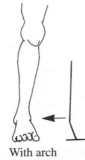

With arch
support

I hated the things!—not because they hurt, but because it was harder for me to walk with them than without them. They pushed up on my arches and bent my ankles outward. I sprained my ankles more than ever.

I tried to protest, but nobody listened. After all, I was a child. "You have to get used to them!" I was told. "Who do you think knows best—you or the doctor?"

So, mostly, I suffered in silence. I hobbled around with swollen, black-and-blue ankles. Whenever I could, I secretly took the arch-supports out of my shoes and hid them. But when I was caught, I was punished. I was made to feel naughty for not doing what was "best" for me.

Metal leg braces: worse still! Several years later, as my walking got worse, I was prescribed a pair of metal braces (calipers). They held my ankles firmly, but they were heavy and uncomfortable, and they made me more awkward than ever. I hated them, but wore them because I was told to.

One holiday, I took a long walk in the mountains. The braces rubbed the skin on the front of my legs so badly that deep, painful sores developed, down to the bone. It took me months to recover. I refused to wear the braces again.

Personal Efforts to Prevent Deformity and Contractures

As the years went by, my feet became increasingly deformed. The inward-turning (varus) dislocations of my ankles got worse, making walking more and more difficult and painful. But, after my childhood experience with hurtful orthopedic appliances, I was unwilling to try braces again.

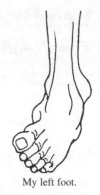

My left foot.

More years went by. I became a biologist, then a school teacher. In my late twenties, I began to work in the mountains of western Mexico as a founder and facilitator of Project Piaxtla, a community health program run by villagers.   Fifteen years later, Piaxtla gave birth to PROJIMO, the Program of Rehabilitation Organized by Disabled Youth of Western Mexico.

Throughout this time, although walking was uncomfortable and difficult for me, I knew that to combat contractures and be able to continue walking, *it was important for me to walk a lot.*

At PROJIMO, we had learned that one way to help children combat varus contractures of their feet was for them to *practice walking on boards placed side by side in an open "V".* This stretches their feet and ankles in the opposite direction of the contractures. For myself, I did a similar sort of corrective exercise by hiking on well-worn mountain trails. Walking on such V-shaped (or U-shaped) trails was easier than walking on flat ground (where my ankles tended to double over side-ways). After walking for 2 or 3 hours on such trails, my feet and ankles were sore from all the stretching—but walking was easier for me, even on a flat surface. (I had discovered this trick of walking on a V-shaped trail in childhood.) In PROJIMO we found it could help other children with weak ankles and varus contractures. So, we included the following suggestions in the book *Disabled Village Children:*

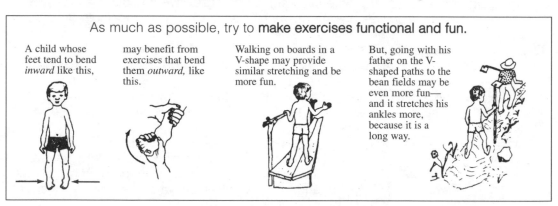

As much as possible, try to **make exercises functional and fun.**

A child whose feet tend to bend *inward* like this,

may benefit from exercises that bend them *outward,* like this.

Walking on boards in a V-shape may provide similar stretching and be more fun.

But, going with his father on the V-shaped paths to the bean fields may be even more fun—and it stretches his ankles more, because it is a long way.

As I began (unwisely, in terms of my physical health) to spend more time writing and less time walking, the contractures and deformities of my feet grew worse. My left foot, especially, became very dislocated at the ankle.

A plywood foot-stretching device

Still unwilling to try braces again, but needing to decrease the contractures of my left foot, I created a device to wear while sitting and writing. It stretched my ankle and foot in the opposite direction of the contracture. Made of plywood and a strip of rubber inner-tube, the device did help somewhat, but it became very uncomfortable if I wore it for long. So I did not use it much. At best, it perhaps helped to prevent the ankle deformity from advancing as fast.

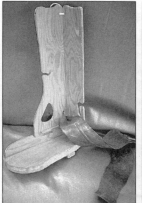
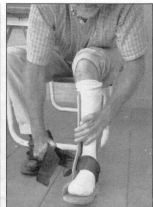

Plywood foot-stretching device. The strip of inner-tube is stretched over the ankle and held by slots in the wood.

Designing Braces that Actually Help: Marcelo as a Partner in Problem-Solving

PROJIMO's first brace maker was **MARCELO** Acevedo, a village youth whose legs were paralyzed by polio as a baby. I first met Marcelo when he was 3 years old, in a remote mountain village called Caballo de Arriba (Upper Horse). Unable to walk, he dragged himself about on his arms. The Piaxtla health team helped Marcelo to get braces and crutches, and arranged for him to go to school in the village of Ajoya, where Piaxtla had its base. (There was no school in his own village.) When he was 14, the Piaxtla team trained Marcelo as a village health worker. So he was able to return to his village with an important skill.

When PROJIMO began in 1981, Marcelo was one of its founding members. Arrangements were made for him to apprentice in a brace shop in Mexico City, where he learned the basics of making orthopedic appliances. Volunteer orthotists (professional brace makers) who visited PROJIMO helped Marcelo to upgrade his skills. A careful and creative worker, Marcelo soon became an outstanding technician and designer. He has since learned how to make artificial limbs, wheelchairs and other assistive devices.

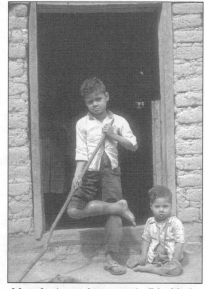

Marcelo Acevedo at age 4. Disabled by polio, he lived in a village 2 days by trail from the closest road. Here Marcelo sits next to his brother, who also was temporarily disabled when a tree fell on his leg.

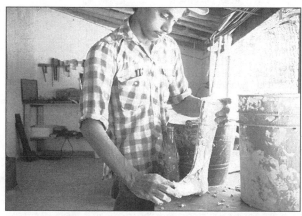

Project Piaxtla helped Marcelo get surgery, braces, schooling, and trained him as a village health worker. Later, he helped found PROJIMO and studied brace-making in orthopedic workshops in Mexico City and California.

One day, Marcelo watched me walking with difficulty across the PROJIMO yard, and approached me on his crutches. "David," he said, "I think you could walk much better if we made you some leg braces."

"Leg braces!" I exclaimed. "Not on your life! I was tortured enough with those things as a child. I know they help some kids walk better. But for me they were *torture!* They made me walk worse."

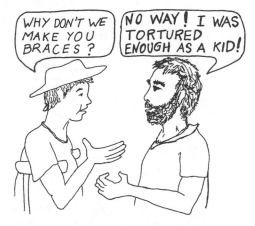

"Maybe the braces you used as a child didn't work because the doctors and brace makers simply prescribed and made them, without including you in developing them," said Marcelo. "What do you say if you and I work together on designing braces for you, and we keep experimenting until we create some that work?"

"And if they don't work …?" I asked.

"Then at least we will have had the adventure of working together and trying our best," said Marcelo. "You helped me to walk. Now it's my turn with you." What could I do but agree?

STAGES IN THE DEVELOPMENT OF THE PLASTIC BRACES: THE FIRST DESIGN

On evaluating my need for bracing, we felt that the two biggest goals were to stabilize the foot-drop (front of the foot hangs down and is too weak to lift) and varus (inward turning) dislocation. Marcelo thought that a plastic brace could help to hold my feet in a better position, allowing a more stable, comfortable gait. He took plaster casts of my lower legs, modified the positive (solid) molds, and stretched hot polypropylene plastic over the molds to form the braces (see p. 90).

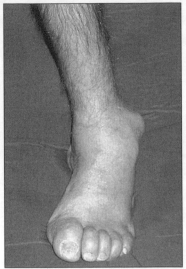

My left foot, more deformed than my right, had a varus contracture with a dislocation that caused a big lump of bone on the side of the ankle.

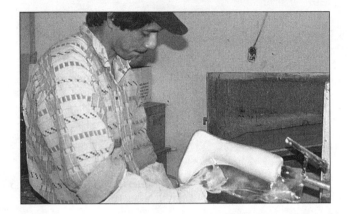

The first design was similar to a standard plastic AFO (ankle-foot orthosis) except that a broad area on the outside of the ankle was left to hold the ankle in place and keep it from dislocating outward.

The plastic just above the ankle was cut back narrow enough to allow the brace to bend upward a little at the end of a step. This permitted a more comfortable, easier gait.

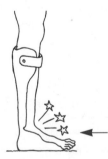

I tried the braces and, at first, liked them. They held my feet in a better position, and I could stand and step more firmly. But, when I began to walk longer distances, I ran into problems. The upward flexibility of the braces caused pain inside the ankle and mid-foot.

Worse still, the pressure of the varus ankle against the plastic became quite painful. Because the sideways contracture at the ankle made complete straightening of the heel impossible, every time I put my weight on the foot, the ankle tried to bend outward.

The dislocated lump on the side of the ankle pressed painfully against the plastic brace. We tried putting a soft pad in the brace over the lump, but that didn't help much.

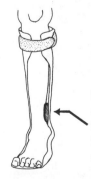

One time, on a long hike, the pressure on my dislocated left ankle against the plastic became so painful that, to relieve it, I pushed a folded handkerchief between the brace and the outer side of my leg above the ankle. This immediately helped to reduce the pressure against the lump and it lessened the pain.

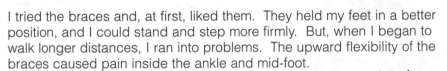

On returning to PROJIMO, I showed Marcelo how I had relieved the pressure on the lump at the ankle. Together, we set about designing a new brace with that modification built in.

THE REVISED DESIGN: PLASTIC BRACE WITH PRESSURE RELIEF ON THE DEFORMED ANKLE

A brace was needed that would exert pressure in 3 areas of the leg, in order to hold the leg and heel in as straight a line as possible.

The first, more standard design put pressure on the:

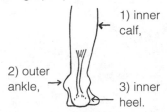

1) inner calf,

2) outer ankle,

3) inner heel.

Because the heel could not be straightened completely, the pressure on the outer ankle was great, and painful with each step.

The new brace was shaped like this with the plastic coming clear around the outer (lateral) side of the leg. This prevented any upward flexing of the foot, thus reducing my mid-foot pain.

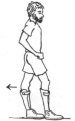

The wide side of the brace at the ankle allowed a long, broad pad to be placed so that it pressed against the whole side of the leg.

This helped straighten the ankle and heel, while taking pressure off the ankle-bone.

The new braces did eliminate the painful pressure against my ankles. But I still had some mid-foot pain. Also the completely stiff ankle of the brace made for an awkward, choppy gait, and pushed my knee backward uncomfortably at the end of the step.

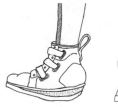

REAR VIEW

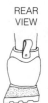

Rocker-bottom, inward-sloping shoes. To overcome the above problems, we experimented with rocker-bottom shoes. To find out how much rocker-effect was needed and at what position on the shoes, Marcelo first taped small blocks of wood to my shoe-soles, and asked me to walk on them. We tried different positions and heights until we found those which were most comfortable.

We also tried wedging up the outer (lateral) side of the shoe. We found that by making the outer edge of the sole thicker than the inner edge, the varus deformity of my feet was better corrected and walking was more comfortable.

A PERSONALIZED PLASTIC BRACE INSIDE A ROCKER-BOTTOM SHOE—FINAL RESULTS:

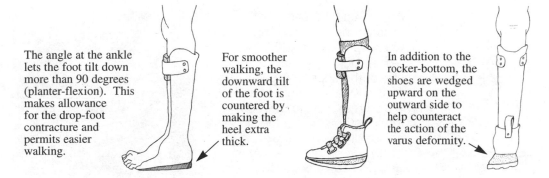

The angle at the ankle lets the foot tilt down more than 90 degrees (planter-flexion). This makes allowance for the drop-foot contracture and permits easier walking.

For smoother walking, the downward tilt of the foot is countered by making the heel extra thick.

In addition to the rocker-bottom, the shoes are wedged upward on the outward side to help counteract the action of the varus deformity.

Results: After a long process of trial and error, in which Marcelo and I worked together through a problem-solving process, we arrived at a combination of custom-made braces and adapted shoes that have given me new freedom. I can now walk up to 15 miles a day with little discomfort. I walk better today than I could 30 years ago. And I owe these successful results not to the interventions of orthopedic specialists in the USA, but to a disabled village brace maker who worked closely with me as a friend and equal.

Simple Tricks for Experimenting with Modified Shoes

ADJUSTABLE ROCKER-BOTTOM. I have been through
many sets of braces and shoes in the years since
Marcelo and I first developed braces that more or less
met my needs. In addition to Marcelo and Armando
from PROJIMO, a young North-American brace maker,
Oliver Bock, has also worked closely with me to help fit
me with suitable braces and shoes. Oliver first visited
PROJIMO as a teenager, became fascinated by brace
making, and later studied in an orthotics training program
in California. But although he now has professional
training, he still makes a point of working closely with his
clients, involving them in an innovative, problem solving
process. Over the years Oliver has also made many
trips to PROJIMO, to help teach brace making to village
rehabilitation workers from other programs, and to help
the PROJIMO brace makers up-grade their skills.
Again, he shares new ideas and techniques more as a
friend and equal than as a formal instructor.

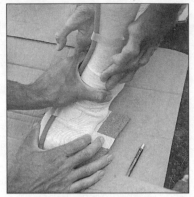

Oliver Bock, an orthotist from
the USA, volunteers periodically
at PROJIMO to share ideas. Here
he helps me (and I help him) to
position my foot in preparation for
casting it to make a plastic brace.

When I need to adapt new shoes or modify old ones, I now use a couple of simple
methods to provisionally try the modifications I think I may want.

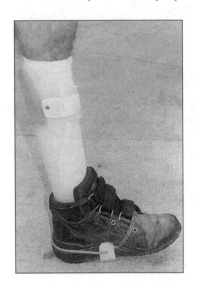

To create the effect of a
temporary rocker-bottom sole,
I used a U-shaped piece of
polypropylene plastic.

The U fits snugly on the
bottom of the shoe, and
can be tied on firmly with a
string that passes through
holes in the arms of the U.

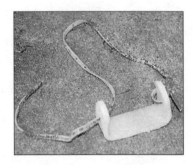

The strings pass over the top of the shoe and behind the
heel, allowing the shoe to be removed without removing
the U. The U can be easily moved backward or forward,
to test for the most beneficial position. (I find that just one
centimeter of change can make a big difference in comfort
and ease of walking.)

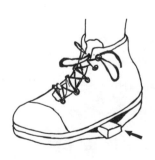

ADJUSTABLE WEDGE. To
experiment with different
wedging on the shoe, I make
a deep horizontal cut in the
sole of the shoe. I pry this
open with a screwdriver and
slip a small wedge of wood,
rubber, or metal into the slot. I
can easily move the wedge
backward or forward, or use
wedges of different thicknesses.

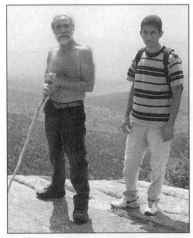

Each of these methods permits me to try out a series of
temporary modifications for hours or days, to decide
which are most helpful.

Thanks to help from peers and friends, today my
disability is less of a handicap than it used to be.

Here, David Werner climbs a
mountain with Efraín Zamora, a
friend who helped with the artwork
and layout of this book.

Leg-Braces for Noé:
from Old Plastic Buckets to Polypropylene

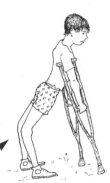

*NOÉ was a cheerful boy with "diplegic" cerebral palsy (meaning that mainly his legs are affected). When he was 5 years old he learned to walk with crutches, but with a lot of difficulty. He stood very stiffly on his slender, spastic legs. The tiptoe (equinus) position of his feet pushed his knees backward (recurvatum). As he grew bigger, his knees bent farther and farther back. When he was 8, a specialist in the city prescribed full-leg metal braces with orthopedic boots. Noé wore them for a while, but hated them. They were heavy and awkward and slowed him down. He protested so much that after a few months his parents gave up trying to make him wear them. The backward bend of his knees gradually grew worse and he began to complain of **knee pain.** When Noé was 10, his family learned about PROJIMO and took him there.*

The team realized that if Noé kept walking with his knees bending so far backward, the ligaments (cords) behind the knees would stretch more and more, until walking would become impossible (see page 128). Perhaps if his feet could angle up slightly (preventing tiptoeing) he might be able to walk without his knees bending so far backward. Light-weight, below-the-knee plastic braces might serve the purpose.

When Noé first came in 1981, PROJIMO was just beginning and they had not yet begun to make plastic braces. Although plastic braces were available at large rehabilitation centers in the cities, they were very costly (around US$200 for a single below-the-knee plastic brace). The PROJIMO team decided to experiment with low-cost methods to make plastic leg braces.

Braces made from Plastic Buckets

PROJIMO had been given some old plastic buckets (that once held soy sauce for restaurants). They experimented with heat-molding pieces of the bucket over plaster casts of Noé's feet. At last they developed a method that gave fairly good results. The basic steps (explained in more detail in the book, *Disabled Village Children,* Chapter 58) are shown below.

Make a plaster cast of the foot in the desired position.	Fill the cast with plaster to make a solid mold.	Mark on the child's leg the shape of the brace.	Cut shape of leg from old plastic bucket. Heat plastic in an oven (on a powdered metal tray) until soft.	Place the hot plastic over the mold and bind tightly until cool.	Smooth and weld the heel joint with a soldering iron.	Trim and round the edges of the brace.	Add straps as needed, and test the brace.

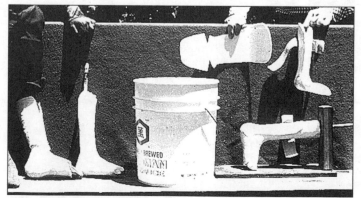

Photo of the steps in making Noé's plastic bucket braces.

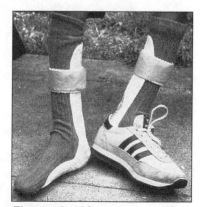

The completed braces.

Results of the Plastic-Bucket Braces

The below-the-knee plastic-bucket braces did, to some extent, help Noé to stand straighter, with his knees bending back much less. However, when he walked rapidly with a swing-through gait, his knees still bent backward.

The biggest problem with the plastic-bucket braces, however, was that with a child as big and active as Noé, the braces did not last long. They developed cracks and broke within a few weeks.

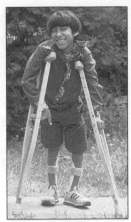

Noé's plastic-bucket braces helped prevent his knees from bending backward.

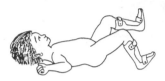 However, the **plastic bucket braces have proved effective for maintaining a good position of a baby's club feet after the clubbing has been corrected**—and for other situations where a child does not walk yet, or puts little stress on the braces.

Polypropylene Braces

Although plastic-bucket braces met some needs at very low cost, for Noé and many persons, stronger plastic was needed. Polypropylene, which is used by professional brace makers, is strong and easier to heat-mold than many other plastics. because it is available in large sheets in a near-by city, PROJIMO began to use it. They made full-leg braces for Noé in the following manner:

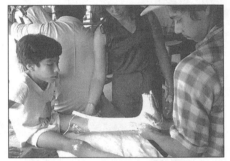

1. Marcelo takes a plaster-cast of Noé's leg. From this, he will make a solid plaster mold.

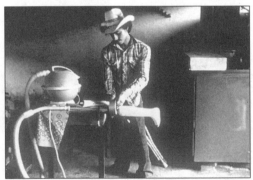

2. To avoid bubbles forming under the plastic, he attaches the leg mold to a vacuum cleaner to suck out the air from under the hot plastic. The plastic sheet is being heated in the metal box on the stove (right).

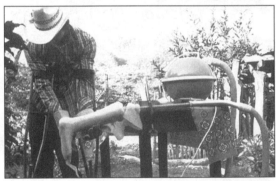

3. He stretches the soft hot plastic over the mold. After it cools, he will cut the plastic to form the brace.

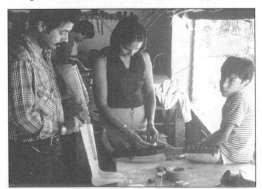

4. Roberto, assisted by Noé's mother, attaches the plastic lower leg piece to the upper leg piece with jointed metal bars. (Here, the upper leg piece was made with leather. Later, the leather was also replaced with plastic.)

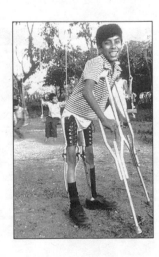

Noé was delighted with his new plastic braces. They were light, comfortable, and kept his knees from doubling backwards. He is now a grown man, but continues to use them, returning to PROJIMO every 2 or 3 years for new braces or repairs.

Different Approaches to Making Plastic Braces and Artificial Limbs

Although many programs in the Third World have made no effort to use plastics, others have made good use of plastics, overcoming many obstacles in order to do so:

In Pakistan, where polypropylene is hard to obtain, a community rehabilitation program in Peshawar made braces from the **plastic windows of wrecked buses.** Instead of an oven, they use **a small mud stove full of hot coals.** (An electric blower was used to keep them very hot.) The brace makers use pliers to hold the plastic over the stove, moving the plastic back and forth to heat it evenly. (They find they get better results this way than in an oven without a thermostat.)

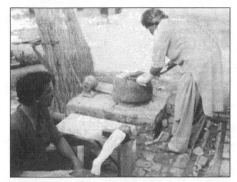

Brace makers in Peshawar heat a sheet of plastic over a small outdoor stove.

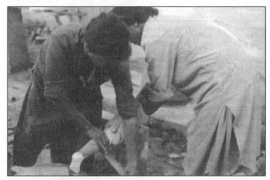

After draping the hot plastic over the plaster mold of the foot, they wrap it firmly with strips of old rubber inner-tube.

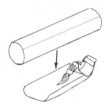

To save on the short supply of polypropylene plastic, the Peshawar workers often mold only the foot-piece out of these. They use plastic **PVC pipe for the upper part of the brace.** This they heat just enough so that it can be spread to fit the shank of the leg. (If heated until it is quite soft and moldable, PVC, like many plastics, tends to crinkle like bacon.)

The molded foot and PVC leg are then riveted or laced together. ⟶

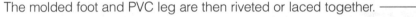

In India, the *Gandhi Rural Rehabilitation Center* near Madras also combines the use of PVC legs and polypropylene feet. They have simplified and reduced the cost of braces by using **pre-molded polypropylene components.** They make these in advance, and keep a stock of components in a range of forms and sizes. The components are **made by molding the plastic over wooden legs and feet of different sizes.** ⟶

This way, they do not need to cast the leg and make a mold for each individual child. The cost of plaster bandage is avoided. (Ironically, this is one of the highest material costs in making plastic braces). Also, fitting is quick. When a child arrives, his needs are evaluated, measurements are taken, components are selected, and the brace is assembled.

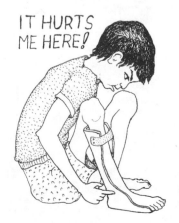

IT HURTS ME HERE!

The disadvantage to using pre-made parts is that **the brace often does not fit the child precisely.** The exact fit of the individually-molded brace is lost. I saw several children with these pre-formed braces who had blisters and callouses (especially over the ankle bones), resulting from an imperfect fit.

Never-the-less, with time and patience, most problems can be corrected. Spots that press on bony areas can often be re-heated and pushed out enough to relieve the pressure.

The most important part of fitting braces is to establish a friendly, trusting relationship with the child. Let her know you want her to make suggestions, and to tell you when something bothers her or hurts. When you include the child as a partner in problem-solving, the results are more likely to meet the child's needs.

A useful book on low-cost brace-making, called *A Plastic Caliper for Children,* has been prepared by *Handicap International* (HI). The book includes many innovations, including the combined PVC and polypropylene braces made at *The Gandhi Rural Rehabilitation Center.* (The Center is assisted by HI.) The steps involved in making braces with pre-formed component parts is summarized at the start of that book as follows:

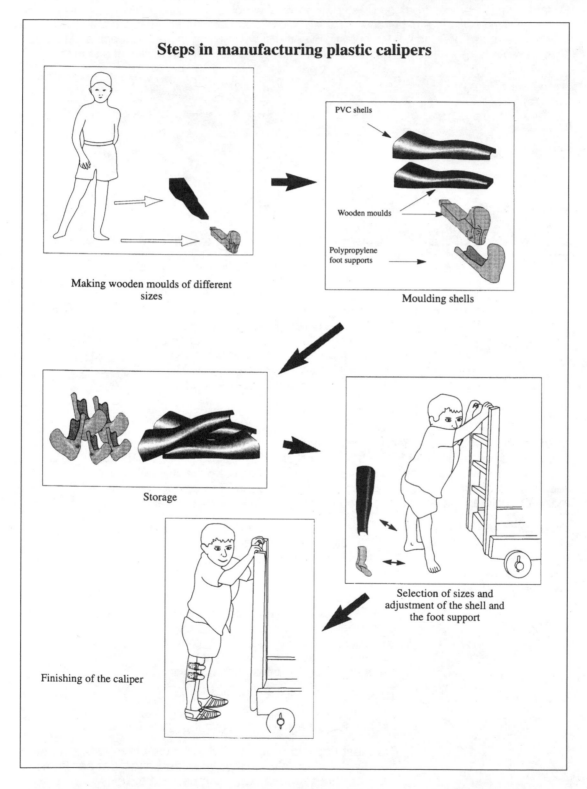

Steps in manufacturing plastic calipers

Making wooden moulds of different sizes

PVC shells

Wooden moulds

Polypropylene foot supports

Moulding shells

Storage

Selection of sizes and adjustment of the shell and the foot support

Finishing of the caliper

A Plastic Caliper for Children, written by HI staff at its Pondicherry, India branch, is available through *Handicap International.* (For the address, see Resource List 2, page 344.)

Plastic Braces to Help Stabilize Carla's, Neto's, and Robi's Knees

CHAPTER **13**

Braces to Help Carla Walk Straighter

CARLA is bright and eager. She wants to do everything other 8-year-olds do. But sometimes her body does not cooperate. Born with cerebral palsy, she has both spasticity (uncontrolled tightening of certain muscles) and athetosis (sudden, uncontrolled movements), which make walking difficult. Her knees bend and bump when she walks. To keep from falling, she uses crutches. Even so, sometimes she falls.

At PROJIMO, Carla made her wishes clear. "I want to stand and walk better. I'm tired of these dumb crutches!" She had seen other children begin to walk better with below-the-knee plastic leg braces. "I want some of those things!" she insisted.

On evaluating Carla's possibilities, Mari and Marcelo were unsure whether braces might help. By positioning her feet and ankles more firmly, braces might give stability and help her stand straighter. But they might also trigger more spasticity.

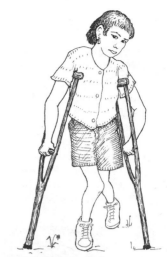
Before Carla had braces: "My knees bend and bump when I walk. I want to walk better, without holding on!"

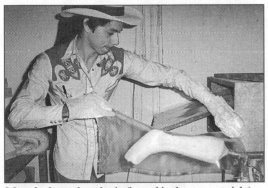
Marcelo drapes hot plastic (heated in the oven, at right) over the plaster mold of Carla's foot, to make a brace.

Some experts used to say "Spastic and plastic don't mix!" But the PROJIMO team has found that plastic braces often work well for such children. Mari explained to Carla that the results would be uncertain. But the girl was still eager to try.

Marcelo found some old braces that more-or-less fit Carla. She tried them. It looked like she stood and walked a bit better with them, and Carla said they gave her better balance. So Marcelo took plaster molds of her feet and made polypropylene below-the-knee braces.

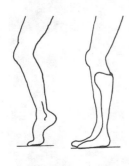
WITHOUT   WITH

Mari and Marcelo asked Carla to walk between the parallel bars—first without the braces, and then with them—to compare how she walked. Without the braces she walked on tiptoes, with her knees quite bent. With them, the braces held her feet flatter and pushed her knees back. She stood more upright. Everyone, including Carla, agreed that with the braces her legs were straighter (more upright, less knock-kneed) and that she stood more firmly, with better balance.

Within a few days, Carla began to walk without crutches. Although she still fell occasionally, she persevered. With her new braces she had more confidence and control—partly, perhaps, from the self-assurance she gained by feeling that people were listening to her ideas and wishes, and were including her in the problem-solving process.

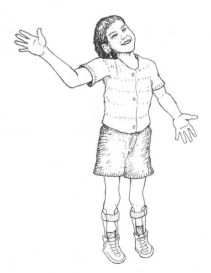
"Look! I can walk better now!"

A Brace for Neto's Back-Bending Knee

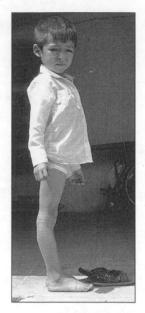

NETO is a shy, clever little boy from a remote mountain village. His grandfather brought him because, he explained, the boy was very small for his age and lacked energy. "He doesn't like to go with me to work in the fields any more," he said. "He's either sick or lazy!"

"Grandpa!" objected the boy. "I keep telling you: **my knee hurts.**"

On examining Neto's right knee, Mari found that it bent further back than the other one. Behind it, there was a fluid-filled swelling (a herniated bursa, or *Baker's cyst*). Neto could not remember having injured his knee. Yet, the ligaments behind the knee appeared to be severely stretched. The knee bent back so far that, when the boy put his weight on it, he strained it and ran the danger of stretching it more.

Mari asked Raymundo, the project's brace maker, to look at Neto's knee. Raymundo thought that Neto needed to wear a leg brace that would keep his knee from bending backwards—to allow time for the stretched tendons to contract enough to hold the knee straighter.

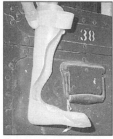

"I don't want a big thing like that!" protested Neto, pointing to a child limping with a long-leg brace. "I can't wear one of those in the mountains. My leg won't bend at all! I'll break my neck!"

"Would a small, light-weight below-the-knee brace, like this one, be better?" asked Raymundo, showing him one.

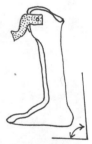

Neto examined the brace doubtfully. "Would it stop my knee from hurting?" he asked.

"We'll have to see." answered Raymundo. "Do you want to try one?" Neto nodded importantly. Raymundo took a cast of Neto's leg, with the foot bent up a bit from a 90 degree angle. Then he made a plastic brace. Neto's grandfather helped the boy to try it on.

When he stood up, Neto's knee stayed straight, without bending backward. "It doesn't hurt now!" he said. "It's great!" But when he tried walking up a slope, he cried out in pain. "This thing's no good for the mountains!" he said.

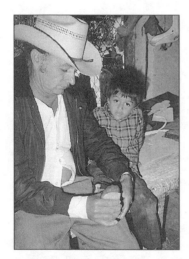

Raymundo cut back the brace at the ankle to give it upward flexibility.

"On an uphill slope, the brace pushes your knee back," Raymundo observed. "I have an idea." He cut back the sides of the brace at the ankle, far enough to let the foot easily flex upward. Yet it still firmly resisted being bent downward more than 90 degrees.

The boy tried it again on a slope. "Its much better!" he said.

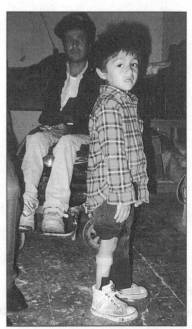

"It doesn't hurt now!" says Neto to Raymundo, the brace maker.

The PROJIMO team continues to see Neto periodically, and his back-knee has gradually became straighter. After one year he stopped using the brace. Now 3 years have passed, and he has had no further problem.

A NEW BRACE DESIGN TO STOP A KNEE FROM BENDING BACKWARD

Many children with a weak leg from polio develop a **back-knee.** A small amount of back-bend of the knee often actually helps the child to walk without a brace, by locking the knee back with each step. But there is a danger that the knee will slowly bend back more and more, stretching ligaments until finally they tear and the child can not walk. (See the skeleton on page 128.)

The old way. Children with a back-knee are often given a *long-leg brace.* But many refuse to wear it because it holds the leg rigid, and is heavy and uncomfortable. Because the child can walk without it, he feels he doesn't need it. As a result, a lot of children develop **permanent damage** to their knees and some lose the ability to walk.

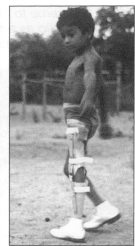
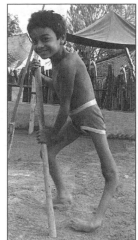

The conventional way to protect the leg of a child with a back knee like this is with a full-length leg brace.

*A **better** way.* In India, Dr. P. K. Sethi, inventor of the Jaipur foot (see page 119), has worked closely with villagers who had polio, to design a below-the-knee plastic brace which is an improvement on the one PROJIMO made for Neto.

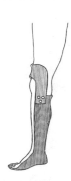

To keep the knee from bending too far back, this new brace extends above the front of the knee, and pushes on the lower thigh. The main disadvantage to this brace is that, when the person sits or squats, the top part of the brace sticks out above the knee. This makes it hard to use with long pants (unless a hole is cut in the knee). But because, in Indian villages, men as well as women traditionally use loose, wrap-around clothing, the brace presents no problem.

BRACE DESIGNS TO PUSH THE KNEE BACKWARD

Some persons with a weak leg walk by pushing on the knee with one hand, to keep it from collapsing. For such persons, Dr. Sethi designed a *floor-reaction orthosis.* The fore-foot is angled downward, so that when the person steps, his weight tips the brace backward, which pushes the knee back.

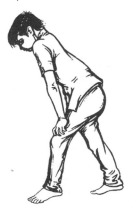

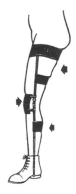

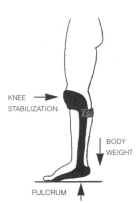

KNEE
STABILIZATION

BODY
WEIGHT

FULCRUM

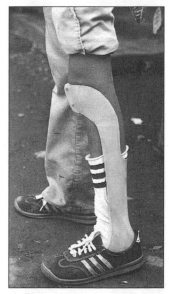

The child who walks like this...

typically gets a brace like this.

But a floor-reaction-brace often works as well or better.

A floor-reaction brace made at PROJIMO.

ADJUSTABLE PLASTIC BRACES TO CORRECT RAÚL'S CLUBBED FEET

Below-the-Knee Braces to Help Straighten Raúl's Feet While Standing

Because serial casting at PROJIMO was not acceptable to the family, PROJIMO'S brace maker, Armando (who is also disabled), designed adjustable plastic braces that could gradually stretch Raúl's club feet into a more functional position. The brace needed up-and-down flexibility at the ankle, with a mechanism to gradually stretch the tight heel cord and correct the downward, tip-toe contracture. But the brace also needed sideways stability at the ankle, to prevent the foot from doubling inward.

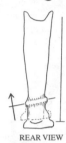

Transverse bar

To provide this vertical (up and down) flexibility and lateral (sideways) stability, Armando modified the plaster mold of Raúl's foot to form a transverse (sideways) bar at the back of the ankle.

After forming a brace by stretching hot plastic over the mold, Armando cut deep notches on each side at the ankle so that the bar behind the ankle would work like a hinge, bending up and down, but not side-ways.

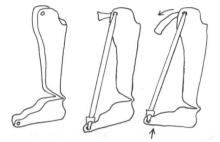

The ankle hinge was higher on the inner (medial) side so that as the foot was pulled upward it also rotated outward somewhat, to help correct the pigeon-toe deformity.

REAR VIEW

A band of rub-ber inner-tube was stretched between small holes at the top and the toe of the brace to

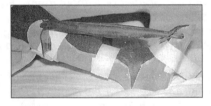

provide a gentle but steady upward pull on the foot. The force of pull could be easily adjusted by pulling more of the tube through the tightly-gripping hole. The effect of this steady pull was similar to serial casting. But, instead of changing the cast to gradually correct the position of the foot, all the family needed to do was to tighten the rubber strap.

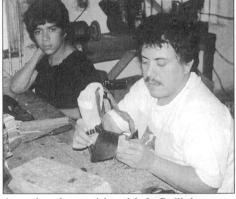

Armando makes special sandals for Raúl's braces.

Using his braces in a standing frame. One of the purposes of these below-the-knee braces was to help Raúl begin to stand with his feet in a good position. If the braces worked as planned while he was standing, the weight of his body on his feet would help to correct his tip-toe contractures.

To start Raúl standing with his legs and feet in a good position, Polo made a simple wooden standing frame for him. He added a V-shaped leg-separator to hold his feet somewhat apart, and his toes angled slightly outward.

Upon trial, Raúl's loosely-jointed knees opened in a bow-legged stance. So it was necessary to add straps to hold his legs straight.

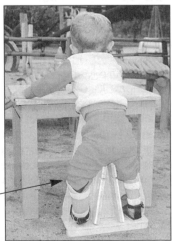

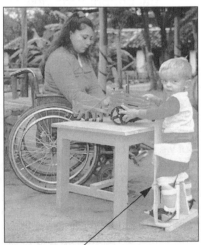

Corrective Plastic Night-Braces Especially Designed for Raúl

In addition to the braces that Raúl could use while standing, he also needed braces that would gradually help to correct the position of his feet during the night. For night use, the braces described on the preceding page had 2 disadvantages:

1. When he was not standing on them, the downward push of his fore-foot caused the brace to slip down his leg, lifting the heel of his foot off the heel of the brace, thus leaving the tip-toe deformity uncorrected. →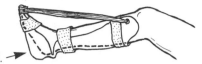

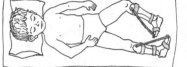

2. When not standing on the standing frame, which held Raúl's feet with the toes angled forward correctly, muscle imbalance caused his feet to rotate into a pigeon-toed position.

To keep the night-braces from slipping downward, these braces were designed for use with knees bent. A strap from the toe of the brace was stretched up over the thigh. This both stopped the brace from slipping downward, and reinforced the corrective action. Every time Raúl tried to straighten his knee, the strap would pull the brace more forcefully against his fore-foot, giving an extra corrective stretch to the tight heel cord.

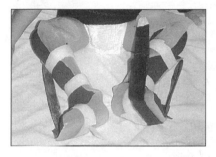

To prevent Raúl's lower legs and feet from rotating inward, the plastic night brace was made with a medial (inward-side) extension above the knee, which rested against the inner side of the thigh. With the knee bent, this thigh-flap prevented the lower leg and foot from rotating inward. The back edge of the thigh-flap had a narrow notch to hold the elastic thigh-to-toe strap in position.

To make the thigh-flap, first the plaster mold of the lower leg was extended by tying a section of plastic bottle to the top of the mold, and filling it with plaster (see photos, page 102). This allowed a plastic brace to be molded with an extension above the knee. The extension was cut free from the lower-leg brace, except on the inner side.

The upper, broad ring of plastic was then heated (with a heat gun), and opened out to form the thigh-flap.

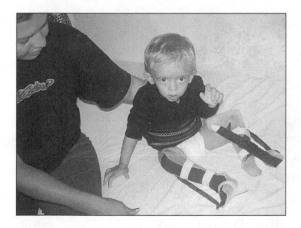

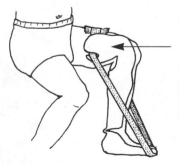

This flap was cut and shaped for the correct angle and comfort by repeated trials on Raúl's leg.

The first night's trial of the deformity-correcting braces was at PROJIMO, soon after the braces were completed. To everyone's delight, Raúl soon fell asleep, with his legs and feet in the corrective position and the inner-tube bands gradually stretching and improving the deformities.

For Raúl to be able to stand by himself and begin to walk, it became apparent that he needed full-leg braces, with a hip band to keep his feet in a forward position. With the below-the-knee braces (AFOs), his feet turned in a lot, and his knees bent sideways and backwards.

Long-Leg Braces for Walking

Mari felt it was important that Raúl begin to walk without further delay—if possible, even while his foot deformities were being corrected. (With feet fairly well-aligned, the weight of his body could help to correct the contractures.) Because his knees were so unstable, Armando thought Raúl needed long-leg braces. So he added knee joints, plastic thigh supports, and a hip band to his below-the-knee braces. Raúl's mother helped Armando to make and fit them. They had them ready for trial in 2 days. After early trials, and some complaints by Raúl, adjustments were made to the length of the braces and angle of leg separation. At last Raúl was happy with his braces.

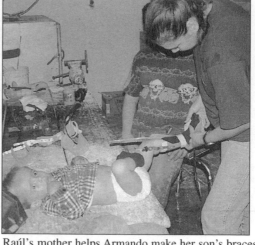

Raúl's mother helps Armando make her son's braces.

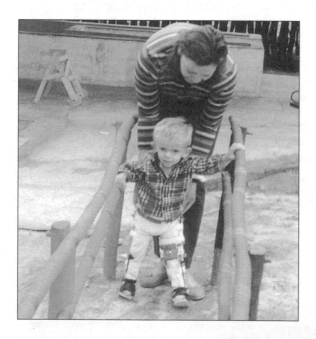

With his new braces, first Raúl tried walking between parallel bars. Then he experimented with a wooden walker that Polo, a village youth, had made for him. The child's first steps were difficult, but little by little he overcame his fear. After a while he began to walk with the walker on his own. Both Raúl and his parents were delighted.

Eventually, Raúl will need further surgery. But, thanks to the corrective action of two sets of braces (one set for standing and walking, the other for night use) any surgery he may need will be less extensive. Most important, Raúl has been able to start walking and exploring his world in an upright position, even while his deformities are being corrected. That gives him a head start.

Equally important was Raúl's change in response to the management of his disability. When he first came to PROJIMO, he was terrified. But after a few days of interacting with Mari, Armando, Cecilia, and Polo—who treated him as a person, not a patient—Raúl began to enjoy the whole process. He would lift his feet and point to them, smiling. For a child his age (under 2 years old), Raúl's cooperation and enthusiasm were amazing. Everyone fell in love with him.

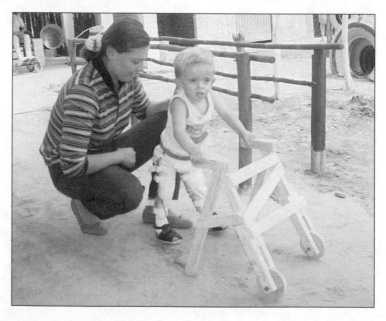

SIMILAR IDEAS ARE DEVELOPED BY DIFFERENT FOLKS IN DIFFERENT SITUATIONS

A Telescoping Brace for Straightening Turned-In Feet

When the PROJIMO team invented the plastic brace with a bent knee to straighten Raúl's in-turned feet, they were unaware that, in the United States, a somewhat similar brace was already available on the commercial market. It goes under the name of the Denis-Browne Telescoping Brace. It is available, pre-made, in different sizes, from *AliMed* Inc., Dedham, MA 02026, USA. The cost is more than US$100.

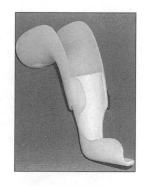

We include the design here because it is in some ways better and easier to use than PROJIMO's bent-knee design for Raúl.

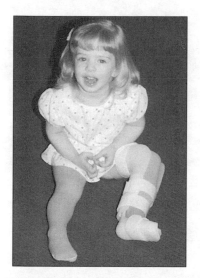

The telescoping brace is made of two molded-plastic pieces. The upper piece holds the knee at a right angle (90 degrees). The lower piece holds the ankle and foot. The two pieces are held together with Velcro (self-stick tape), so length and angle can be easily adjusted.

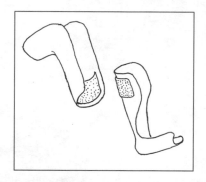

The main advantage of the telescoping brace is its adjustability. The length can be changed for different children, or for the same child as she grows. The angle of the foot in relation to the lower leg bone (tibia) can also be changed. Thus, a foot that turns in due to clubbing or "tibial torsion" (a twist in the lower leg-bone) can be slowly corrected by gradually rotating the lower half of the telescoping brace. The photographs on this page are taken from the AliMed Catalogue, with permission.

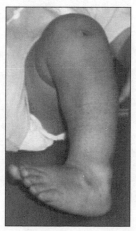
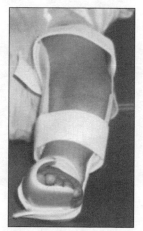
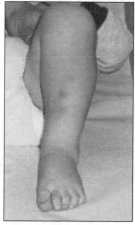

Telescoping brace—before, during and after treatment.

Preparing the Plaster Molds of Raúl's Feet to Make him Braces

To make Raúl's braces, first plaster casts were made of his legs. Then solid molds were made by filling the cast with plaster of Paris, as shown below.

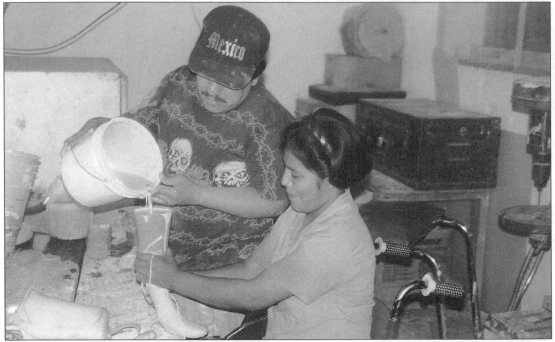

Rosaura, who is paraplegic, helps Armando make a mold for Raúl's braces (see page 99).

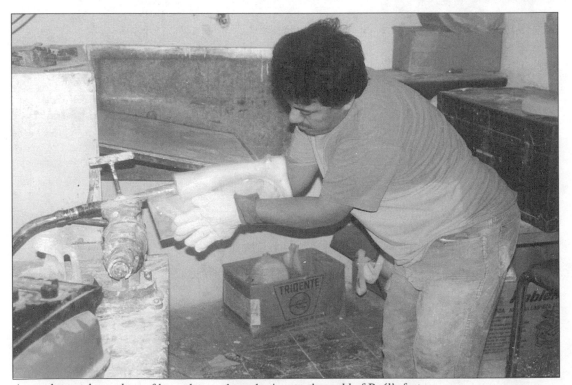

Armando stretches a sheet of hot polypropylene plastic over the mold of Raúl's feet.

Positioning the feet correctly while casting them is often difficult. The next chapter demonstrates a device that makes positioning of the foot while casting much easier.

A Foot-Positioning Device for Taking Plaster Casts

Plaster Casts

At PROJIMO, the village rehabilitation workers put plaster casts on the legs and feet of many disabled persons, for different reasons.

Sometimes casts are taken to form molds for making leg braces (orthopedic appliances).

Or a series of casts is used to gradually correct deformities of the feet or ankles. An example is the correcting of a baby's club feet.

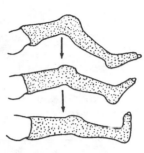

A series of plaster casts:

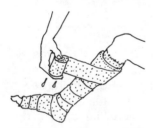

Correcting Teresa's contractures with casts.

A COMMON PROBLEM. Whether for brace-making or correction of deformities, often it is hard to hold the foot in the correct position while wrapping it with plaster bandage. The assistant who holds the foot must keep shifting her hands to permit the wrapping. As a result, the foot is often casted in a poorly corrected position. As soon as it is wrapped, it may be positioned more correctly. However, this repositioning can create wrinkles in the plaster which, after it hardens, can cause painful pressure, and can even damage the skin and underlying tissues.

Ann Hallum, a physical therapist who visited PROJIMO, told of her own bad experience with a cast:

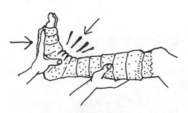

After Ann had foot surgery, her foot was casted by wrapping plaster on it in a partially corrected position.

Then the position was forcefully corrected. The resulting wrinkles and pressure caused growing discomfort and pain.

In a few days, the pressure against the top of her ankle caused permanent nerve damage (with weakness, numbness, and tingling).

PROJIMO workers have often found it hard to hold the foot in a good position while casting it. This is especially difficult in persons with strong spasticity or stubborn contractures.

Sometimes, several attempts at casting are needed to get the position correct. Or the cast must be removed to relieve pressure or pain. Especially in persons who lack feeling in their feet (spina bifida, spinal-cord injury, leprosy), it may be hard to prevent pressure sores. Casts must be removed often to check the skin.

In such persons, adjustable braces are sometimes safer than casts to correct deformities.

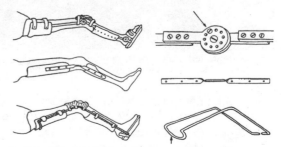

In these 3 brace designs, the knee angle can be adjusted to gradually correct the knee contracture.

A GOOD SOLUTION FOR EASIER CASTING. In February, 1996, I (the author) had surgery on my foot, to fuse my ankle bones. The cast was changed in 2 weeks. To position it correctly, the surgeon put my foot on a flat metal bar in the form of an up-side-down "L", which was mounted in the cement floor. He placed my foot and leg in exactly the desired position and asked me not to move. He wrapped a plaster bandage around my lower leg and foot, also covering the flat bar under the foot. When the plaster was fairly hard, he slipped the casted foot backwards off the bar. Then he gently pressed the plaster on the bottom of the foot to close the slit that was left from the bar.

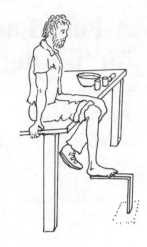

With this simple device, the foot can be positioned correctly and held firmly during casting, without the hands of an assistant getting in the way. When I was next at PROJIMO, I described this innovation to the team. Marcelo and Polo began to make one right away.

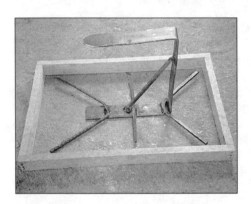

Rather than mounting the device in the floor, they decided to mount it in a rectangular slab of cement so that it could be moved from place to place. To make the bar, they used a 1½-inch-wide steel strut that they found in the wheelchair shop. This they hammered into a "U". On one arm of the U, they welded cross-bars of re-bar (construction rod) so that it would be held firmly within the cement base. Then they made a 2-inch high rectangular wooden frame. They set the steel-bar U within it, and then filled it with cement.

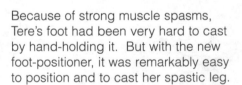

TERE was the first person to have a foot casted with the new device. She is a young women whose spastic foot pushes downward and sideways when she tries to stand on it. She needed a strong below-the-knee plastic brace to keep her foot flat on the ground, and to push her knee back, while standing. (She was just beginning to stand using parallel bars. See page 208.)

Because of strong muscle spasms, Tere's foot had been very hard to cast by hand-holding it. But with the new foot-positioner, it was remarkably easy to position and to cast her spastic leg.

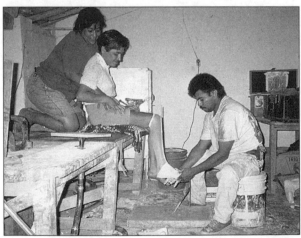

The device was especially helpful for persons with spasticity, like Tere, whose knees needed to be kept bent while casting.

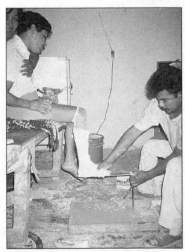

It was a bit hard to pull the casted foot off the device after the plaster hardened. This problem was corrected by smoothing and rounding the edges of the bar with a file and sand-paper.

The new foot-casting bar is a great success. And so simple! Folks at PROJIMO wonder why they didn't think of it before.

After casting, Juan pushes Tere's foot backward to slide it off the device.

Plastic Bottles to Correct Margarita's Turned-In Feet, and to Heal Jesús' Pressure Sore

CHAPTER 16

A PLASTIC BOTTLE FOOT-TUBE FOR MARGARITA

MARGARITA was born with club feet (equino-varus). When she was one month old, her parents took her to PROJIMO. The village team put her feet in plaster casts for 6 weeks, and gradually corrected the deformities. Then they made plastic braces to hold her feet in a slightly over-corrected position.

One year later, Margarita began to walk. When she was 1 year and 4 months old, she was walking fairly well. However her mother was concerned about her "pigeon-toed" feet. Indeed, when she walked, her feet turned inward a lot. On examining her, this appeared to be due in part to the position of her feet in relation to her legs, and in part to inward rotation of her hips.

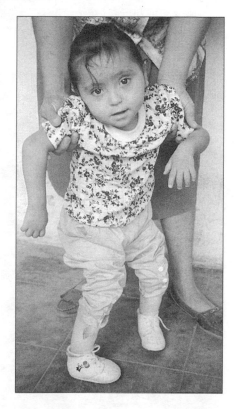

Margarita's parents had taken her to an orthopedist who prescribed a device, for use at night, that would hold her feet turned outward (externally rotated). This involved a metal bar attached to outwardly-rotated orthopedic shoes. The bar and shoes would cost the family over 800 pesos (US$100.00). Short of money, the family returned to PROJIMO to see if a less costly solution could be found.

A Simple, Low-Cost Alternative

To create a night-appliance that would hold Margarita's feet in an outwardly-rotated position, the PROJIMO team improvised a simple device using a half-liter plastic bottle. It only took about 5 minutes to make, and it cost nothing. The same high-top shoes and plastic braces that the child wore during the day could be used with the foot-tube at night. No other equipment or costs were required.

To make the foot tube, a long, slender plastic bottle can be cut with a knife (or an electric grinder). Remove both ends, and cut an oval in the middle of the bottle, just large enough to fit both feet through it.

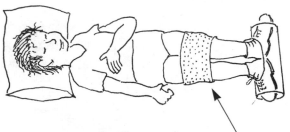

Cut the plastic bottle on the dotted lines.

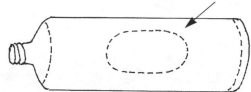

Upon trial, it was found that a band around the legs might be needed to keep the child from pulling her feet out at night.

When the new device was tried, Margarita seemed comfortable. However, her parents worried that she would fret and be unable to sleep at night with her feet confined.

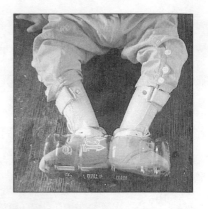

The PROJIMO team advised them to start by putting the appliance on Margarita's feet for short periods. As she got more used to it, the time could gradually be extended.

RESULTS: After two months of using the "foot-tube" appliance at night, Margarita's parents agreed that she was walking with her feet in a more normal, less turned-in position.

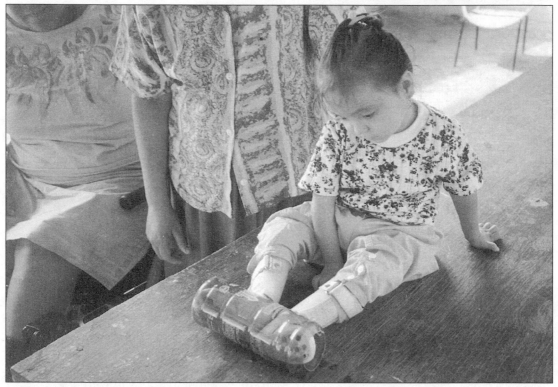

DUPLICABILITY AND ADAPTABILITY: This appliance has since been made for another child, with a piece of soft-plastic water pipe (stiff, but with moderate flexibility). With the plastic pipe, the feet can be separated, as well as outwardly-rotated.

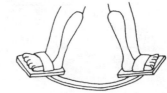

YES

CAUTION: **This plastic bottle method cannot be recommended for all children with in-turned feet.** It worked for Margarita, whose feet could easily be opened widely. But if a child's feet do not open easily, or if the rotation appears to be forcing the hips or knees into a distorted position, don't use it.

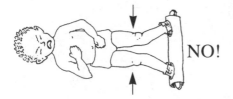

NO!

If the feet cannot be rotated outward easily by hand, it is better to use a device that will rotate them more gradually. The shoes can be screwed to a wood or metal cross-bar like this. ⟶

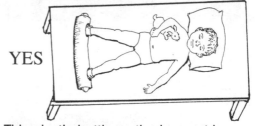

If you have to use force, or if it hurts, don't do it.

A PLASTIC-BOTTLE FOOT PROTECTOR FOR JESUS

JESÚS is a boy who was born with spina bifida, a defect in the spinal-cord that causes paralysis and reduced feeling in his legs and feet (see page 131). Chapter 45 explains how Jesús became involved in Child-to-Child activities with other children and school teachers. Here, we look only at the problem of chronic sores on his foot.

Jesús' loss of feeling from his hips to his feet has caused repeated problems. As a young child he was able to walk, although with considerable difficulty. Sores developed on his right foot and because he had no feeling in his foot he continued walking on it. Infection set in, spread to the bone, and eventually the whole foot was dangerously infected. When he was 6 years old, his lower leg had to be amputated (cut off).

When Jesús first came to PROJIMO, he had pressure sores on his backside, which were the result of reduced feeling. From crawling around on all fours, he also had sores on his stump and on the toes of his left foot.

To keep pressure off the sores on his bottom, the PROJIMO team had Jesús spend time on a wheeled cot (called a gurney, see Chapter 37). Inez cleaned his sores daily, and treated them with honey. The pressure sores on his backside were healing well. But the sores on his toes grew bigger and deeper. The problem was that Jesús was very active. He kept bumping or scraping his toes, or lying with them pressed against the gurney. The bandages quickly got dirty and matted. Mari told him to be more careful, but since he felt no pain in the open sores, he was careless. Unless a way could be found to protect Jesús' foot, Mari was afraid that his left leg might also eventually have to be amputated. What to do?

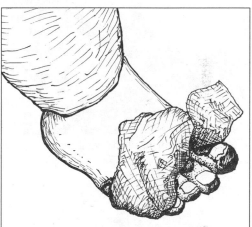

In spite of frequent washing and bandaging, the sores on Jesús' toes were often exposed, dirty, and full of flies.

A **simple device** was needed that would protect Jesús' injured toes from all sides, yet would let air circulate freely (especially because the weather was extremely hot). Marcelo, the brace and limb maker, found a solution. He riveted the bottom half of a square plastic bottle to Jesús' plastic lower-leg brace. It fit around the end of Jesús' foot and shielded the toes without touching them.

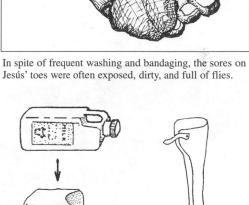

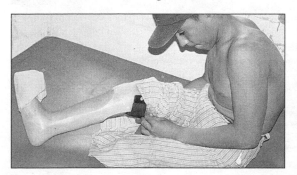

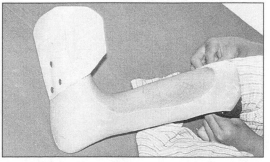

RESULTS. Pleased with his new device, Jesús took care to use it all day long. The results were impressive. In 4 days the sores were dry, clean, and well on their way toward healing.

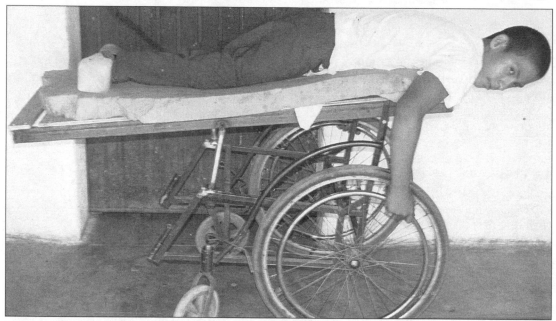

His toe protector in place, Jesús does a "wheelie" on his gurney.

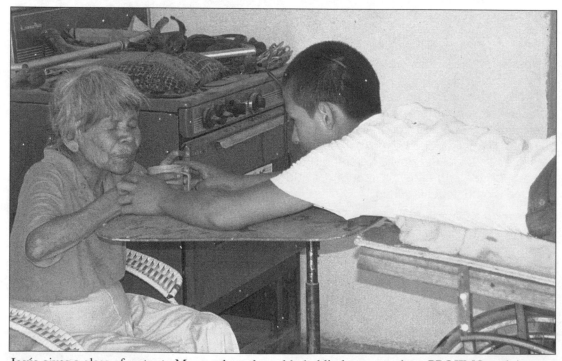

Jesús gives a glass of water to Mona, a homeless elderly blind woman whom PROJIMO took in.

Twist Hoses (and Foot Tubes) to Help Diego Walk

CHAPTER **17**

Foot Tubes That Didn't Work

DIEGO *is a bright, enthusiastic 8-year old boy with spastic cerebral palsy. When his family first took him to PROJIMO, he could walk with a walker, but with difficulty. Without his walker, he could not walk at all. A combination of in-turned feet, scissoring legs, and jerky, exaggerated movements made it extremely difficult for him to take steps. With each step, as he brought his back foot forward, the toe of his shoe would begin to hook around the heel of his weight-bearing foot, and he had to drag and jerk it free.*

Nonetheless, Diego made a great effort to walk, jerking himself back and forth across the room. "If only my feet … didn't bump … together!" said Diego, his voice jerky and high pitched from the spasticity in his throat and tongue.

"We'll see what we can do so your feet don't bump together so much when you walk," said Mari. "Great!" said Diego.

FOOT TUBES THAT ROTATE AND SEPARATE THE LEGS. To help Diego's feet turn outward, and to help his legs separate more when he walked, the team first tried a modification of the foot-tube design (see Chapter 16). They felt this might work because, when the boy relaxed, they could easily point his feet in opposite directions.

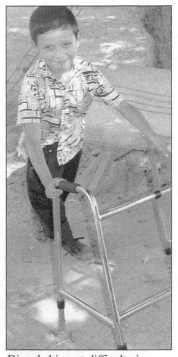

Diego's biggest difficulty in walking was that the spastic scissoring of his legs caused one foot to hook behind the other when he walked.

To both rotate and separate Diego's legs during the night, Polo made a device with 2 plastic bottles mounted on a thin board. Diego tried it and thought it might be OK.

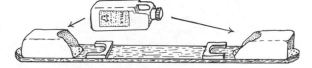

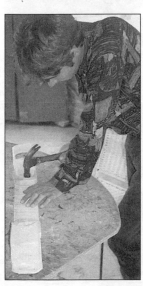

Eager to walk better, he promised to use it often. Mari suggested he wear it part of the night, and when he relaxed or watched TV.

But when the family returned to PROJIMO a few weeks later, Diego was discouraged.

"The thing is uncomfortable for him," said his mother.

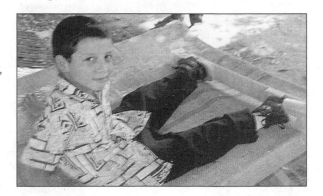

"It's killing me!" said Diego with a shy smile. "Isn't there a better way to straighten my stupid feet?"

"We could try torsion cables," suggested Mari.

"Try *what?*" asked Diego, doubtfully.

"Rubber tubes from your shoes to your waist, that twist your feet outward," Mari explained. "Interested?"

The boy frowned importantly. "Why not!"

A Trial with Elastic Spiral Leg Bands

Because the plastic bottle foot-tubes had not been successful, Mari wanted to do an experiment to see if twist cables were likely to work. She attached strong elastic straps to the tops of Diego's shoes and wound them up and around his legs, stretching them enough to pull his toes outward. She attached the upper ends behind his back. Then she asked Diego to walk with his walker. She found he walked without his toes turning in as much. And he stumbled less.

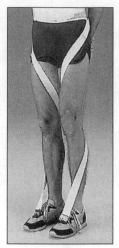

An example of elastic spiral leg bands to help turn the toes outward.

Plug-in Twist Hoses (Torsion Cables)

Reassured that the cables might help, Mari called Armando from the brace shop to see Diego. She asked him if he could make twist-cables for the boy.

"I think so," said Armando. "We have some old rubber hose from the gas-welder in the wheelchair shop. That should work for the cables."

Diego already had a new pair of shoes that fit over his below-knee orthopedic braces. "Do you think you can make the cables so that Diego can attach and remove them from his shoes easily?" Mari asked Armando. "That way he can break them in bit by bit, without much discomfort." Diego nodded with approval.

"I'll see what I can do," said Armando.

Armando designed and made twist-cables that could easily plug in and out of Diego's shoes. First he made a metal waist band, to which he riveted a leather belt with a buckle of self-sticking tape (Velcro). On both sides of the belt he fastened a metal tube that held the upper ends of the pieces of welding hose.

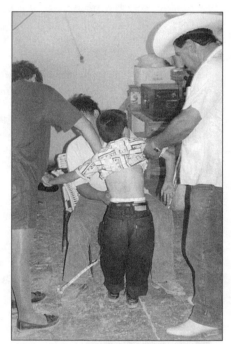

Armando (seated) measures Diego's waist in order to fit him with twist hoses.

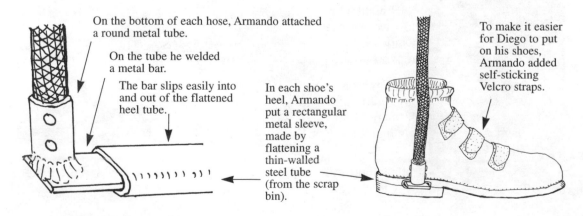

On the bottom of each hose, Armando attached a round metal tube.

On the tube he welded a metal bar.

The bar slips easily into and out of the flattened heel tube.

In each shoe's heel, Armando put a rectangular metal sleeve, made by flattening a thin-walled steel tube (from the scrap bin).

To make it easier for Diego to put on his shoes, Armando added self-sticking Velcro straps.

SURPRISING RESULTS. When the twist tubes were finished, Diego tried them. They were easy to put on. First he put on his braces and shoes, next the waist belt, and then he plugged the cables into his shoes. Armando showed him how to twist the cables before plugging them in, so that they rotated his feet outward.

An unplanned advantage to the plug-in feature was that the boy himself could experiment with the amount of twist he wanted. The twisting force on his feet depended on how many turns he gave the cables before plugging them into the heels of his shoes.

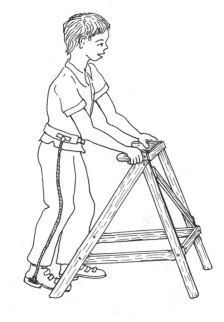

As soon as the cables were attached, Diego began to walk with his walker. To his own and his parents surprise, almost immediately he was able to swing one foot past the other without the toe of that shoe bumping into the heel of the other. This made walking a lot easier.

Mari watched carefully as Diego walked. She was pleased to see that although his feet now turned outward slightly, his knees pointed straight forward. (If the cables had caused the knees to twist outwardly [valgus], this could mean that they were causing a harmful twist at the hips.)

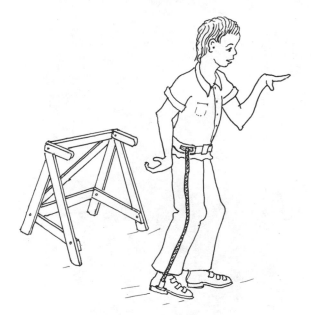

Diego walked back and forth with his walker a few times. Then, to everyone's amazement, **he let go of the walker and began to walk without it!** At first he wobbled and almost fell. But soon he figured out how to balance, and proudly walked back and forth on the porch. Diego grinned ear-to-ear as he walked. His mother wept with delight. Everyone applauded both for Diego and Armando.

Diego's middle name also happens to be Armando. In the adventure of building and trying the new device, the two Armando's formed a sort of a bond. (Armando, the brace maker, had polio as a baby and had begun to walk only when he, too, was 8 years old—also with PROJIMO's help.) When Mari asked Diego Armando what he wanted to do when he grew up, the boy replied, "I want to make braces and help other kids learn to walk, like my *tocayo* does." (*Tocayo* is Spanish for name-sake.)

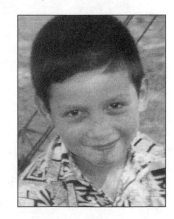

If Diego follows through on his dream, he will be the fourth youngster who first came to PROJIMO to be fitted with braces, and who then became a community-based brace maker himself.

A Walker with a Foot Separator—in Bangladesh

Different programs find different ways to deal with similar problems. At the *Center for Rehabilitation of the Paralyzed*, in Bangladesh, there was a little girl named *JANAKI*, who had cerebral palsy. Like Diego, she had difficulty walking with a standard walker. Her spastic legs tended to scissor, and would bump against each other when she tried to take steps.

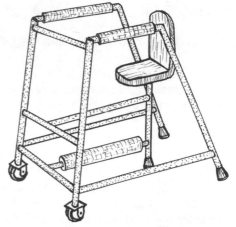

After experimenting with a number of alternatives, the staff made a simple metal walker for her which had bars positioned between her legs. The lower bar was covered with a sponge roll. The roll was upholstered with smooth plastic, so that her lower legs would slide against it as she walked. With this device, Janaki was able to walk much better. Because the bar held her feet somewhat apart, she also had better balance.

The walker also had a small seat on which Janaki could sit when she wanted to rest.

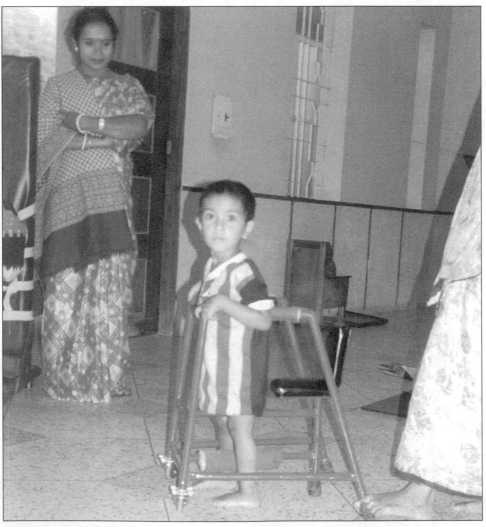

Delighted with her new walker, Janaki proudly walks in front of her mother.

A Low-Cost Stump-Cast Clamp for Making Artificial Legs

Experimenting with Village-Made Limbs

In Mexico, there are thousands of people who need an artificial leg, but don't have the money to buy one. A modern above-the-knee prosthesis often costs a farm laborer or factory worker twice his or her yearly wages.

The PROJIMO team has experimented with different kinds of low-cost legs. They sent a villager to Thailand to be an apprentice for making bamboo limbs, molded leather sockets, and wooden knee-joints. (All of these are pictured in the book, *Disabled Village Children*.) Some of the "appropriate technology" legs worked very well. But—alas!—most people did not like them: they said they looked too primitive. They had seen fancy limbs made of fiberglass, and they wanted something "modern."

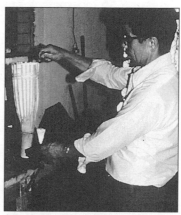

Salvador, making a bamboo limb, which he learned to do in Thailand.

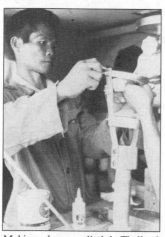

Making a low-cost limb in Thailand.

In response to users' wishes, PROJIMO arranged for a team member, Florentino, to apprentice for two weeks in a limb-making shop in a distant city. There he learned the basics of making fiberglass-and-resin limbs. When he returned, Florentino improved his skills by trial and error. He shared what he knew with Marcelo Acevedo, who in time became a master limb-maker. Marcelo, in turn, taught Guadalupe (himself an amputee), Conchita (see Chapter 42), and others.

PROJIMO has been able to fit persons with modern fiber-glass legs at a much lower cost than they could find elsewhere. While quality varies, these limbs tend to be better than those made at much higher cost by professionals in the cities. Two government rehabilitation programs have contracted with PROJIMO to fit their clients with these artificial legs.

The PROJIMO leg-makers (mostly disabled) have had little formal training. They learn by doing. **Although their technical skills may not equal those of highly trained technicians, it is their relationship with the persons receiving limbs that makes all the difference.** Often the person stays several days, and becomes involved in fitting and building the limb. After it is done, she spends the next days at PROJIMO learning how to walk with it. Efforts are made to fix any problems, even when this means remaking the leg.

A good limb is the result of a close working relationship between builder and user.

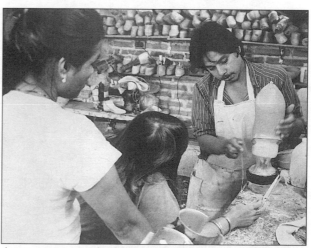

A young woman watches Marcelo and Conchita make a fiberglass-and-resin socket for her artificial leg. This modern technology is done at the small village center, at relatively low cost (less than one fifth the cost she would pay in the city).

LOW-COST MATERIALS AND SECOND-HAND PARTS

Marcelo and the other limb makers at PROJIMO have devised several techniques for making modern fiberglass-socket limbs at lower cost. Whenever possible, they try to get high-quality knee-joints from discarded limbs (often those of elderly persons with diabetes who have died). Support persons and groups in the USA and elsewhere are on the lookout for second-hand joints, foot pieces, and other parts. Where such recycling is possible, top-quality limbs can be provided at affordable prices.

To make a limb that fits well, the first step is to cast the person's stump. First, the technician makes a "negative" (hollow) cast of the stump by wrapping a plaster bandage over the stump. Next, the technician makes a "positive" (solid) mold, by filling the hollow cast with plaster.

First, make the negative cast of the stump.

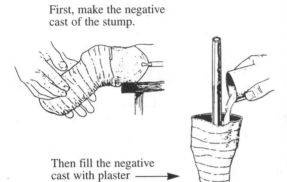

Then fill the negative cast with plaster to make the positive cast. ⟶

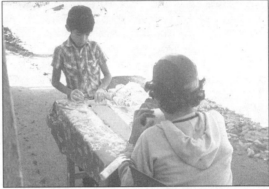

By rolling their own plaster bandages, the cost is reduced to a fraction of that of commercial plaster bandage rolls.

The team has found ways to keep down the costs. First, they have experimented with **roll-your-own plaster bandages,** rather than buying expensive commercial plaster bandages. With these home-made plaster rolls, casting the stump is somewhat more difficult, but the cost is only about one tenth that of the commercial equivalent.

The time it takes for the plaster to set (that is, to get hard after wetting it with water) can be controlled in 2 ways. To speed up the setting time, add a small amount of salt (ordinary table salt) to the unset plaster powder. Or add a little powder from old plaster that has already set. (The dust that collects from filing plaster molds works well.) *CAUTION: Hot weather or warm water also speeds up the setting time,* so local experimenting is necessary.

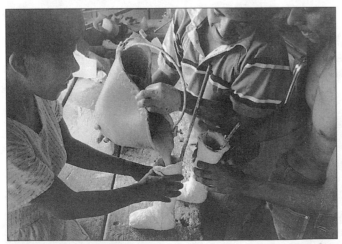

The mother of a child who needs plastic leg-braces helps Marcelo and Armando to make the positive casts. The same methods of casting are used as for amputations. Here, a post of re-bar is being mounted in the plaster.

For making positive casts, the village leg-makers use low-cost plaster sold for building houses, instead of costly orthopedic plaster-of-Paris.

Most limb makers, when they make a positive cast, put into it a ½ inch metal water-pipe. The pipe is used to grip the heavy stump-cast in a vise while it is being "modified" (shaped into a form for molding the socket).

Instead of the metal pipe, PROJIMO uses **re-bar** (reinforcing rod, used in the cement walls of buildings). It is cheaper.

A Clamp to Hold the Stump-Cast

Problem: To position and reposition the heavy stump cast while modifying it to form the mold for the socket of the artificial limb, a clamp is needed to hold it securely. Most high-class prosthetic (artificial limb) shops have a strong, factory-made clamp. But this is expensive (the equivalent of about US $130). For this reason, PROJIMO's leg-makers simply used a bench-vise to grip the metal rod which they had molded into the cast.

However, with the force used in filing and shaping the cast, the bar often slipped in the vise. Also, the cast needed to be rotated repeatedly during modification. To do this, the vise had to be loosened, and the heavy cast had to be held in the right position while tightening the vise. For a big heavy cast this often took two persons.

Solution: One time a North American limb-maker, John Fago, was visiting PROJIMO to help the team up-grade their skills. John is an amputee who first came to the project as a photographer. (Several photos in this book are by John.) After visiting PROJIMO, John decided to get training as a prosthetist, in order to help in the development of low-cost, high-quality limbs. (He now runs a small, non-profit program called *New Legs for Nomads*.) Marcelo explained to John the difficulty he had in trying to hold the stump-cast in a bench vise.

Together, Marcelo and John set about designing a simple stump-cast clamp which would hold the cast securely, yet also allow it to be easily and quickly repositioned.

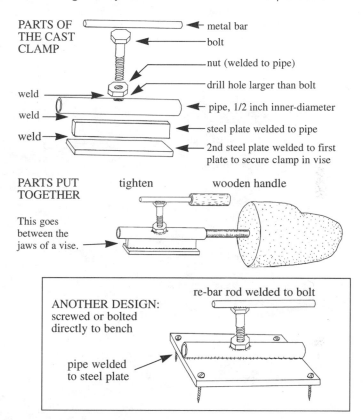

PARTS OF THE CAST CLAMP
- metal bar
- bolt
- nut (welded to pipe)
- drill hole larger than bolt
- pipe, 1/2 inch inner-diameter
- steel plate welded to pipe
- 2nd steel plate welded to first plate to secure clamp in vise

weld
weld
weld

PARTS PUT TOGETHER   tighten   wooden handle

This goes between the jaws of a vise.

ANOTHER DESIGN: screwed or bolted directly to bench

re-bar rod welded to bolt

pipe welded to steel plate

Usefulness elsewhere. The clamp was put together out of scrap metal in about 1 hour. It works remarkably well, allowing the cast to be effortlessly rotated and re-clamped.

The innovation proved so popular that Javier, who worked in the brace shop, took one look at it and immediately made one to hold casts for making orthopedic appliances.

A few months later, John Fago took his photos of the clamp to Cambodia (where tens of thousands of people have lost their legs from stepping on land mines— see page 173). Limb-makers in small shops there faced similar problems and, on seeing the photos, at once made their own cast clamps—adapting the PROJIMO design to local materials. So PROJIMO, which had originally taken some of its appropriate technology ideas from grassroots limb shops in the Far East, was able to return a useful innovation.

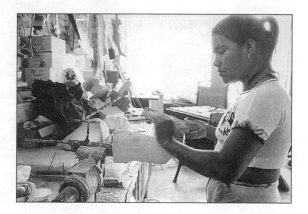

How Good Ideas Spread

From Mexico . . .

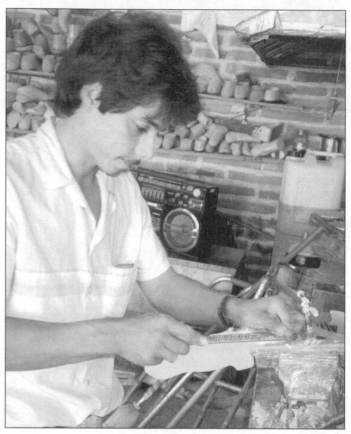

John Fago showed photos like these of PROJIMO'S stump-cast clamp to village limb makers in Cambodia.

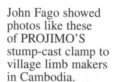

. . . to Cambodia

When the Cambodian limb-makers (who also had disabilities) saw John's photos, they realized how much easier it could make their work, and promptly made their own, as shown here.

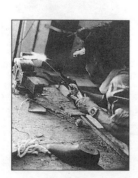

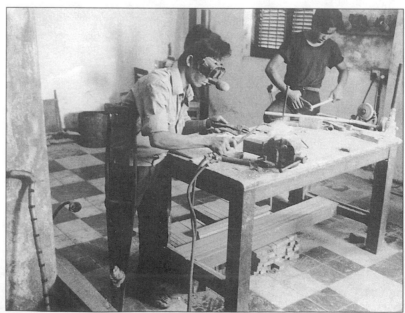

Photos: John Fago

The Key to Making Legs is Making Friends

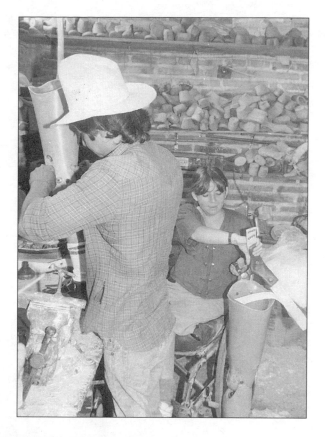

Conchita and Marcelo have worked hard to learn how to make modern fiber-glass-and-resin limbs, because this is what people say they want.

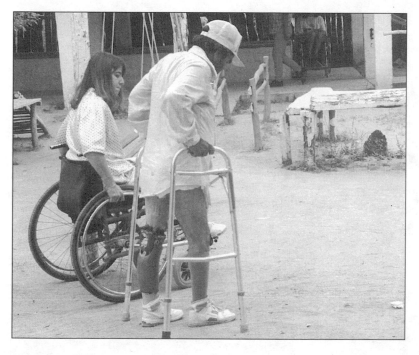

Before she finishes a limb, Conchita makes sure it fits well.

Here, a man tests his new leg while Conchita assists him in learning to walk.*

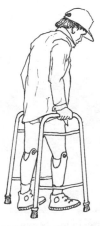

Walking is easier with the arms straighter.

*CAUTION: Reviewers of this book have rightly pointed out that this man's walker is too high (as are the crutches of the smiling boy on page 273). His elbows are bent far too much. For easier walking on walkers, crutches, or parallel bars, usually the arms should be nearly straight (see page 11). Conchita, of course, could argue that the high walker encourages its user to bear more weight on his new leg. What do you think?

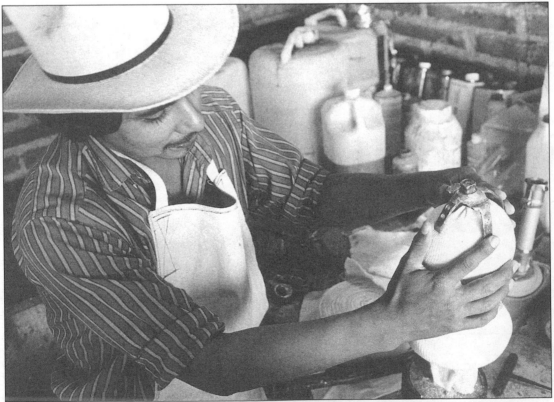

Marcelo has become skilled at making "modern" artificial legs of fiberglass and resin—but does so at a much lower cost than at the rehabilitation centers in the cities.

Photo: John Fago

The Mukti Limb:
Fast, Cheap Legs from Plastic Pipe

CHAPTER **19**

CULTURALLY-ADAPTED LIMBS IN INDIA

The Jaipur Foot

India is the home of some remarkable innovations for and by disabled persons. The **Jaipur Foot,** now world famous, was developed by an orthopedic surgeon, Dr. P. K. Sethi, in response to a disturbing realization. A kind-hearted person, he had gone to great efforts to provide the best, most modern fiberglass-and-resin Western prosthetics to the neediest of amputees. Weeks or months later, he would see these same amputees hobbling on crutches, without their limbs. Humbly, he asked them *why.* Apologetically, they told him. He began to realize that *limbs well-suited to a Northern city are completely out of place in rural India.* Indian villagers need a leg with which they can go barefoot into homes and temples, squat at their toilet, sit cross-legged on the floor while eating, and work knee-deep in the mud of rice paddies.

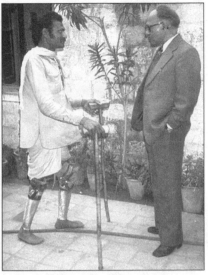

Dr. P. K. Sethi talks with a double amputee who has been fitted with Jaipur limbs at the Center in Jaipur, India. Many ideas for improving the limbs come from the users.

THE JAIPUR FOOT

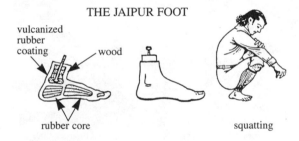

vulcanized rubber coating

wood

rubber core

squatting

Through a process of trial and error, with a lot of feed-back from village amputees, Dr. Sethi developed a design that was more suited to the traditions, poverty, and environment of rural India. The Jaipur foot-piece is heat-molded in iron forms in which pieces of wood are covered with vulcanized rubber. It is very flexible, water-proof, and looks real (with toes, veins, and skin color). The foot is fixed to a lightweight aluminum shank crafted by traditional tinsmiths. The above-the-knee limb has a swivel knee joint that permits comfortable squatting and cross-legged sitting.

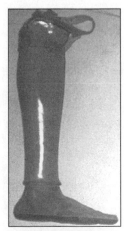

The Jaipur limb has a rubber foot and aluminum shank.

The Jaipur foot is so practical and low-cost, that it is now produced in many countries of Asia, Africa and Latin America. At many community centers that make these limbs— including a large center in Colombo, Sri Lanka—most of the limb-makers are themselves amputees.

Because the Jaipur technology is already widely known, here we will limit our description to only a few photos. The limb was developed working closely with local disabled persons and with local crafts-persons. Much can be learned from this cooperative learning process.

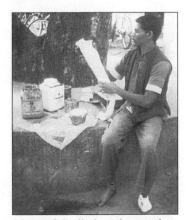

Many of the limb-makers at the Jaipur Center are amputees, like this young man, or they are local, traditional craftspersons.

STEPS IN MAKING A JAIPUR LIMB FOR GOPI, WHO LOST HIS LEG JUMPING A TRAIN

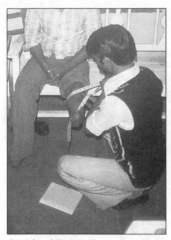

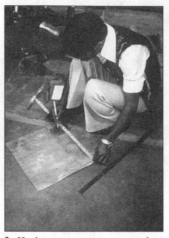

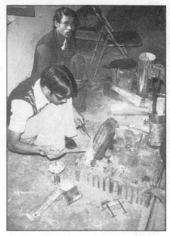

1. A local limb maker measures Gopi's stump.

2. He draws measurements on a sheet of aluminum and cuts them out.

3. He welds the aluminum sheet into a tube.

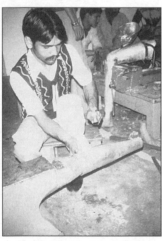

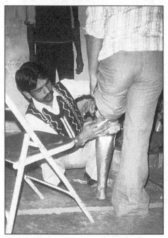

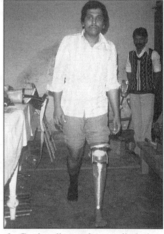

4. He hammers the tube to look like a leg and to correctly fit the stump.

5. After attaching the foot to the tube, he adds padding and a strap, and tries it on Gopi's leg.

6. Gopi walks on the new limb the same day it was begun.

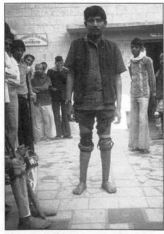

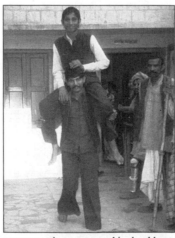

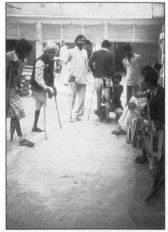

Here, a double amputee with Jaipur limbs runs carrying a man on his shoulders.

More folks waiting for limbs.

A Mukti Limb—Made from Plastic Pipe

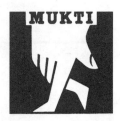

The Jaipur foot is not the only user-centered breakthrough in prosthetic limbs from India. In 1986, Meena Dadha, a remarkable woman from Madras, became concerned that there were hundreds of thousands of amputees in India who needed a limb and could lead more fruitful, happier lives if they had one. A method of leg-making was needed where limb-making teams could "go to the people," even in remote villages, and make good quality legs quickly at low cost.

Mukti is the name of a limb-making program that has its main base in Madras, and runs a mobile outreach program to rural areas. The limb-making equipment is transported in a van to small towns that invite Mukti's service and agree to bring together amputees from nearby villages. A 5 or 6 day workshop is organized in a temple, meeting hall, or school.

As part of a United Nations training program, I (the author) had the privilege of observing a Mukti workshop in a remote village. To my amazement, a team of 5 craftspersons produced 60 limbs in 5 days. I watched as they made a limb for a poor farm worker. He began to walk on his new limb just 2 hours after the first measurements were taken! (He, of course, stayed longer for gait training and adjustments.)

The key to this fast, low-cost technology is the use of plastic water pipe for the socket and the shank of the limb. The pipe is 3 inch diameter "HDPE" (high density polyethylene) irrigation pipe, with a melting point of 134 to 137 degrees C. It is produced by Polylefins Industries, which makes skin-colored pipe especially for Mukti. (The pipe is somewhat different from PVC pipe, and easier to mold.)

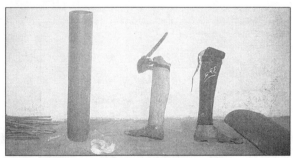

Plastic pipe is converted into prosthetic legs, as shown here.

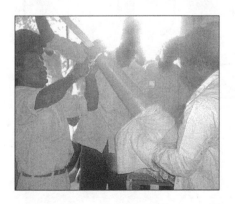

To make the limb, a plaster mold of the stump is made. To the bottom of this mold, plaster of Paris is added to form a mold of the entire shank. To do this, a cardboard cone is attached to the bottom of the stump mold, and filled with plaster-of-Paris (see drawings on next pages). A measured section of plastic pipe is put over a stout wooden stick, and is heated in an oven until it begins to droop.

◄—— Then, the hot pipe is stretched over the cast of the leg.

On cooling, the plaster is removed from the inside of the mold. A pre-made rubber foot, similar to a Jaipur foot (produced in different sizes in Mukti's center in Madras), is fixed to the bottom of the shank. Straps are attached to the top of the limb to hold it firmly on the stump.

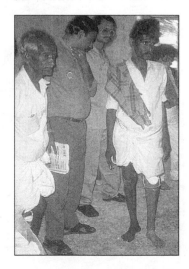

The results are impressive. The elderly farm worker whom I saw fitted was able to walk surprisingly well with his new, light-weight leg on that same afternoon. He was overjoyed.

A series of drawings on how to make the limb, from a booklet by Mukti, are reproduced on the next 3 pages.

STEPS TO MAKE A MUKTI LIMB

adapted from a booklet by Mukti, titled *A Limb of Utility Is a Joy Forever*

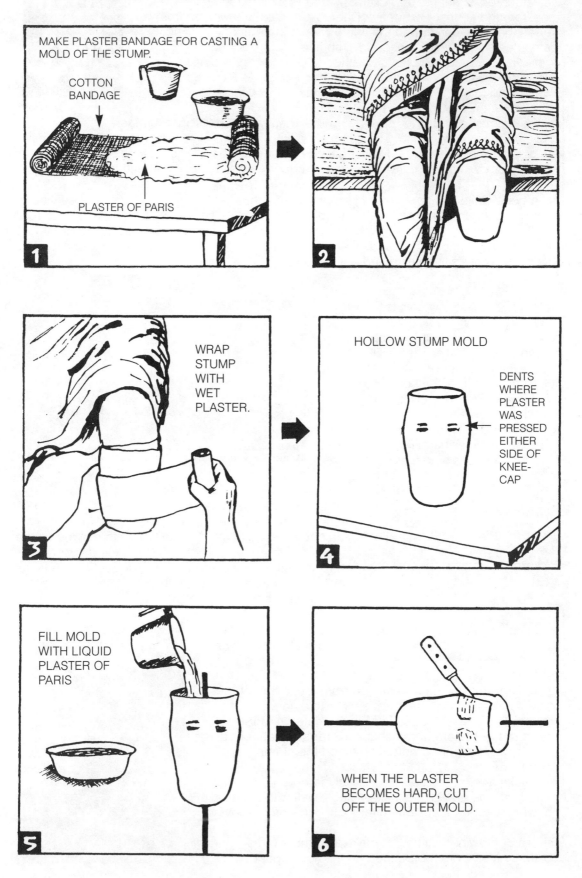

1 MAKE PLASTER BANDAGE FOR CASTING A MOLD OF THE STUMP.

COTTON BANDAGE

PLASTER OF PARIS

3 WRAP STUMP WITH WET PLASTER.

4 HOLLOW STUMP MOLD

DENTS WHERE PLASTER WAS PRESSED EITHER SIDE OF KNEE-CAP

5 FILL MOLD WITH LIQUID PLASTER OF PARIS

6 WHEN THE PLASTER BECOMES HARD, CUT OFF THE OUTER MOLD.

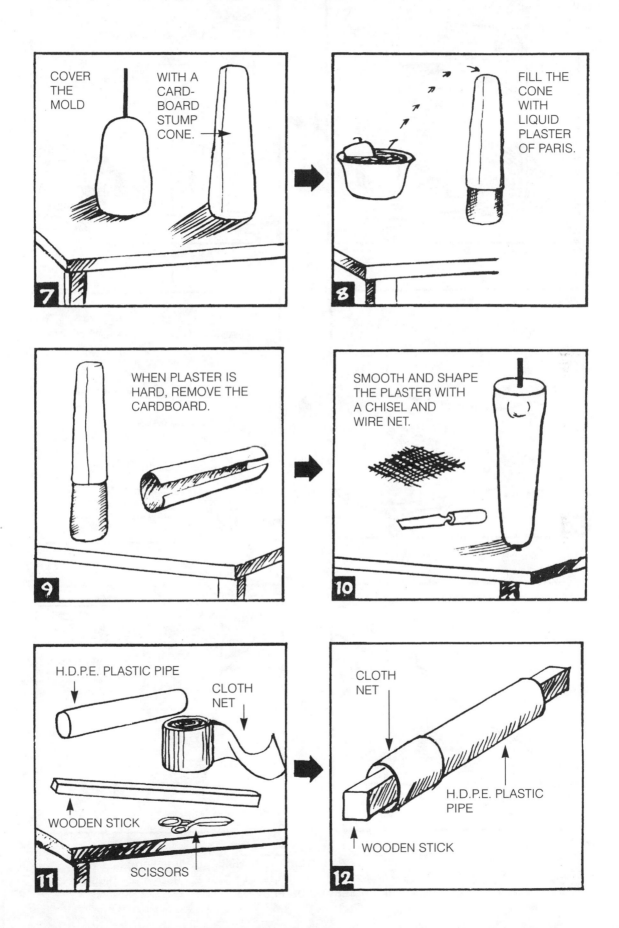

COVER THE MOLD WITH A CARD-BOARD STUMP CONE.

7

FILL THE CONE WITH LIQUID PLASTER OF PARIS.

8

WHEN PLASTER IS HARD, REMOVE THE CARDBOARD.

9

SMOOTH AND SHAPE THE PLASTER WITH A CHISEL AND WIRE NET.

10

H.D.P.E. PLASTIC PIPE

CLOTH NET

WOODEN STICK

SCISSORS

11

CLOTH NET

H.D.P.E. PLASTIC PIPE

WOODEN STICK

12

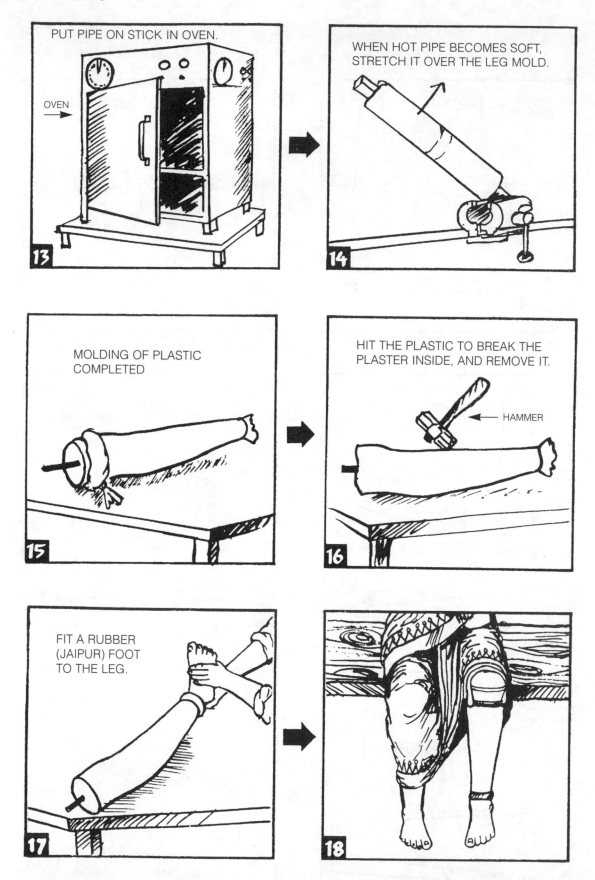

PUT PIPE ON STICK IN OVEN.

OVEN

13

WHEN HOT PIPE BECOMES SOFT,
STRETCH IT OVER THE LEG MOLD.

14

MOLDING OF PLASTIC
COMPLETED

15

HIT THE PLASTIC TO BREAK THE
PLASTER INSIDE, AND REMOVE IT.

HAMMER

16

FIT A RUBBER
(JAIPUR) FOOT
TO THE LEG.

17

18

More information on Mukti Limbs can be obtained from Mukti, (address on page 342).
Many other groups are also experimenting with limbs and braces made from plastic pipe,
including Handicap International (address on page 341).

A Wooden Skeleton for Teaching Functions of Muscles and Bones

The Human Body: Understanding its functions, rather than memorizing big words. *For rehabilitation workers—whether at the home, community or professional level—it helps to have a basic understanding of the human body, and how it works. Community based rehabilitation tries to de-mystify scientific knowledge, and to share it in a simplified form anyone can understand and use. To learn about the structures of bodies (anatomy), **it is important to understand what muscles and bones do, and how they interact to make the body work,** rather than to learn a lot of big Latin names for body parts.*

The FLEXIKIN—a Good Teaching Tool, but with Limitations

Years ago, PROJIMO invented a jointed cardboard doll called a Flexikin to help teach families about body joints and how they work. Its main use was to motivate the family of a child with *contractures* (joints that do not straighten) to patiently keep doing the necessary stretching exercises.

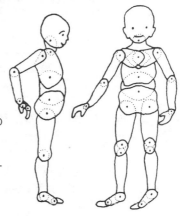

Stretching exercises can slowly help to correct a knee contracture.

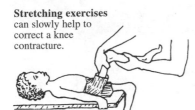

Unfortunately, progress is often very slow. So the family tends to stop the exercises. But with a flexikin, the family can measure and record the gradual straightening of joints. This motivates both the child and family to keep doing the exercises.

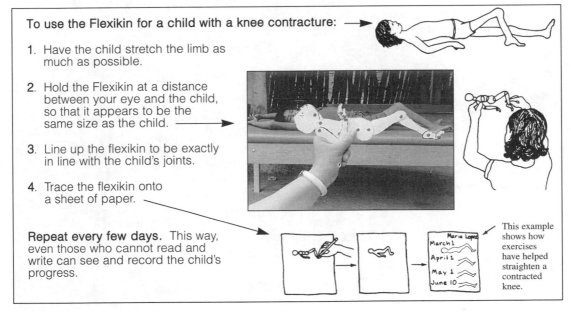

To use the Flexikin for a child with a knee contracture: ➜

1. Have the child stretch the limb as much as possible.

2. Hold the Flexikin at a distance between your eye and the child, so that it appears to be the same size as the child. ➜

3. Line up the flexikin to be exactly in line with the child's joints.

4. Trace the flexikin onto a sheet of paper.

Repeat every few days. This way, even those who cannot read and write can see and record the child's progress.

Maria Lopez
March 1
April 1
May 1
June 10

This example shows how exercises have helped straighten a contracted knee.

The flexikin can be used to teach about and record the different body positions and deformities related to a variety of disabilities. The arrows in these pictures show possible problem areas.

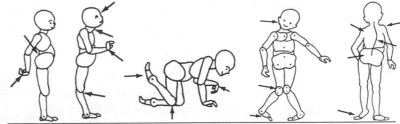

MAKING THE FLEXIKIN MORE EASILY—WITH HOME-MADE PLASTIC RIVETS

The original design for Flexikins used small metal rivets to join the movable joints. However, community based rehabilitation workers in many countries complained that they did not have such rivets. This problem was solved by a CBR workshop participant in Brazil, who created **home-made plastic rivets** from small plastic rods (those used for stirring drinks).

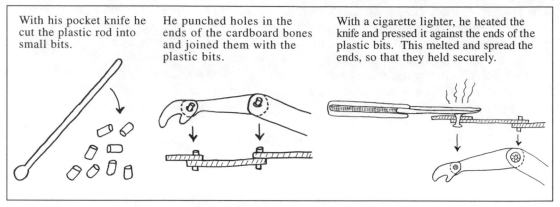

With his pocket knife he cut the plastic rod into small bits.

He punched holes in the ends of the cardboard bones and joined them with the plastic bits.

With a cigarette lighter, he heated the knife and pressed it against the ends of the plastic bits. This melted and spread the ends, so that they held securely.

With these plastic rivets, CBR programs almost anywhere can make and use flexikins.

A Plywood Skeleton to Learn about How the Body Works (Functional Anatomy)

If it is true that **a drawing is worth a 1000 words,** it is also true that **a model that moves and simulates real life can be worth a 1000 drawings.**

To help learners "see for themselves" how muscles and bones move and work, PROJIMO has developed a plywood skeleton, complete with joints that bend and straighten.

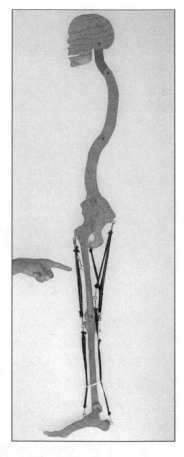

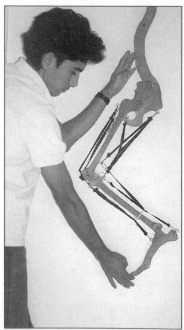

Strips of rubber inner-tube, which stretch and contract like muscles, are attached to the plywood bones by string tendons. (Like real tendons, the string does not stretch and contract as do the rubber muscles.)

The model skeleton can be used to teach basic principles which are useful for planning appropriate therapy, bracing, and special seating.

Efraín shows how the different muscles of the leg contract to bend the knee and raise the foot.

Learners can move the joints and discover how muscles stretch and contract to move different parts of the body. By replacing some muscles with weak ones, or with contracted ones (using strips of leather instead of rubber), they can see how muscle-imbalance and/or contractures cause abnormal positions or deformities.

To understand why **it is more effective to do certain exercises with the body or limb in one position and not another**, it helps to know something about important muscles and tendons, and where they attach to the bones. This knowledge can also be helpful for daily activities, like dressing. For example, consider this mother of a child with spastic cerebral palsy.

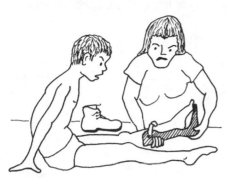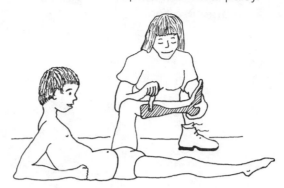

This mother finds it hard to put on her child's brace. When his leg is straight, the foot points down so forcefully that she cannot bend it up.

She would probably find it much easier to bend his foot up and put on the brace, if she were to hold his knee bent rather than straight.

How can you help the mother (or a rehabilitation worker) understand *why* it is easier to put on the brace with the knee bent? You can explain that **1)** Bending the knee helps to break the spastic pattern and relax the leg muscles; and **2)** When the knee is bent, the foot bends up more, because some of the muscles that pull the foot down are attached to the lower end of the thigh-bone. When the knee is bent, a tight calf-muscle becomes looser, because the distance from the thigh-bone to the heel is shorter.

Pictures can make this clearer.

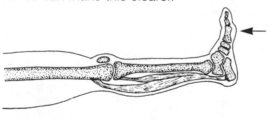

The calf muscle, by pulling on the heel bone, pushes the foot down. This muscle is attached to the heel bone on one end and to the thigh bone on the other end.

When the knee is bent, the distance between the thigh-bone and the heel-bone becomes shorter. This makes a tight calf-muscle looser and therefore it is easier to bend the foot upward.

A moving model can make it clearer still.

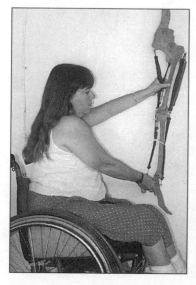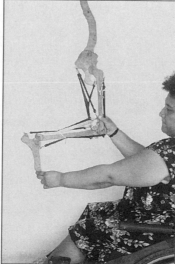

The above drawings help. However, **people learn better when they see and handle a model with bones and muscles that move.**

In these photos, Conchita and Mari use the plywood skeleton to teach stretching exercises to the mother of a girl with cerebral palsy. The girl stands and walks on tiptoe due to tight heel cords and early contractures. Mari shows the mother why it is easier to lift the foot when the knee is bent.

In addition to muscles and tendons, the model has *ligaments* (non-stretching cords that connect bone to bone) made of string. Important ligaments behind the knee bind the thigh-bone to the lower leg-bone. These cords prevent the knee from bending too far back. **By lengthening or cutting the string-ligaments on the model, learners can see what happens when the real ligaments get stretched or torn** (see pages 89 and 94).

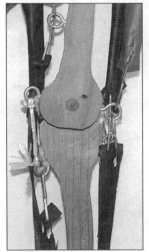

Healthy ligament.

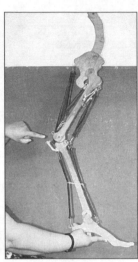

Torn ligament.

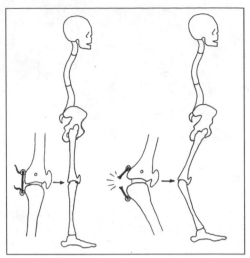

Drawings of back-of-knee ligament, whole and torn.

The skeleton can also be used to show how hip-flexion contractures can be caused by tight muscles between the front edge of the hips and the thigh bone. To demonstrate this, the rubber band which represents the muscle is replaced by a strip of leather that represents a tight muscle that no longer stretches.

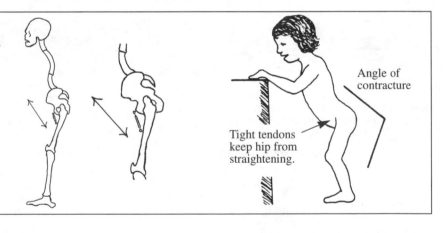

When the muscles between the front of the hips and the thighs are tight, the hip girdle tilts forward, causing a sway-back when standing. Such contractures should be avoided through stretching exercises and good positioning. (See pages 16 and 220.)

Angle of contracture

Tight tendons keep hip from straightening.

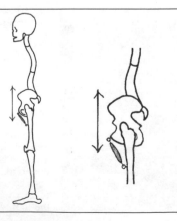

When the muscle between the front of the hip and the thigh bone is normal, the hip girdle stands up straight and the child's back is in a straight line with her legs.

A wealth of useful knowledge can be gained by this hands-on model.

Because this methodology involves people making their own observations and drawing their own conclusions, it falls into the category known as **discovery-based learning.**

Part Three

OVERCOMING DIFFICULTIES WITH BODY FUNCTION THAT RESULT FROM DAMAGE TO THE NERVOUS SYSTEM

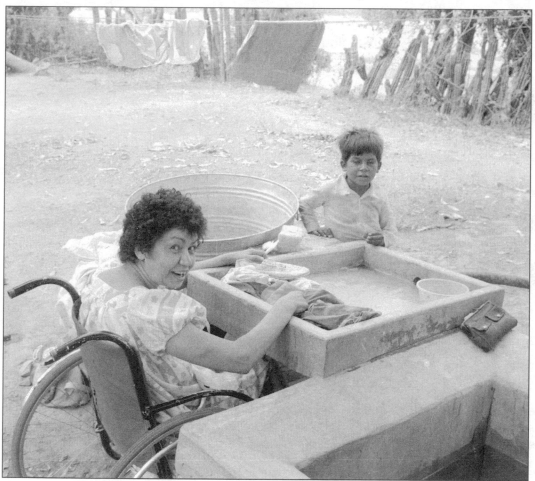

Photo by John Fago

INTRODUCTION TO PART THREE

Creative Solutions to Personal and Situational Needs

The human body is a marvelous system of complex structures and processes that work in harmony to sustain and protect a living, active person. Many disabilities that affect certain functions of the body upset the balance which preserves a person's health and well-being.

Consider pain. The ability to feel pain is an important protective mechanism of the body. In disabilities where the sense of feeling and pain is reduced or lost in parts of the body—such as leprosy, spinal cord injury, spina bifida, or advanced diabetes—minor injuries happen more easily, and they run a risk of becoming major or life-threatening problems.

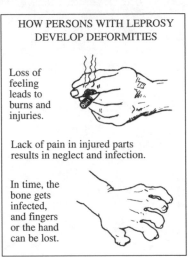

HOW PERSONS WITH LEPROSY DEVELOP DEFORMITIES

Loss of feeling leads to burns and injuries.

Lack of pain in injured parts results in neglect and infection.

In time, the bone gets infected, and fingers or the hand can be lost.

For example, many deformities that come with leprosy (Hansen's disease) such as loss of fingers, hands, and feet, are not caused by leprosy itself. They come from secondary (and preventable) injuries and infections that happen because of **loss of feeling**. (Leprosy germs attack nerves that transmit feeling.)

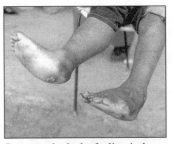

Because she lacks feeling in her feet, this child with spina bifida developed sores which led to bone infection. She may need to have her right foot amputated.

Children with spina bifida, who often have no feeling in their feet, also can develop sores and bone infections similar to those seen with leprosy. Jesús, whom you meet in Chapters 16, 26, and 45, lost a leg from such a problem, and also had severe pressure sores on his backside.

Pressure sores and urinary infections are common and often life-threatening problems in persons with spina bifida and **spinal cord injury.** Two chapters in Part 3 (Chapters 27 and 28) look at innovative ways of protecting against and treating pressure sores. Chapters 25 and 26 look at techniques for avoiding and combating urinary infections.

Persons who are quadriplegic (spinal-cord injured in the neck) usually have hands paralyzed as well as legs. In Chapter 24, a young man tells how he made his own **device to hold a pen.** In Chapter 28, a youth learns to **use spasticity to dress.**

Persons with uncontrolled movements or limited control of their hands (or whole bodies) often have trouble with carrying things, especially liquid food and drink. Chapter 22 shows how a man with cerebral palsy designed a **non-spill carrying tray.**

Chapter 21 describes the creation of devices for **straightening the back of a baby** with spina bifida who had an extreme spinal curve. Chapter 23 looks at innovations that helped a man who had a **stroke** to **relearn to talk and walk.**

In sum, Part 3 looks at a range of innovations to improve function and safeguard health, primarily for persons with complications of injuries to the brain or spinal cord. Often the concerned person plays a key role in the problem-solving process.

CHAPTER 21

A Back-Brace Crib and Bounce-Bed for a Baby with Severe Spinal Curve

YURI was born with a sack-like lump on her lower back. Her mother, Eva, sold the family donkey and took Yuri to a city hospital. She was told that her daughter had spina bifida, a deformity of the spinal cord that often causes paralysis of the lower body. Surgery was done to cover the delicate sack of nerves with healthy skin.

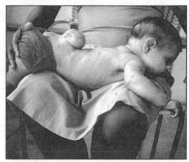

During her first months of life, Yuri grew well and seemed healthy. However, her mother was concerned that her body was bending more and more to one side. When she was 4 months old, her mother took her to PROJIMO.

A baby with spina bifida

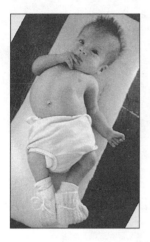

The PROJIMO workers found that the baby had scoliosis (a sideways spinal curve) of almost 90 degrees.

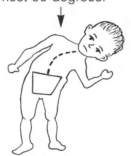

The curve could be partly straightened using gentle manual pressure.

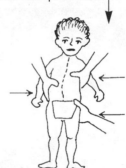

The team encouraged Eva to take Yuri to the city for X-rays and evaluation. But that would cost too much for the family. Eva asked if something could be done in the village at a lower cost to help correct the spinal curve, or at least to keep it from getting worse.

This led to a discussion about different possibilities. First the team suggested some sort of a **body jacket** to hold the baby's body straighter. But it was summer and the weather was extremely hot. Yuri's mother was worried that the baby would cook to death in a confining plastic jacket. She already suffered from heat rashes.

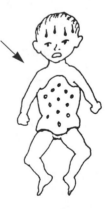

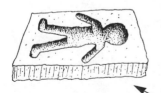

The next idea was a kind of **molded mattress.** The baby was still quite small and spent a lot of time lying on her back. Juán, one of PROJIMO's brace-makers, thought he could make a mattress out of foam-plastic. He would mold or carve out the foam to hold the baby in an improved position.

However, both the body jacket and the molded mattress would have a serious limitation. The position would be fixed, and not easily adjustable. Some sort of an **adjustable positioning device** was needed that could be modified as the baby's body gradually straightened.

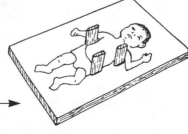

One suggestion was to use 3 **adjustable padded posts,** → positioned so as to help straighten the baby's body.

An Adjustable Back-Straightening Bed

Out of the suggestion of 3 padded posts, a better idea grew: to use 3 rows of thin wood rods (dowels). The rods fit snugly into holes in a wooden bed-board.

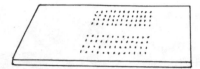

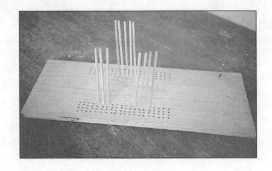

By drilling rows of closely-placed holes, the posts can be positioned so as to press against the baby's body and to match her contours—almost like hands. The position of the rods can be adjusted and readjusted easily to meet the child's changing needs.

The team and Yuri's mother, Eva, decided the idea was worth trying.

They placed a foam-rubber pad over the board as a mattress.

Squares of foam rubber were placed between the rows of rods and the child's body.

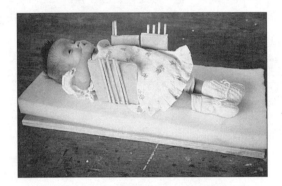

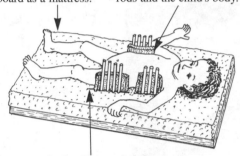

Long cuts in the foam pad allowed it to fit over the 3 groups of rods.

This back-bracing bed was made in about 2 hours, and then tried with the baby. The position of the wooden rods could be easily adjusted, even with the baby lying between them.

To everyone's wonder, not only did the crib hold Yuri in a much improved position, but did it so gently that the baby appeared to be comfortable. The team advised Eva to at first leave her baby in the device for only 15 or 20 minutes, and then—as long as the baby seemed comfortable—to gradually lengthen the time, until the baby could spend 2 to 3 hours in it at a time.

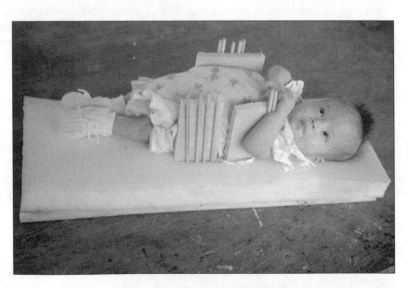

The importance of often removing the baby for play, movement, feeding, and affectionate handling was emphasized. Yuri's mother smiled warmly in response to this advice.

A Bounce-Bed for Self-Stimulation Through Movement

To a limited extent, the back-brace crib served its purpose. Yuri's mother, Eva, used it for her baby several hours each day. Three months later, the curve in the baby's back had not increased, and it appeared to have decreased somewhat.

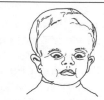

However, it was clear that Yuri's overall development was quite slow. As often happens with spina bifida, she had been born with **hydrocephalus.** With this condition, liquid builds up in the brain and the head becomes larger than normal. Brain damage can result. To prevent brain damage, the doctors in the hospital had put a drainage tube, or *shunt,* into Yuri's brain. Nevertheless, brain damage was apparent. Partly

Hydrocephalus (water on the brain) often occurs with spina bifida and, unless corrected early with a "shunt," can cause brain damage, and sometimes blindness.

because of her large head, she did not begin to lift her head, to roll over, or to sit, at the age when most children do. Except for a little motion of her arms, she almost did not move at all.

Body movement is important for the overall development of a young child, especially for the growth of balance and body awareness in a baby who is mentally and physically delayed.

The PROJIMO team, together with a visiting physiotherapist, Ann Hallum, encouraged Eva to handle the baby often, to encourage a variety of movements, and to help her to develop the neck strength needed to control her large head.

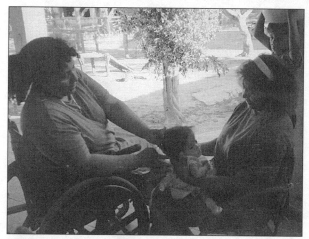

Mari teaches Yuri's mother, Eva, to help her baby gain head control by gently supporting Yuri's head with her fingertips when her head begins to fall.

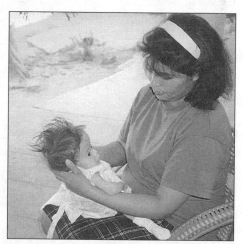

Eva helps Yuri develop head control by catching her head with her fingertips when it starts to fall.

A BED WITH A BOUNCE. To encourage increased body movement, PROJIMO's special-equipment maker, Juán, made a small rocking bed for Yuri. He bent a piece of 1/4-inch re-bar (reinforcing rod) to form a sloping metal frame, supported at the lower end. Over this, he fitted a canvas sling. On the sling, he attached a soft cloth sewn in the shape of diapers, to hold the baby.

The advantage of this bed is that, with the baby's slightest movement, the whole bed rocks up and down. This change in the baby's angle, and her position in relation to her surroundings, stimulates the child to move. Encouraging motion in response to movement helps the baby gain greater body awareness.

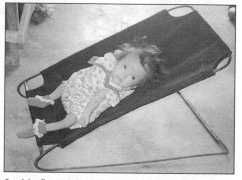

In this first trial model of the bounce-bed, the cloth was stretched fairly tightly over the metal-bar frame. This permitted Yuri's body to twist a lot to one side.

Loosening the bed-cloth to help correct the spinal curve.

On trying out the new bounce-bed, it seemed to work well. At the baby's slightest movement it dipped up and down, and the baby seemed to enjoy this. But, while observing Yuri on the spring bed, Mari and the baby's mother, Eva, were concerned about the sideways curve in the baby's back. The curve was still quite marked, and the bed did little to correct it.

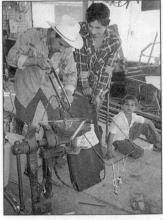

Mari had an idea. If the canvas were allowed to sag more from side to side so that the baby would lie in a cloth trough, this might hold her in a straighter position. So the shop workers made the cloth sag more. When Yuri was placed in the modified bed, its trough-like form did, indeed, hold her body in a straighter position.

To cause the cloth of the bounce-bed to sag more, the frame was narrowed by cutting out pieces from the cross bars and rewelding them.

When the cloth was stretched tightly over the frame, the curve in Yuri's back was very pronounced.

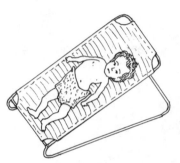

When the cloth was loosened to sag like a trough, it held Yuri's body (and spine) much straighter.

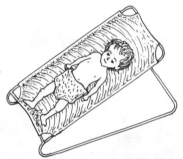

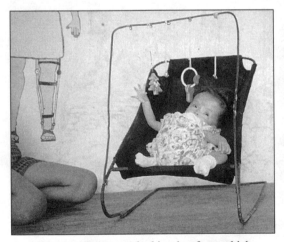

Arching over the bounce-bed is a bar from which rattles and brightly colored toys are hung to stimulate the baby's use of her eyes, ears, and hands.

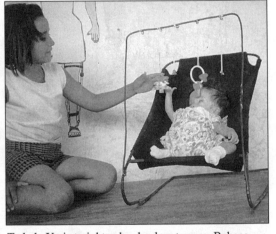

To help Yuri straighten her back yet more, Rebeca attracts her attention from the right side, so that she bends her head and body in that direction.

The modified bounce-bed thus serves a double purpose. The gentle pressure of the cloth trough helps to correct the sideways curve of the child's spine, yet allows freedom of movement. The bed dips up and down in response to the child's slightest movement. The hanging rattles and toys above her head catch her attention. She reaches out to play with them. This causes still more movement of the bed, which, in turn, provides visual and bodily stimulation that may help to speed the child's development.

In conclusion, Yuri's development will probably continue to be slow because of the brain damage caused by hydrocephalus. But, with the help of a wide range of stimulation, including the bounce-bed, she is making progress.

Non-Spill Trays: A Personal Invention Shared with Others

Some disabled persons have a problem carrying jars, glasses, and pots of food and drink. If a container falls, it can be dangerous. The difficulty is greater for persons with only one arm, with half of their body paralyzed (paraplegia), or any condition that causes shaking or uncontrolled movements.

*PETER AND MARIANNE WEST are a married couple in England. Both have cerebral palsy. Both have trouble carrying drinks because of what they call the **wobble factor.** In their search for solutions, they learned of a large, commercially-made fiberglass tray with an overhead handle, which was advertized as spill-proof. But it was no longer available.*

Peter designed a simple, wooden non-spill tray to meet his own and his wife's needs. He got the idea for the design from a tray used for carrying coffee in Arab markets. The tray can carry a lot of cups and glasses, and packs flat for storage in a small kitchen.

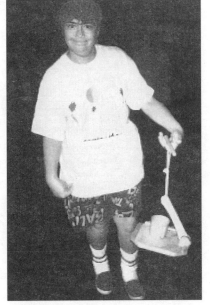

A girl with cerebral palsy carries a drink on a non-slip tray.

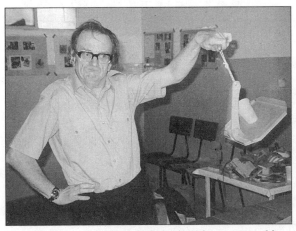

Peter West, in a workshop in Palestine, demonstrates his non-spill tray. (Photos by Kennett Westmacott.)

Peter now teaches people how to make the tray in a community workshop called *People Potential* (see page 342) where he and Kennett Westmacott give disabled persons and family members courses in "Resources and Creativity," and "Appropriate Disability Design." He and Kennett have taught many others to make the tray in various countries.

I first saw the tray being made and used in a disability skills workshop in Angola (see Chapter 29).

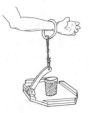

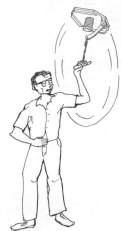

The non-spill capacity of the tray is quite amazing. It can be swung from side to side, and even whirled in a circle overhead, without spilling the liquid in a cup.

The tray can be adapted to meet individual needs. For example, for a person who has difficulty gripping (because of arthritis, leprosy, etc.), you can attach a handgrip of clay, plaster, or putty to the handbar. Also, the tray can be fitted onto a holding device on a wheelchair, to carry containers over uneven ground.

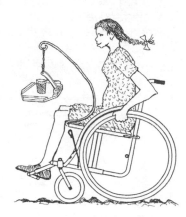

How to Make a Non-Spill Tray

(These instructions are adapted from *CBR News* No 17, May-Aug., 1994. Drawings by Celia Till/AHRTAG. Text by Peter West.)

1. The base of the tray starts with a square (as large or as small as will meet your needs). Cut off corners, as shown. Glue small piece of wood to 3 sides.

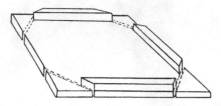

2. The wood lever is slightly shorter than the tray. Make sure the bottom edge is angled so that the lever sits on the base at a 45 degree angle.

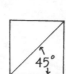 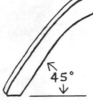

3. Place 2 small pieces of wood upright in the center of the fourth side, leaving space between them for the lever.

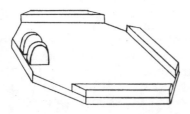

4. With the lever in place (at 45 degrees), drill a hole of about 6 mm (1/4 inch) in diameter through the middle of the 3 pieces. Enlarge the hole in the lever slightly (so it will move easily). Make a peg from a rod of hard wood, so that it fits tightly between the 2 side-pieces. If fitted correctly, the lever should move easily and stop at 45 degrees. When satisfied, glue the peg in place and trim off the ends. Now fasten the remaining edge pieces on either side of the lever.

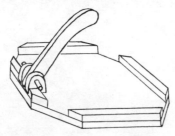

5. Make a handbar from a small piece of wood. It should be big enough for a hole to be drilled through its center. Thread a piece of strong thin rope through the hole.

6. Drill a hole through the free end of the lever. **Be sure the hole is exactly over the center of the tray when the lever is fully raised.**

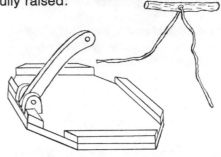

7. Knot the center of the rope. This is very important. Without this central knot, the objects on the tray will move in a different direction to the tray, and fall off or spill. Pull the rope through the hole in the handbar and tie it firmly, so that the handbar is connected firmly to the lever.

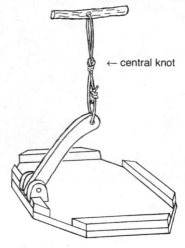

← central knot

Note: To make the tray more fun, the lever can be cut in the shape of another design— for example, a fish.

 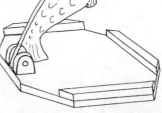

CHAPTER 23

Helping José Walk and Talk after His Stroke

JOSÉ, who is 48 years old, was brought to PROJIMO by his concerned wife and son. Six months before, he had had a stroke (cerebral vascular accident) that paralyzed his right side. At first he could not walk or talk. Weeks later he began to walk with much difficulty, using a cane. But his speech did not return. He had trouble expressing his wishes. He got angry with his wife when she did not understand him—and she would get angry with him. She thought his inability to speak came from weakness of his mouth, and that if he could learn to move his lips and tongue better he would be able to talk. She was sure he understood everything she said to him, and was irritated that at times he didn't respond appropriately.

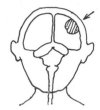

The part of the brain that controls language is on the left side of the head.

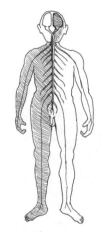

Fortunately, when José first visited PROJIMO, Ann Hallum, a visiting physical therapist, was there facilitating a course to help up-grade the village team's knowledge and skills.

CAUSES OF LANGUAGE PROBLEMS. Ann explained that, after a stroke, difficulty with speech and communication can be caused by a combination of problems, depending on the area of the brain that was injured (by stroke, illness or injury). Injury to one area of the brain's "language center" can prevent the person from understanding the spoken or written word *(receptive aphasia).* Damage in another language area can prevent her from recalling or forming words or phrases correctly, either in spoken or written form *(expressive aphasia).* Persons with severe language problems may have losses both in receiving and in expressing language *(total aphasia).*

José's right-sided paralysis meant that his left brain (with the "language center") was damaged. Simple testing was needed to find out the causes of his difficulties with communication.

Because the nerves coming from the brain cross to the opposite side of the body, a stroke on the left side of the brain tends to paralyze the right side of the body.

TESTING JOSÉ'S UNDERSTANDING OF LANGUAGE. To test how well José could associate words with the things they represent, a PROJIMO worker, Andrés, put a number of objects—a carrot, a spoon, a tomato and a cup—in front of him. Andrés said, "Give me the carrot." José looked at the different objects a long time, then picked up the carrot. Everyone clapped and praised him. However, with the other objects he had more difficulty, and often made mistakes. When Andrés said, "Give me the tomato," José pondered a long time, then handed him the spoon.

Further testing showed that although José had a lot of trouble with nouns (things), he was much better with verbs (action words). Often he would understand a noun when it was used in a phrase involving a familiar action. For example, when Andres asked him to pick his sombrero (hat) from several objects on the table, he was confused. But when Andres said, "Take off your sombrero," José gave a sigh of understanding and at once took off his hat.

These findings gave **clues to how his family might communicate more effectively with José.** It helped his wife understand why he often did not respond appropriately to her questions; why he would grunt "Yes!" when she asked, "Do you want a cup of coffee?" and then get upset and frustrated when she brought him coffee.

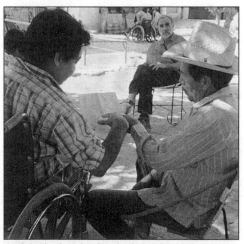

Andrés (in the wheelchair) helps José relearn to associate pictures of common objects with words.

Sometimes, when José wanted to say something, he would repeat the word "Burro!" (donkey) many times. This used to make his wife angry. But when, during the testing, she saw his confusion with names of things, she gained more understanding of his problem.

During the testing, it became clear that José had difficulty with names of things. But when his mistakes were clearly pointed out, he learned fairly quickly. When he was asked to pick up the spoon, but took the tomato, Andrés would say to him, "No, that is not a spoon. It is a tomato." After 2 or 3 repeats, José would usually pick up the spoon when asked.

Helping José to Talk

A PICTURE BOARD FOR BETTER COMMUNICATION. Because one of José's biggest difficulties with language was recognizing the names of things, Andrés and others sat down with José and his wife and drew up a list of the things that were most important for communication in the home. This included a variety of foods and other objects.

They drew pictures of these things on sheets of paper. To make it easier, they started by drawing a single object on a sheet, and showed José one drawing at a time. They asked him to point to the thing he wanted to have or to say at that moment.

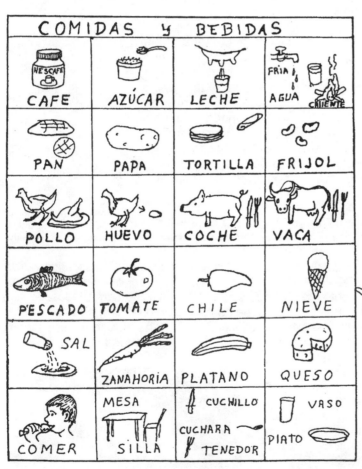

After practice with this, the team made **communication boards** for different groups of things. One of the first boards they made was of foods.

When considering which foods to include, Mari's daughter, Lluvia, insisted that a drawing of *ice cream* be included. Mari thought ice cream would not be one of José's priorities. "But what if he wants it?" Lluvia insisted. So, ice cream was included.

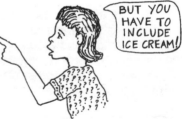

BUT YOU HAVE TO INCLUDE ICE CREAM!

When he began using the list, one of the first things José pointed to was ICE CREAM. When it was brought to him, he laughed with delight.

With practice, José learned to identify most of the objects on the boards and to recognize their names when spoken. He learned to use the board to point to something he wanted, especially when he had trouble associating it with the right word.

Later, to make it easier for him to carry his sheets of pictures, the team reduced and reassembled the most useful drawings into **a small notebook that he could carry in his pocket.** ➤

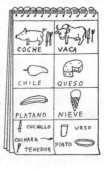

During the days that José was at PROJIMO, his wife and Andrés used both the picture boards and real objects to help him associate words with things and actions. Although progress was slow, his communication skills improved. Most important, perhaps, was that José and his wife were less frustrated with one another and began to realize that they were both doing their best.

A DEAF MAN HELPS JOSÉ COMMUNICATE WITH SIGNS

In helping José to re-learn to recognize words, it became clear that he was quick to notice and interpret gestures and signs.

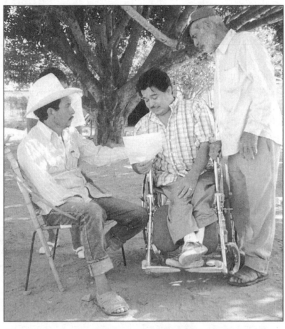

One day a deaf carpenter named Chon, who sometimes helps at PROJIMO, saw Andrés teaching José with the picture board. Quickly understanding José's difficulties with words, Chon began to explain things to José, using signs and gestures. (Chon's sign language was not a standardized formal system. It had been developed out of necessity, by him, his family, and the villagers since he was a child. But Chon managed to communicate and understand almost everything with remarkable clarity.) José picked up on Chon's signs very quickly. This gave José's wife new ideas for communicating with her husband. Everyone thanked Chon for his valuable assistance, and he was delighted to have been able to help with his expertise.

Chon, who is deaf, helps José, who lost his speech from a stroke, learn to communicate with signs and gestures.

Helping José Learn to Walk Better

When José first came to PROJIMO, he walked with difficulty, using a home-made cane made from a bamboo-like plant called *otate*. The curved top of the cane was formed by the main root of the plant. Two smaller side-roots provided additional supports for a firm grip.

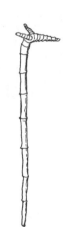
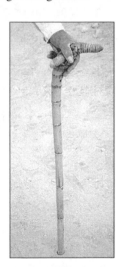

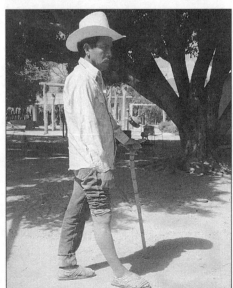

José had a very fixed habit of walking with his stroke-weakened leg in a "back-knee" position.

For several weeks after his stroke, José's right leg was almost completely paralyzed. Then, little by little, it began to recover strength. José learned to walk again by bending the weak right knee slightly backward, in a locked position that supported his weight without using his weak thigh muscles. This back-kneed gait caused him to walk awkwardly with short shuffling steps, and with danger of falling hard if he lost his balance. (After his stroke, José's balance was poor. Walking with his knee locked backward made his balance and stability worse.)

Improvement with Time. On testing José at PROJIMO 8 months after his stroke, the team found he had regained much of the strength in his weak leg. He was able to partially squat on that leg alone. With daily squatting exercises, the leg would probably get stronger still.

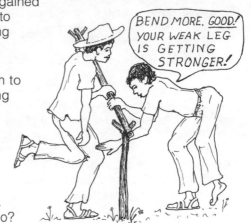

BEND MORE. *GOOD!* YOUR WEAK LEG IS GETTING STRONGER!

Problem. José's right leg was now strong enough to let him walk fairly normally. But the habit of locking his knee backward at the start of each step was, by now, strongly fixed. Inez, a physical therapy assistant at PROJIMO, encouraged him to bend his right knee while walking. He had José practice shifting weight from one bent knee to the other while he held onto a bar. Once José understood the request, he did this willingly. But he still walked with a "back-knee." What to do?

A Partial Solution. Something was needed to help José break his habit of back-kneeing and to relearn to bend his knee when stepping with his leg. The team decided to experiment with **a leg-brace that would push his knee forward when he put weight on his foot.**

Before making the plastic brace, Inez did **a trial with a plaster cast.** The cast lifted the front of the foot slightly upwards, so that when the foot was flat on the ground, the knee would bend. However, this was not enough to prevent José from walking with his knee pushed back (on his heel with his toes in the air). Therefore, Inez mounted a metal bar in the cast under José's foot. The bar projected backwards, behind the heel. This way, when José took a step with his right foot, the heel bar would push the foot to make it land flat on the ground. This would cause the knee to bend forward with each step.

To make the heel bar removable and adjustable, Inez inserted a flat iron bar into a thin-walled metal tube. He then hammered the tube into a rectangular shape around the flat bar.

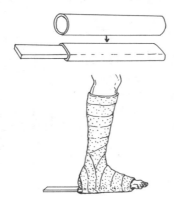

The experimental cast worked fairly well. Although José felt awkward in it, he at once began to walk bending his knee, and soon he had a more normal gait. The cast had the additional advantage of correcting the foot-drop (front of the foot hangs down when the foot is lifted) which remained after his stroke ... Within an hour or so of practice, José put aside his cane and began to walk with larger, more even steps. He was delighted, although still somewhat disturbed by the cast.

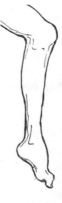

FOOT-DROP

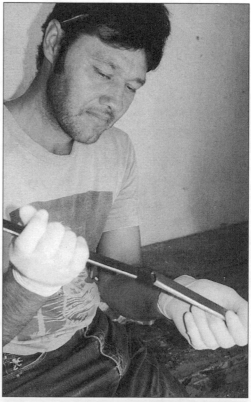

Inez, jack-of-all-trades, uses a metal tube to form a sheathe round the heel-bar, which he will mount first on the cast, then on the brace for José's foot.

Casting José's Leg

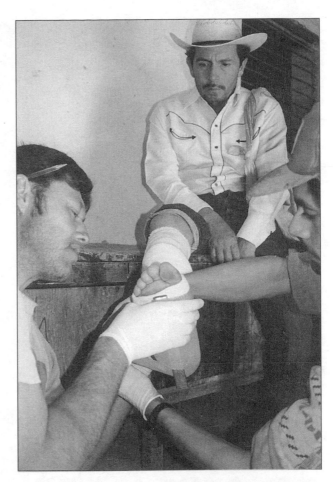

Inez and Marcelo cast José's leg, mounting the metal bar under his foot.

To keep the bar from breaking loose, they use donated casting material made of resin and fiberglass.

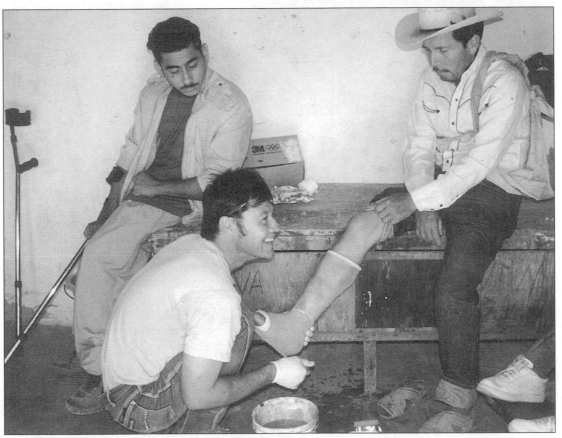

A *plastic brace with an adjustable heel bar.*

After demonstrating that the cast with the heel-bar helped José bend his knee while walking, Marcelo made a plastic brace in which he mounted the same bar. Because the experimental cast had bent José's knee forward only slightly—and sometimes the knee started to bend backward—when making the brace, Marcelo increased the ankle-angle so that the front of the foot was somewhat higher.

José practiced with his new brace at PROJIMO for a few more days before he and his wife went home. It is still too early to know the final results. For the time being, José walks more evenly and with larger, more regular steps. The team hopes that after a few weeks (or months?) with the brace, José will become so accustomed to bending his knee when he walks, that he will continue to bend it when he no longer wears the brace.

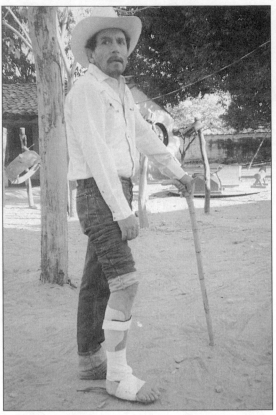

José walks with his new heel-bar brace. The bar projecting backward from the heel helps him bend the knee of his weaker leg when he walks.

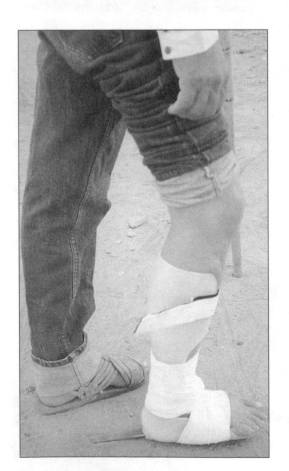

Adjustments. At the time of this writing, José had returned home with his brace. As he gets used to walking with his knee bent, the heel-bar can gradually be pushed deeper into the brace to make it shorter.

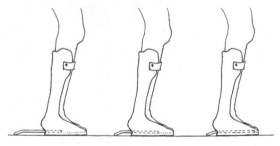

Depending on his progress, José may soon be able to stop using the bar brace. For a while, he may need a modified shoe with the heel that sticks 2 or 3 centimeters out behind. This, too, will push his knee forward gently, though less powerfully than does the long heel bar.

CHAPTER 24

Gene Invents a Writing Brace for His Paralyzed Hand

In this chapter, Gene Rodgers, a disabled North American activist, describes how he designed a pen holder to write with his paralyzed hand.

GENE, who is quadriplegic, was editor of the newsletter of The New Mexico Technology Assistance Program (NMTAP), an organization managed by disabled folks "to address the assistive technology needs of individuals with disabilities in New Mexico." The story of his brace is included, in his own words, because it is a good example of how technologies are often more appropriate when the users are involved in designing them.

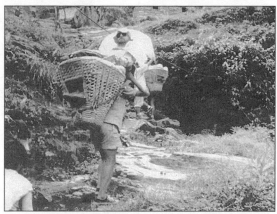

Gene is an adventurer. Here he treks in the mountains of Nepal, carried in a basket on the back of a Sherpa. (Sherpas are Nepalese mountaineers renowned for their strength.)

WRITING BRACE by Gene Rodgers

It has been said that "necessity is the mother of invention." If that is the case, then common sense must be the father.

I am a C-5 quadriplegic, paralyzed from the shoulders down. I can't use my hands to grip a pen, but I have enough movement in my shoulders to use a writing brace. When I went to college, I used a writing brace that was designed for me by an orthotist (a professional brace maker). The brace was heavy, long, and it cost several hundred dollars. It was impossible to put on and take off by myself. I got tired using it.

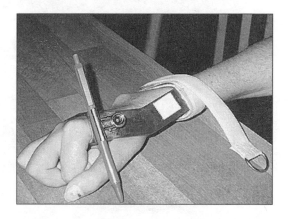

I decided to make a brace that would work well for me. I started by listing the functions of the brace. It had to hold a pen or a pencil. It had to hold my wrist in place so my wrist wouldn't push around the writing paper. It had to be light, and easy to put on and take off.

The old brace used metal to hold all my fingers in a position to hold a pen. I decided that a simple bulldog-type paper clip could hold a pen just as well; I didn't need to have my fingers held in place.

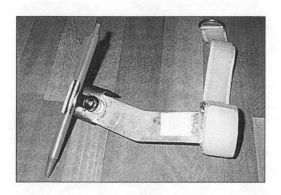

I used a piece of scrap metal, bent around my wrist and forearm to hold my wrist in place. I wanted to use 2 Velcro straps on the brace, to wrap around my forearm, but my friend who was making it only had time to put on one strap. As it turns out, one strap works fine. I put the brace on and take it off (with my teeth) in less than 5 seconds.

Gene puts on his writing brace using his teeth:

Gene describes how he puts on the brace:

"To pick it up, I hook my fingers around the writing brace, and then put the pen in my mouth—which, in effect, allows me to grip the brace via the pen. I position my arm under the brace, push the brace onto my arm with my chin, and rub the Velcro strap against the armrest to attach the strap to the brace."

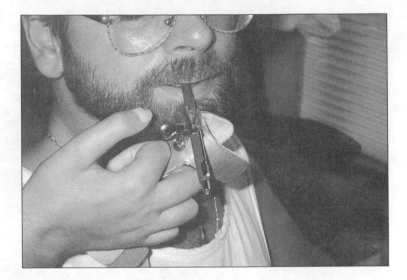

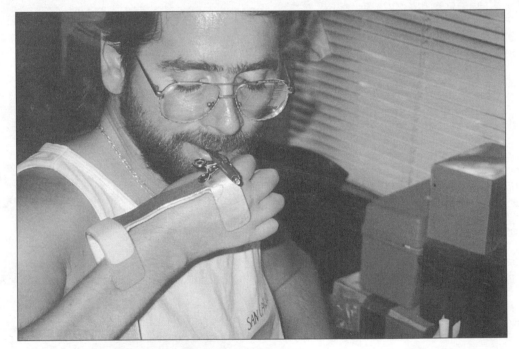

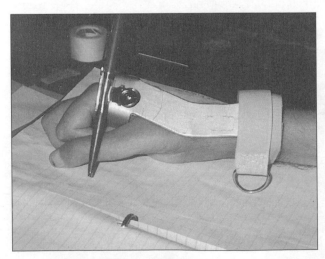

"To take it off, I grip the metal ring in my mouth and remove the strap."

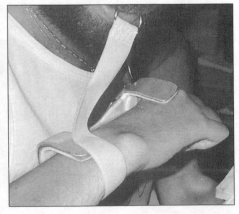

Disability is No Limitation to Adventure

Long before he became quadriplegic as result of a fall from a cliff, Gene loved to climb mountains. As you can see from this photo, he has not let his disability prevent him from climbing even the most difficult mountains. Here, a fellow climber helps him to rope-climb up a cliff-face in New Mexico. For Gene, the sky is the limit!

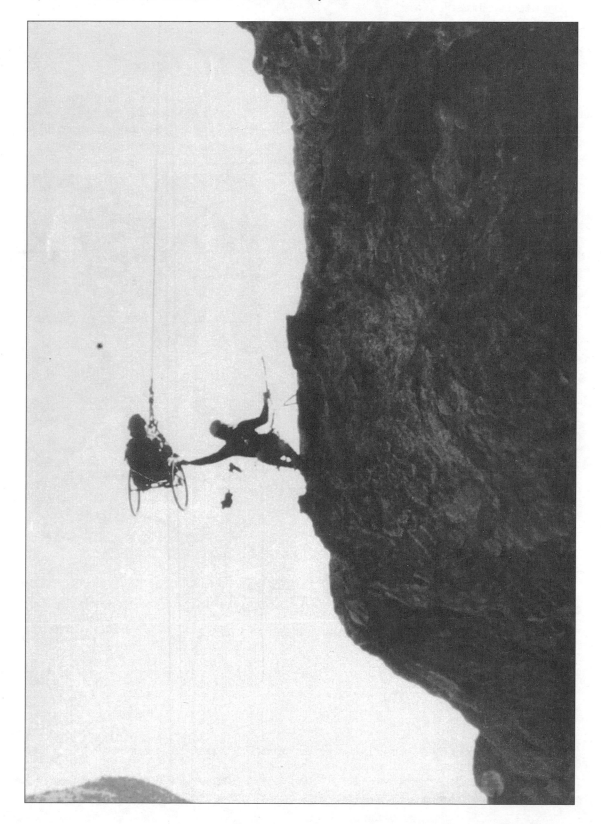

OTHER INNOVATIVE IDEAS FOR HOLDING THINGS

In designing a hand brace, Gene Rodgers had the idea of using a "bulldog clip" to grip the pen or pencil. Similarly, other persons have used clothes pins (the kind with a wire spring). Here is a design, from an excellent book of simple assistive devices called *More with Less* (see page 344).

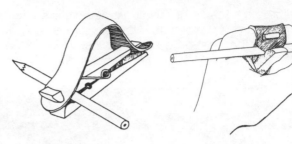

Many other very simple devices for holding pens, pencils, spoons, forks, and other instruments have been designed by disabled persons, their helpers and their friends. The following device for holding a spoon and other utensils was designed by a man in Hawaii who had lost his fingers with Leprosy. (Courtesy of Jean and Kennett Westmacott.)

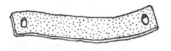

Cut a strip of old bicycle inner-tube, about 3 x 20 cm. Make a small hole, big enough to stretch over the handle that you want to hold.

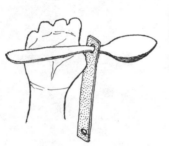

Measure the width of your hand across the palm, and use this as the distance to the next hole.

To put the device on the hand, put the handle of the instrument through one hole and place it on the palm.

Use your teeth to pick up the other end of the rubber, and stretch it a little so that it goes over the other end of the instrument. It should be tight enough to give a firm grip.

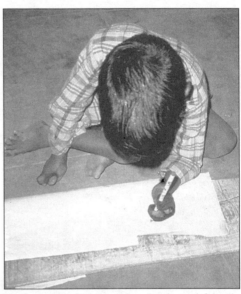

Writing at last! This boy, whose hands are deformed from birth, holds a pen with the help of a strip of bicycle inner tube.

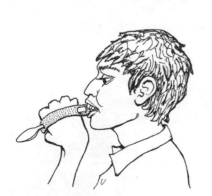
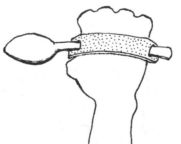
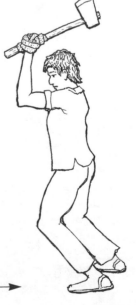

To hold larger tools like a hoe, this same man wrapped long strips of bicycle inner tube around his hands and the handle of the hoe many times. The elastic rubber allows a bit of "give" that is needed for the quick action and sudden jolt of hoeing—or for chopping with an axe. ⟶

Life-Saving Innovations in Bladder Management by Spinal-Cord Injured Persons

CHAPTER **25**

The 2 biggest causes of death in spinal-cord injured persons are **pressure sores** and **urinary tract infections.** Most persons lose urine control. They may dribble uncontrollably or be unable to relax the muscles that let urine pass. Specialists mostly agree that often the best way to reduce the frequency and severity of urinary infections is to use **intermittent catheterization.** That is to say, every 4 hours or so the person puts a thin rubber tube (catheter) through the urine opening (in the penis or vulva) and into the bladder to drain the urine. This is a lot safer than using a catheter that stays in place. A **permanent (Foley) catheter,** which is normally changed every 2 weeks, runs a higher risk of introducing infection.

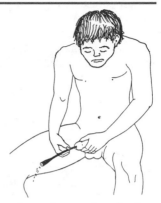

Intermittent catheterization

Nevertheless, in some countries, doctors caring for spinal-cord injured persons often keep them on a permanent catheter, perhaps because they think that they will not live long in any case. **It is very important that spinal-cord injured persons and their families communicate with and learn from one another, and not simply follow what their doctor tells them.** Some doctors consistently give good advice; others do not.

As we will discuss in Chapters 27 and 28, spinal-cord injured persons need to learn new ways of listening to their bodies. Because they usually have no feeling or pain below the level of their injury, they must discover other ways to spot difficulties. For example, when a person's legs begin to jerk uncontrollably, or spasticity increases, or

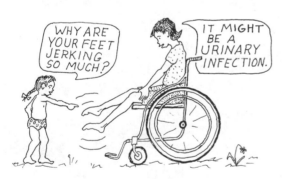

she feels feverish, dizzy, or sweaty, these are warning signals. Somewhere, pressure on her skin may be causing a risk of pressure sores. Or a urinary infection may have started. The person learns to watch for these signs and to look for the causes. This **new body language** can be life-saving. Just as deaf people learn to "listen" in new ways, so do spinal-cord injured persons. There are no better teachers than other spinal-cord injured persons, especially the long-time survivors.

THE STERILIZATION DEBATE. Doctors used to insist that spinal-cord injured persons must sterilize their catheter by boiling it before each use. As a result, users often went long periods without catheterizing. This led to more frequent infections and to kidney damage.

Then, spinal-cord injured persons began to discover that **clean catheterization** gave results that were as good as **sterilized catheterization.** Because it was easier, people tended to do it more often and regularly, and so they were healthier. Clean sterilization became an underground art, taught to newly injured persons by survivors.

In the USA, doctors have at last begun to recommend clean rather than sterile catheterization. Not long ago, I was delighted to hear a urinary specialist (urologist) approve clean catheterization technique for a paraplegic boy, explaining, **"If you want people to catheterize regularly, you have to encourage the method that is simplest and easiest."** Still, international rehabilitation professionals have criticized the book *Disabled Village Children* for giving "dangerous recommendations" for catheterization without boiling the catheter. **The spinal-cord injured community needs to pressure such experts to learn from disabled persons' experience.**

Using Double Catheters in a Plastic Bag to Reduce Infection

Even a boiled or sterile catheter can introduce infection. This is because there are always bacteria (germs) in and around the urinary opening of the penis or vulva, regardless of how well they are cleaned. More than 25 years ago, after years with frequent infections, Ralf Hotchkiss and other paraplegic friends in California began looking for safer ways to catheterize themselves.

One innovation was to **keep the catheter in a plastic "zip-lock" bag with a bit of antiseptic solution.** Hydrogen peroxide works well and is non-irritating. It can be very dilute; a 3-percent solution is fine. To use the catheter, push its tip out of a corner of the bag and into the urinary opening. Make sure the fingers touch only the plastic bag, not the catheter.

Another innovation is to **use 2 catheters, one inside the other.** The first (outer) catheter is inserted 1 or 2 cm into the urinary opening, past the area with the most germs. Then the inner catheter is inserted through the outer one.

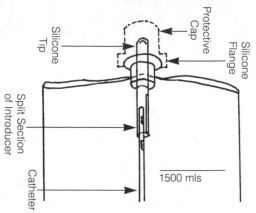

By combining both the above innovations (using double catheters and keeping them in a plastic "zip-lock" bag with antiseptic solution), Ralf has greatly reduced his urinary infections.

THE COMMERCIAL PRODUCT. This combined method proved to give excellent results. It is now factory-produced as the *MMG O'Neil Urinary Catheterization System.* Unfortunately, it is outrageously expensive. But with a little creativity, people can make their own. Or **the commercial system, though sold for a single catheterization, can be used repeatedly for several weeks, like this:**

Diagram from the package of the *MMG O'Neil Urinary Catheterization System,* showing the top of the plastic bag.

1. Insert outer catheter into the urinary opening.

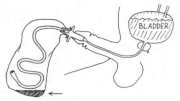

2. Insert untouched inner catheter, and empty the bladder.

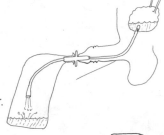

3. Pull inner catheter back into the bag. Take outer catheter out of urinary opening.

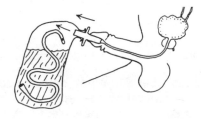

4. Remove outer catheter from bag, and empty urine from bag.

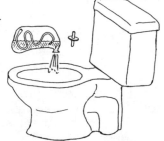

5. Rinse the bag and outer catheter. Dump out rinse water. Repeat. Leave about one tablespoon of water in the bag.

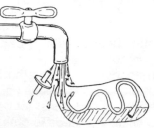

6. Put 1 teaspoon of 3 percent hydrogen peroxide in bag. Fold the bag and catheter in a small, clean zip-lock plastic bag for the next use.

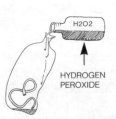

Leg Splints and a Standing Post to Stop Alicia's Urinary Infection

CHAPTER 26

UNUSUAL SOLUTIONS FOR URINARY PROBLEMS

Meeting a disabled individual's needs often requires creatively combining physical, medical, emotional, and social measures. Sometimes a medical problem can be avoided or corrected through certain physical measures.

For example, spinal-cord injured persons often develop kidney stones. This problem can be largely avoided by (1) **drinking** lots of water, and (2) **standing** for a while each day. Persons with an injury at a relatively low level of their spine (whose arms are not affected) may be able to stand (and walk) with leg braces and crutches (see Chapter 36). Those with higher-level injuries (arms also affected) may need to stand in a standing board. This can simply be a wide plank onto which the person is strapped and then tilted upright. An added advantage to standing daily is that supporting the body's weight on the legs helps to keep the bones growing, prevent osteoporosis (weakening of bones due to loss of calcium), and reduce the chance of fractures.

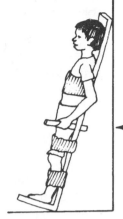

A very basic standing board can help prevent kidney stones and broken bones.

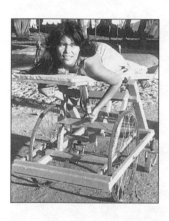
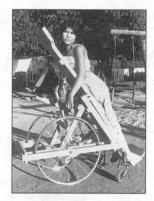

To facilitate standing, PROJIMO has experimented with different types of standing boards. It has also developed a low-cost **standing gurney** (wheeled-cot) that can be tilted to an upright position by the rider herself. (A standing wheel-chair is shown on page 183.)

Chepa adjusts her wooden standing gurney at different angles by pulling on a knotted rope. The knots slip into a slot to hold the board at the desired angle.

ALICIA, whose story is told in this chapter, is a warm-hearted older woman now living at PROJIMO. Her physical ability is quite limited, but she helps out, both with self-care and with several work activities that she is able to do with her spastic arms and hands. Although she works slowly and with difficulty, she is very patient and loves feeling useful.

*Our main focus will be on an unusual series of measures to help Alicia overcome a chronic urinary infection. As you will see, the problem had **a complexity of causes,** ranging from **hot weather** to **spastic ankles,** and from some personal **embarrassment** to a **shortage of staff.** Solving the problem required measures beyond what health workers usually consider when trying to manage urinary infections.*

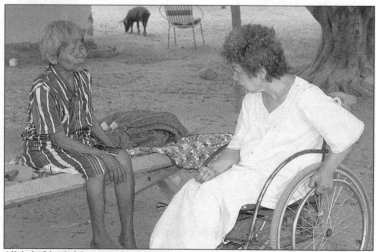

Alicia befriends Mona, an elderly blind woman who recently arrived at PROJIMO.

Alicia's life has not been easy.   Until the age of 8, she lived as most village girls do, attending school and helping with house work and other tasks. Then she fell ill with measles, which led to meningitis. This caused a physical disability similar to spastic cerebral palsy. She could not walk, and it was hard for her to sit up or attend to her personal needs. Although her spastic mouth and tongue affected her speech, her mind was alert. Her mother took good care of her, exercised her as best she could, and carried her lovingly from place to place.

But, when she was 18 years old, her mother died. Alicia was dutifully but reluctantly taken in by an older sister who was overworked caring and providing for her own children. The sister kept Alicia on a cot covered with a plastic sheet. She slept, ate, went to the bathroom, and spent her days and nights lying on the cot. Her sister fed, bathed, and changed her. When folks at PROJIMO first learned of Alicia, she had already spent 16 years lying all day and all night on the cot, her body and limbs becoming stiffer and stiffer.

The PROJIMO team visited Alicia, gave her a wheelchair, and met with the family. They explained the importance of taking Alicia outside and having her eat and interact more with the family. But each time they visited, they found the wheelchair unused and Alicia still lying on the cot. Finally, the team invited Alicia to stay at the village center.

At PROJIMO, with the help of exercise and simple activities, Alicia's body and arms gradually became more flexible, although her severe spasticity still prevented her from doing many things. Some of the best therapy was achieved by encouraging her in different aspects of self care. Little by little, she learned to slowly push her own wheelchair.

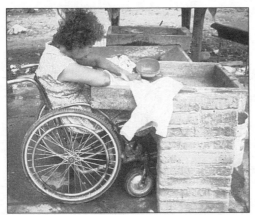

Alicia learned to wash her clothes at the outdoor laundry area, designed for persons in wheelchairs. This improved her control of her arms and hands.

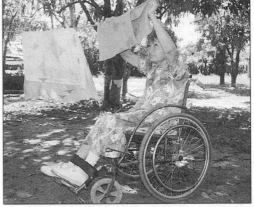

Hanging clothes on an overhead clothes line was at first very difficult for Alicia. But it helped her regain flexibility and the use of her arms and back.

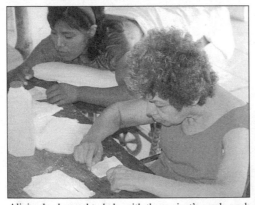

Alicia also learned to help with the project's work, such as folding bandages for treatment of pressure sores.

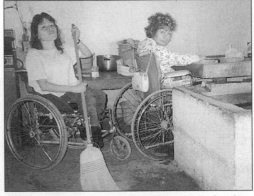

She began to help in the kitchen. Here, she washes the dishes in a wash area suited for wheelchair riders.

Alicia is still quite limited in what she can do, and needs help with many daily activities such as dressing, bathing, and transferring from her wheelchair to the bed and toilet. But compared to her previous situation, she says, "I feel like I have been set free from prison!"

Helping Alicia transfer by herself from her wheelchair to a bed. . .

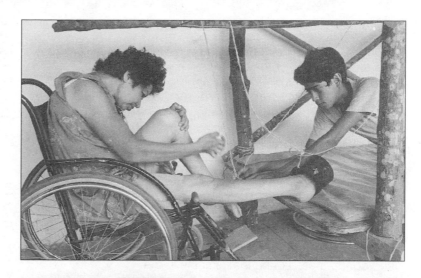

One of Alicia's wishes was to be able to move from her wheelchair to a bed by herself. A visiting physical therapist thought this would be impossible, because of Alicia's extreme spasticity. However, the PROJIMO team decided to give it a try. They built a rack of poles over a bed that they improvised.

Lalo, a village therapy assistant, helps Alicia to find a way to lift her legs onto the bed. She did this by putting her feet in plastic rings, and pulling on a rope.

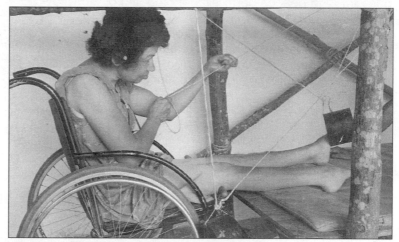

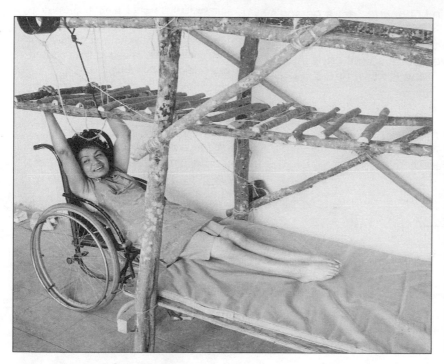

After several weeks of practice, Alicia learned to pull herself onto the bed. It was a lot of work for her, but she enjoyed the attempt to become more self-reliant. Also, the exercise helped all of her body functions, including her bladder and bowels, to work better.

Hot Weather as a Cause of Dehydration, Fever, and Urinary Infections

In early summer, the temperature in the village of Ajoya rises to a sweltering 115 degrees Fahrenheit (45 degrees Centigrade).   This is especially hard on spinal-cord injured persons, whose bodies usually do not sweat below the level of their spinal injury (in the part of the body that is paralyzed). To prevent dangerously high fever, such persons must drink very large quantities of fluids. Also, their bodies must be kept at a normal temperature by wetting them continuously and fanning them almost constantly.

In very hot weather, urinary infections are more common, even in non-disabled persons. They lose so much water through sweating (and breathing) that very little urine is passed. The dark, concentrated urine that remains in the body for long periods permits rapid breeding of infection-causing bacteria. Again, **during hot weather: spinal-cord injured persons, children with spina bifida, and others who tend to have frequent urinary infections, are at especially high risk of bladder or kidney infections.**

Although the body of a spinal-cord injured person may sweat less than normal, in hot, dry weather he still can lose lots of water, just through breathing. Breathing, like sweating, is one of the body's cooling mechanisms. Each time we breath in, water evaporates from our lungs into the air. *Evaporation cools.* The lungs cool the body, just as does a home air cooler that blows air through wet cloths.

Through breathing, in hot dry weather a person's body can lose two or more liters of water a day. **To reduce the risk of high fevers and urinary infections, in hot weather a spinal cord injured person must drink many liters of liquid a day.**

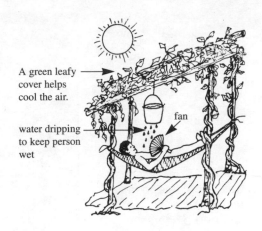

A green leafy cover helps cool the air.

water dripping to keep person wet

fan

The bodies of persons who are quadriplegic (spinal-cord injured at neck level) do not sweat. In hot weather, they risk dangerously high fevers and urinary infections. Here, a boy *sweats artificially* by spraying himself with water while he fans himself. He must also drink many liters of fluid every day.

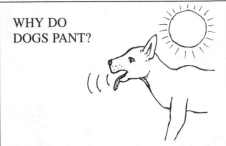

WHY DO DOGS PANT?

In hot weather dogs pant because they do not sweat. To cool their bodies, dogs "sweat" through their tongues and their lungs. Panting moves the air rapidly over their moist tongues and lungs, speeding evaporation and cooling.

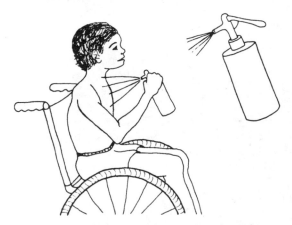

A plastic spray bottle, used for watering plants, is excellent for providing "artificial sweat" for helping to cool the person who does not perspire normally.

A good way to be sure that you are drinking enough fluids is to frequently *check the color of your urine.* It should be almost as clear as water, or only slightly yellow. **Dark or cloudy urine is a sign of danger.**

Spinal-cord injured persons, who do not sweat normally, need to sweat artificially by frequently spraying their bodies with water and fanning themselves. **Especially for quadriplegic persons, who suffer greatly in very hot weather, continuous wetting and fanning during a heat wave can be life-saving.**

The "Chain of Causes" Leading to Alicia's Chronic Urinary Infection

Last summer when the heat became oppressive, Alicia began to complain of low-back pain. She said her feet were more swollen than usual, and the stiffness of her body had increased. Mari suspected a urinary infection. She thumped Alicia's back along each side of her spine. When she thumped on the mid-lower back, over the kidneys, Alicia gasped with pain. Her urine was dark and cloudy. These are signs of urinary infection.

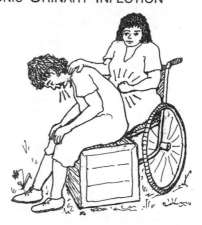

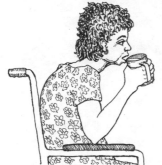

"Drink lots of water!" was Mari's first recommendation. "A large glass, every 15 minutes, as if it were medicine."

Mari knew that many urinary infections clear up, simply by drinking large quantities of liquids. The abundant flow of water (dilute urine) through the body's plumbing system washes out most of the microbes that cause infection. Then the body's defense system gets rid of most of the rest of these microbes.

Obstacles. Getting Alicia to drink lots of water was easier said than done. A series of obstacles—physical and psychological—needed to be resolved.

- First, Alicia drank very little water because when she drank she needed to urinate more often. Due to her urinary infection, she had to urinate often in any case. And urinating was often painful. Even when people offered her different tasty drinks, she would say, "I'm not thirsty." **She did not want to urinate often because she needed help to use the toilet.** Someone strong enough, usually Rosa, had to lift her spastic body from her wheelchair and shift her to the toilet.

- Rosa was always busy washing clothes and doing other chores. **Alicia felt bad to repeatedly have to ask Rosa for help with toileting.**

- Still worse, transferring to the toilet was now more difficult, because Alicia's urinary infection increased her spasticity. To transfer, Alicia would put her arms around Rosa and Rosa would help her to stand and pivot her sideways to sit her on the toilet. But now, with the urinary infection, Alicia's body, arms, and legs were stiffer and less manageable than usual. When she tried to stand, some-times her ankles would twist sideways, and Alicia would suddenly fall over, dragging Rosa with her. **Alicia was worried that either she or Rosa might be injured.** Rosa, too, was concerned that she could no longer transfer Alicia safely.

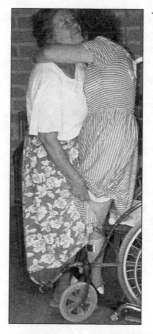

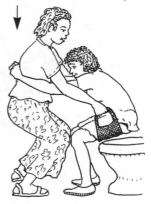

◄— Rosa used to help Alicia transfer to the toilet like this, but it was hard for both, and hurt Rosa's neck and back. At times they fell.

Then Rosa learned a safer, easier way. She held Alicia in a canvas sling, with Alicia's arms clasped around Rosa's body.

For all these reasons it was hard to convince Alicia to drink more water, despite the discomfort and poor health caused by her urinary infection. What to do?

Unusual measures to combat Alicia's urinary infection. The most important step to help Alicia overcome her chronic urinary infection was convincing her to **drink more fluids.** But for this, she needed to be able to transfer to the toilet without fear of falling or being a burden to those helping her. To achieve this, the team came up with a broad spectrum of measures:

1. Ankle splints. To avoid the falls caused by Alicia's spastic ankles when she stood to transfer, the team made simple orthopedic ankle splints of molded plastic. (The methods are described in detail in the book, *Disabled Village Children.*)

2. Massage. To help Alicia reduce the stiffness of her body and stand more easily, Manuella, a village girl who learned some massage therapy from a visiting therapist, gave Alicia a daily session of relaxing massage.

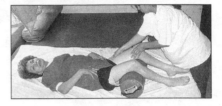

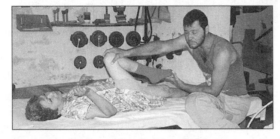

3. Physical therapy. Inez, who assists with therapy, did a range of daily exercises with Alicia to help her to reduce her spasticity and improve her control of body movements.

4. Standing post—for exercise for more independent standing. To help Alicia to stand up more with her own force, and therefore to require less strength and skill from her assistant, Polo made a wooden standing post in the form of a cross. He mounted it firmly in the ground under a giant fig tree. After early trials and adjustments, he padded the cross to represent the body of an assistant.

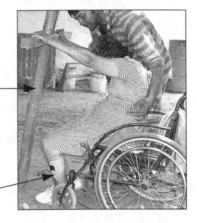

Inez helped Alicia to learn to pull herself to standing. Her stiffness and spasticity made this difficult, but Alicia gradually gained greater control. The ankle splints helped to stabilize her feet and prevent falling.

5. More persons to help Alicia transfer. As Alicia's ability to stand and shift her weight improved, less strength and skill were required to help her transfer. Therefore more people were able and willing to help. Mothers and wives of disabled persons visiting the program were especially helpful. With more people ready to help her to the toilet, Alicia did not mind needing to urinate so frequently, and was more willing to drink more fluids.

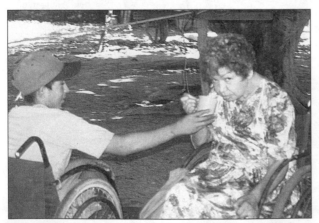

Now that she can use the toilet with less fear of falling and with less need for skilled assistance, Alicia is willing to drink more water. Still, she needs to be encouraged to drink a lot. Here Jesús, who is blind, brings her water and coaxes her to drink.

6. Drinking more water. While all these procedures were taking place, everyone joined forces to coax Alicia to drink more liquids. So, every few minutes, someone brought her a glass of water, tea, or juice. Now that her toileting was less worrisome, Alicia began to drink more. Soon, her back pain went away, her feet became less swollen, and her spasticity was less debilitating. This made transfers to and from the toilet easier still.

Healthy results. Thanks to all these measures—ankle splints, massage, a standing post, guided exercise, and more persons to help her to the toilet—Alicia recovered from her infection.

Cushions and Pressure Testers to Help Avoid Pressure Sores

CHAPTER **27**

PRESSURE SORES: A PREVENTABLE CAUSE OF DEATH

Several chapters of this book (Chapters 10, 16, 27, 28, 31, 37, 38, and 47), concern persons who have developed bed sores or pressure sores. Although the disabilities of these people range from **multiple sclerosis** to **spina bifida,** severe pressure sores are perhaps most common in persons with **spinal-cord injury.** *In many Third World nations, most persons who become spinal-cord injured die within a year or two. The main cause of death is pressure sores.*

What Causes Pressure Sores? Pressure sores usually form on parts of the body that have lost feeling. Because she does not feel and has difficulty moving, the person lies or sits too long in one position. The body's weight cuts off the blood circulation over bony areas. So the skin and the underlying flesh die, and sores form.

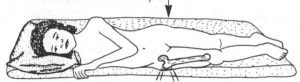

PRESSURE SORES THAT FORM WHILE LYING DOWN often appear over the base of the spine, ⟶ or on the sides of the hips.

A common sore area is over the upper end of the thigh bone.

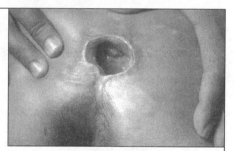

A deep pressure sore over the base of the spine, from lying too long on the back without moving.

PRESSURE SORES THAT FORM WHILE SITTING often appear under the butt-bones.

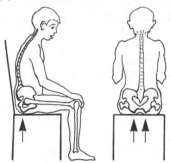

The most common pressure sores that come from sitting are located under the two butt bones (ischial tuberosities).

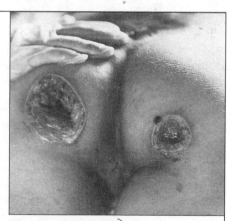

These pressure sores over the butt-bones of a spinal-cord injured person come from sitting too long without moving.

In Project PROJIMO, nearly 400 spinal-cord injured persons have arrived in the last 10 years. Of these, only about 3% have not had pressure sores. Usually, the sores began in the hospital where the person received initial care or surgery for their injury. By the time the person reaches PROJIMO, often their sores are large and deep, and sometimes they are infected.

In PROJIMO, spinal cord injured persons have learned to care for one another, to treat each other's pressure sores, and together to look for better ways to prevent them.

Treatment of Pressure Sores

BEES' HONEY. PROJIMO has experimented with different ways to treat pressure sores. Excellent results are often achieved by using a treatment that dates back to ancient Egypt: *bees' honey.*

First, wash the sore carefully with clean water. Then press a paste of honey, mixed with granulated sugar, into the sore. Do this daily, or twice a day if the sore oozes a lot. This treatment works thanks to the fluid-sucking action (osmosis) of concentrated sugar, which both kills germs (by drying them out) and speeds healing (by reducing swelling).

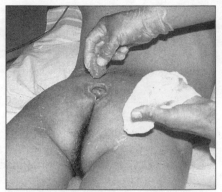

Treating pressure sores with a paste made by mixing bees' honey with granulated sugar.

Even very large, deep sores that specialists say require surgery have responded well to this honey and sugar treatment. (See the results with Osvaldo on page 252.)

PAPAYA. When the sore has a lot of dead flesh in it, it can be packed 3 times a day with a clean cloth soaked in the "milk" from the trunk, or green fruit of papaya. This helps loosen and dissolve the dead flesh. (Cooks use papaya as a meat tenderizer.)

Prevention of Pressure Sores While Sitting

Pressure sores from sitting can mostly be prevented in 2 ways:

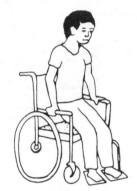

1. **Lift the body** off the seat every few minutes ———▶
   or in other ways change the body's position to reduce
   pressure on the backside. See Chapters 10 and 28

2. **Use a cushion** that reduces pressure against
   bony areas.

CUSHIONS

A good cushion can make a big difference in the prevention of pressure sores. Very costly cushions, either gel-filled or with bubbles of air, are commercially available in some countries. However, **very effective cushions can be made at home at low cost.**

At the *Center for Rehabilitation of the Paralyzed* in Bangladesh, many persons simply use an **inner tube from a motor-scooter tire** (see page 194). The hole in the center is big enough to take the pressure off the butt bones.

This same Center makes an excellent cushion by coating a coconut-fiber mat with rubber. To prevent bed sores when lying down, the person removes the fiber cushion from his wheelchair, and puts it into a square hole in the middle of the bed mattress.

The rubber-coated coconut-fiber cushion is soft but very resilient (dense and strong enough to lift the body's weight).

Both waterproof and porous, the mat can be cleaned simply by pouring a bucket of water through it.

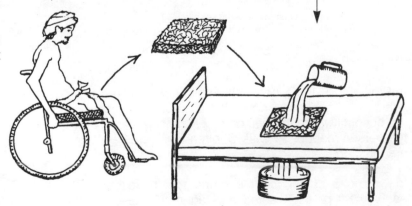

Cushions made from bicycle inner tubes.

Disabled wheelchair builders at *Tahanan Walang Hadanang* (*House With No Stairs,* see page 342) in the Philippines found a way of making air-filled cushions by tying together bicycle inner-tubes.

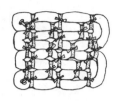

They bind the loops of the tubes together with strips of inner-tube. Enough air is pumped into the tubes so the whole butt is held off the seat.

Cardboard cushions.

PROJIMO has experimented with a variety of cushions. A low-cost cushion that gives excellent results (when properly shaped and fitted to the individual) can be made with **layers of cardboard glued together.** (See Chapter 8 on Appropriate Paper Technology.) Ralf Hotchkiss (Chapter 30) has scientifically tested these cushions and found they can give **protection as good as the most expensive air-filled (*Roho*) cushions.**

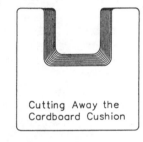

Jacinto demonstrates a cardboard cushion he made for himself.

To make the cushion:

1. From old cardboard cartons, cut enough squares of corrugated cardboard to make a stack 2 inches (5 cm) high, and glue the layers together with water-resistant glue.

2. Cut out a hole for pressure relief under the rider's butt bones.

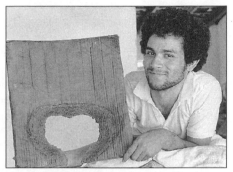

Cutting Away the Cardboard Cushion

3. Wet the top of the cushion so that water soaks into the top layers. Put the cushion in the user's wheelchair, and have him sit on the damp cardboard for several hours, so that it molds somewhat to the shape of his butt and to the wheelchair seat. *(CAUTION: Be sure he lifts his backside off the cushion every few minutes, to avoid new pressure sores.)*

4. When completely dry, coat the cardboard with water-proof varnish. (Polyurethane varnish works well.)

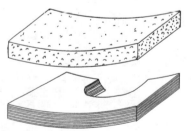

5. Put a thick square of high-density foam rubber on top of the cardboard cushion. (This can be glued on, or kept separate for easy washing.)

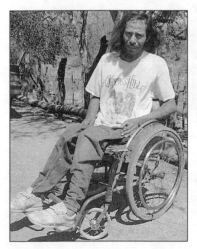

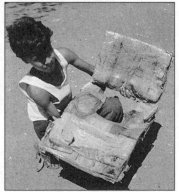

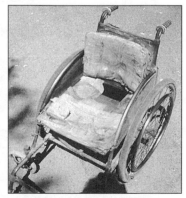

Mario was plagued by pressure sores on his bottom and back until he made this cardboard cushion and backrest, which he has now used for 3 years. He puts a thick foam-rubber pad over the cardboard cushion.

AN INSTRUMENT TO MEASURE THE PRESSURE ON BONY AREAS

ELECTRONIC PRESSURE TESTERS. Even with a good cushion, pressure sores are sometimes hard to avoid. It would be helpful to be able to check whether a cushion (or bed padding, or mattress, etc.) keeps the pressure low enough under the danger spots (bony areas) to avoid sores. In the USA, a few hospitals now have "high-tech" electronic equipment for measuring pressure against the skin. The person sits on a pad that is wired with many small pressure-sensitive cells. The pressure in different spots is read on a monitor, similar to a television screen. But these pressure-measuring devices cost thousands of dollars. They are so expensive that almost none exist in the Third World.

NEED FOR A LOW-COST TESTER. The need for an "appropriate technology" pressure testing instrument was discussed by a small group at the annual conference of *RESNA (Rehabilitation Engineering Society of North America)* held in Toronto, Canada, in 1991. Ralf Hotchkiss, Mari Picos, and David Werner—all involved with the innovative research project at PROJIMO—brain-stormed with special-seating specialist, Michael Heinrich. Michael thought that **a low-cost pressure tester might be made by using small balloons and columns of water.** He decided to visit PROJIMO to work with the team to improvise such an instrument.

The tinkering process (or logical steps) that led to the innovation were as follows:

1. To help prevent pressure sores, there is a need for a simple, low-cost instrument to measure whether pressure on certain parts of the body is dangerously high.

2. Pressure sores occur when the pressure against the skin over a bony area is so high that the blood vessels are squeezed shut. When that happens, blood can not flow through the tissues (the skin and flesh) and the tissues die.

3. An average person's normal blood pressure is enough to lift a column of mercury about 100 millimeters (120 mm during a pulse and 80 mm between pulses). If the pressure on a bony area is higher than the person's blood pressure, the blood flow in the area is obstructed and pressure sores can form.

4. Blood pressure is generally measured using a **pressure cuff** around the upper arm. Air is pumped into the cuff until the pressure in the cuff rises enough to cut off the circulation (at which point the pulse can no longer be heard with a stethoscope).

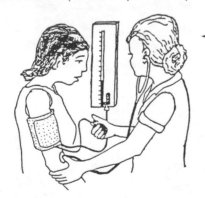

In older cuffs, pressure is measured by observing how high it lifts a column of mercury (quicksilver) in a glass tube.

Hence, **blood pressure is measured in millimeters (mm) of mercury.**

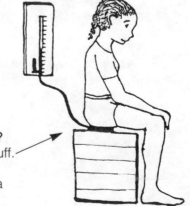

! • IDEA! Why can't we use the same instrument, or one based on the same science, to measure pressure on the skin? The person can sit on top of the pressure cuff. Depending on the amount of pressure that pushes on the cuff, the mercury will rise to a measurable height in the glass tube.

DIFFICULTIES IN USING A STANDARD CUFF:

1. A standard blood-pressure cuff is too big to accurately measure pressure on the small areas directly under the butt bones (ischial tuberosities).

2. Mercury is expensive, hard to get, and dangerous (poisonous).

• **IDEA!** Instead of a pressure cuff, why not use a small elastic bag—maybe a balloon?

• **IDEA!** Instead of mercury, why not colored water?

But using water will require a very tall measuring instrument. This is because mercury is 13.5 times heavier than water. The same pressure that will lift mercury in a tube 12 centimeters (normal blood pressure during a pulse) will lift water 162 centimeters (cm), or over one and a half meters!

But, why not? Plastic tubes can be used instead of glass. When not in use, the whole thing can be rolled up and put in a pocket.

So we thought, "Let's try it!"

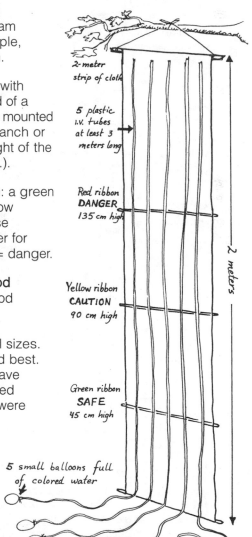

Solution:

In one week, Michael Heinrich and the PROJIMO team designed, made, and tested the first model of a simple, low-cost instrument to measure pressure on the skin.

The instrument is made with **5 small balloons** filled with **colored water**. Each balloon is tightly tied to the end of a **thin plastic tube** about 2 meters long. The tubes are mounted on a long **strip of cloth**. This is hung from a tree branch or a beam, so that the bottom of the cloth is at the height of the seat of the wheelchair (or the mattress of a bed, etc.).

Three horizontal ribbons are sewn across the cloth: a green ribbon at 45 cm. from the bottom of the cloth, a yellow ribbon at 90 cm., and a red ribbon at 135 cm. These ribbons mark the 3 pressure zones in terms of danger for pressure sores: green = safe; yellow = caution; red = danger.

To better see the water level in the plastic tubes, **food coloring** was added to the water. A local natural food coloring, saffron, was found to work well.

The team experimented with plastic tubes of several sizes. Very thin tubing (about 2 mm inner-diameter) worked best. With it, quite small balloons could be used, which gave more exact pressure readings over small areas. Used **"I.V." (intravenous fluid) tubes** worked well. They were available in the village health center.

Several sizes of small balloons (bought in the village store) were tried. **Balloons about 2 x 5 cm when filled** were picked. They held just enough water so that when squeezed flat, the water would rise near to the top of the long plastic tubes.

Note: Before using the tester, put enough water in the balloons and tubes so that the water level reaches the bottom of the cloth.

TESTING THE EXPERIMENTAL DESIGN

The new skin-pressure tester was tried out with disabled children and adults with various disabilities, using different seats and cushions.

To use the pressure tester, the 5 balloons (or fewer) are carefully positioned on the seat or cushion under the person's backside. Typically, 2 balloons are placed directly under the butt-bones (ischial tuberosities): one just above the tail-bone (or base of the spine), and the other two under softer, fleshier areas (for comparison).

POSITION OF BALLOONS

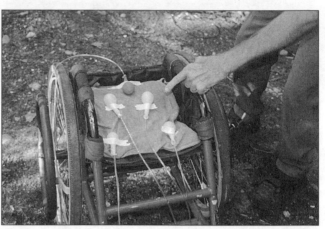

Most of the balloons are placed in spots where pressure is likely to be highest.

Balloons of the pressure tester are positioned on the wheelchair seat. They can be held in place with strips of sticky tape.

Results: The measuring instrument clearly showed differences in the amount of pressure (from low to high) on non-bony and bony areas—with or without a cushion:

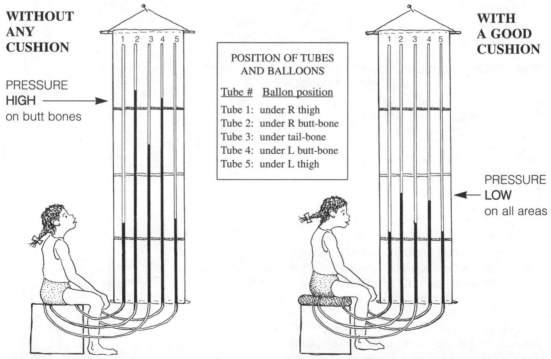

WITHOUT ANY CUSHION

PRESSURE **HIGH** on butt bones

POSITION OF TUBES AND BALLOONS

Tube #	Ballon position
Tube 1:	under R thigh
Tube 2:	under R butt-bone
Tube 3:	under tail-bone
Tube 4:	under L butt-bone
Tube 5:	under L thigh

WITH A GOOD CUSHION

PRESSURE **LOW** on all areas

When a person sat on a flat, hard surface, the pressure on the balloons under the butt-bones lifted the water above the red ribbon into the danger zone, while the pressure under fleshy areas of the butt stayed low.

In contrast, when using a special cushion (whether air, gel, or molded cardboard) pressure on the butt-bones often measured in the yellow or even green zone. However, this varied from person to person and sometimes from one buttock to the other.

PRACTICAL APPLICATIONS:

The pressure tester can be used in a variety of ways. These range from teaching the disabled person how to relieve pressure, to testing and trouble-shooting cushions.

1. *Teaching wheelchair riders the importance of frequent weight shifting.*

The pressure-tester can be used as a way of helping the person learn more about the responses of the body—a process called **bio-feedback.**

When persons being "pressure tested" bend their upper body from side to side, they can see in the plastic tubes how the pressure shoots up into the red (danger) zone under one butt bone, and drops into the green (safe) zone under the other butt-bone.

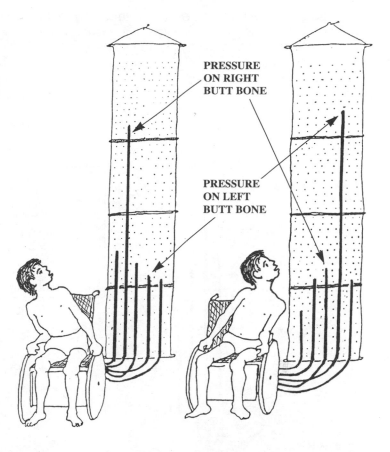

PRESSURE ON RIGHT BUTT BONE

PRESSURE ON LEFT BUTT BONE

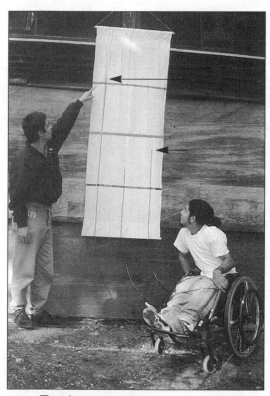

When **TOMÁS** turns to look at the tester, his weight shifts over his right hip, pushing up the pressure as shown in the first column.

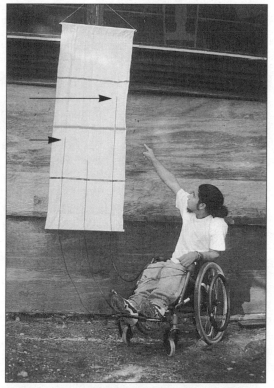

When he leans far to the left, the pressure on the right hip drops (bottom arrow), and on the left hip rises sharply (top arrow).

The pressure tester is an excellent teaching tool to show persons with loss of feeling how important it is—for prevention of pressure sores—to shift weight frequently by bending from side to side, and by leaning forward.

For example, spinal-cord-injured persons who tend to slump back in their wheelchairs can see how this can cause high pressure over the tail-bone (or sacrum).

They can observe how leaning forward lowers the pressure over the tail-bone area, and also over the 2 butt-bones.

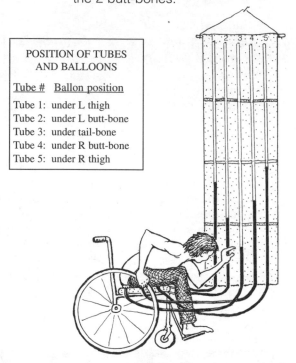

POSITION OF TUBES
AND BALLOONS

Tube #   Ballon position

Tube 1: under L thigh
Tube 2: under L butt-bone
Tube 3: under tail-bone
Tube 4: under R butt-bone
Tube 5: under R thigh

2. Spotting high-pressure spots in persons who sit in a lopsided position.

Example: **ISABEL,** a leader in Brazil's Independent Living movement, has all four limbs weakened by polio. She has a lot of **spinal curve** and sits in a lopsided position. She complained of discomfort when sitting in her wheelchair, and thought a better cushion might help.

During a recent training program in community based rehabilitation (see Chapter 50), students practiced making simple technical aids. One group made a simplified pressure tester, with only one balloon and tube. On testing Isabel, they found she had **very high pressure under one buttock,** and lower pressure under the other.

A second group made her a special cushion to better equalize the pressure under her butt bones. First they experimented with different thicknesses of padding below each buttock. Then they made a **personalized cardboard cushion,** as described on page 157. They retested the pressure and modified the cushion until the pressure under both buttocks was low and nearly equal. **With her new cushion Isabel sat straighter with less discomfort.**

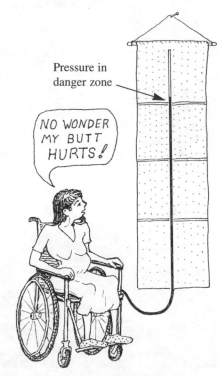

Pressure in danger zone

NO WONDER MY BUTT HURTS!

When Isabel sat on the pressure tester, it showed very high pressure under one buttock. Later, with her new cardboard cushion, there were no areas of high pressure.

3. *Trouble-shooting faulty seating and cushions.*

VICTORIO is a paraplegic wheelchair builder at PROJIMO who took interest in making and testing the "pressure tester." Victorio uses a molded cardboard wheelchair cushion that he made himself. For several months it served him well, but then he began to develop a small pressure sore under one of his butt bones (ischial tuberosities). Although he was careful to lift himself in his wheelchair often, and worked to heal the sore, it had shown little sign of healing for more than two months.

On reading the pressure measurements with the balloons in different positions under his backside, Victorio discovered the cause of his sore. Directly below the butt-bones the pressure was normal. But under the front edge of these bones the pressure was in the red zone (dangerously high).

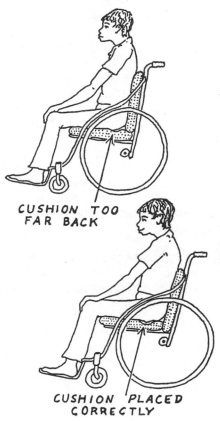

CUSHION TOO
FAR BACK

Now he understood the reason for his problem! Two months before, after enjoying the good results of his cardboard cushion, he had decided also to make a cardboard back support. The new back support—about 3 cm thick—shifted his body forward in the wheel-chair. This caused his butt-bones to press against the front border of the hollows in the cardboard seat cushion (which he had carved to prevent pressure under the butt-bones).

In short, with his new back rest, Victorio was sitting too far forward. On discovering this, he moved his seat cushion 3 cm forward and retested the pressure. Now it was well below the danger zone. Three weeks later, Victorio's sore was healed.

CUSHION PLACED
CORRECTLY

IMPROVING THE INNOVATION

Several problems arose during the initial trials with the pressure measuring instrument, and attempts were made to solve them:

1. *Difficulty in filling the balloons with the colored water.*

It proved difficult to fill the balloons through the long thin plastic tubes. Using **a large syringe** to inject the water down the tubes made it easier. To make it still easier, **small plastic T-connectors** were inserted in each tube a few cm from the balloons. For filling, short side-tubes were attached to these connectors. Plugs were put into these side-tubes to prevent the water from running out when the tester was in use.*

* Both the T-connectors and the tube plugs are available from medical supply houses that sell IV administration kits. (While the side tubes make filling and draining easier, they are not absolutely necessary.)

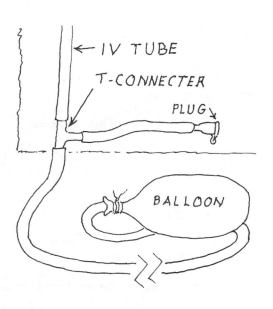

← IV TUBE

T-CONNECTER

PLUG

BALLOON

2. The colored water does not flow easily, and forms bubbles in the thin IV tubes.

The narrow diameter of the plastic IV tubing causes a drainage problem. When the water level in the tubes drops, some water tends to cling in the tubing, causing patches of water separated by air pockets. Tapping the tubes often helps.

It was found that this problem could in large part be overcome by adding a little detergent (a kind of soap) to the colored water. This makes the column of water hold together and helps prevent water droplets from sticking to the walls of the plastic tubes.

3. *Five balloons may be too many.*

On evaluating the tester, most people felt that 5 balloons and tubes were more than are usually needed. It takes a lot of time and precision to set up the 5-balloon equipment. Even with the T-connectors, filling the balloons and getting air bubbles out of the tubes can be troublesome. Also, trying to position all 5 balloons correctly under someone's backside at the same time is not easy. **Persons doing the test often prefer to use 3 balloons or fewer.**

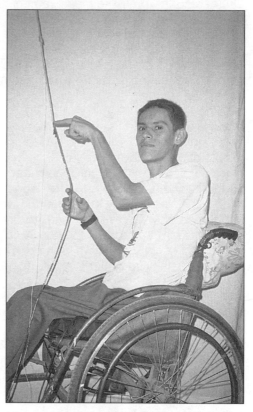

PROJIMO and Michael Heinrich (who made a return visit a year later) have been experimenting with simpler models using 3 balloons and tubes, or even only one or two balloons. The **one-balloon model** ⟶ can be successfully used to trouble-shoot high-pressure areas. The balloon can be positioned under one trouble spot and then another. On the single tube, 3 colored strings or threads can be tied to mark the safe, caution, and danger zones.

As a teaching tool, using one balloon only is not as effective as using more balloons, to show how pressure over different areas rises and falls differently with shifts of position. For a simplified model, **the 2-balloon equipment may be the best compromise.**

The simplest form of the pressure tester consists of a single balloon attached to a long IV tube, with marks or colored ribbons to show the safe, caution, and danger zones of pressure. The whole device can be carried in a pocket.

POSSIBILITIES FOR WIDER USE

Fortunately, the skin-pressure tester was developed, tested, and improved during one of the many "appropriate technology in rehabilitation" courses that PROJIMO has conducted during the past two years. This meant that participants from several different programs in Mexico and Central America were able to take part in all phases of the development and experimentation of this new device. Two of the visitors made their own pressure testers to take back to their respective programs, and others took home drawings, photographs, and designs. (We have yet to get feedback on how this equipment is being used in the different programs.)

PROJIMO has continued to use the pressure tester, both as a trouble-shooting and teaching tool, with good results and often with enthusiastic response from users.

We feel that this low-cost, easy-to-make instrument for measuring pressure against the skin may prove to be a real breakthrough in helping to reduce the vast amount of suffering and death (and the devastating costs) caused by pressure sores in the Third World. **This is one of the most important innovations developed at PROJIMO.**

Julio Uses His Spasticity to Prevent Pressure Sores

CHAPTER **28**

JULIO was 15 years old when his six-year-old sister, playing with their father's pistol, accidentally shot him in the neck. From this injury Julio became quadriplegic (paralyzed in all 4 limbs). When he was taken to PROJIMO several months later, he had a deep, infected pressure sore over his sacrum (the bottom end of his backbone). The sore had already destroyed the end of his spine. It took months of treatment with bees' honey mixed with sugar for the sore to heal. (For information on treatment of pressure sores with honey and sugar see page 156.)

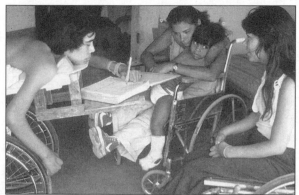

Because Julio was the person with the least power *physically* at PROJIMO, he was given a job that gave him more power *socially:* recording the hours worked and wages earned by each worker. Here, he writes with a plastic pen-holder strapped to his hand.

Preventing More Sores. After Julio's pressure sore had healed and he could sit in a wheelchair, the PROJIMO team wanted to make sure that further sores were prevented. They provided Julio with a good cushion, and helped him explore ways to take the pressure off his backside at frequent intervals. For Julio, this was not easy.

For a person with **paraplegia** (paralysis of the lower part of the body), pressure relief is easy. He simply uses his arms to lift his buttocks ⟶ off the seat every 10 or 15 minutes. This allows blood to circulate in the skin and flesh of the backside, thus preventing sores.

But for someone with **quadriplegia,** whose arms, too, are partly or completely paralyzed, lifting the body to reduce pressure is more difficult. **The following positions can relieve some pressure on the backside:**

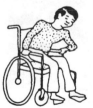
When doing this, one buttock lifts in the air.

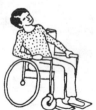

These positions reduce pressure on both buttocks.

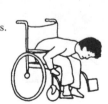

However, for a quadriplegic person, none of the above positions is simple or comfortable. Without great care and self-discipline, such persons often develop new pressure sores.

Spasticity: Hindrance or Help. Many spinal-cord injured persons have a lot of spasticity (involuntary tightening of muscles), especially in their lower body and legs. Spasticity can be very bothersome and make some actions more difficult, such as bending forward to tie shoes, or to relieve pressure on the backside while seated.

However, many spinal cord injured persons learn to use their spasticity to good advantage. For example, some persons use the spastic straightening of their legs to transfer from their wheelchair to a bed, a car, or a toilet. Others use it to stand or walk with crutches but without leg braces. Each spinal-cord injured person should be encouraged to experiment with new ways to move, position, and control their bodies, and to see if they can find ways to put their spasticity to good use.

USING SPASTICITY FOR LIVING INDEPENDENTLY.

Through experimenting, Julio has learned to use his spasticity to be more self-reliant, despite his paralyzed hands and weak arms. (He has developed strong shoulder muscles, which help compensate for his weak arms.)

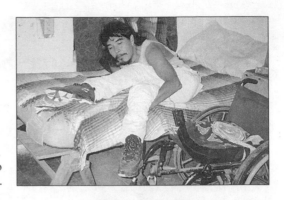

Julio uses his spasticity to transfer to his bed. He shakes his thigh, which causes his knee to straighten stiffly so he can lift it onto the bed.

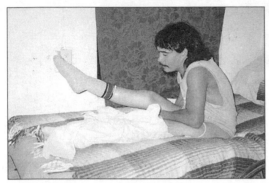

Julio shows how to use his spasticity to straighten his knee.

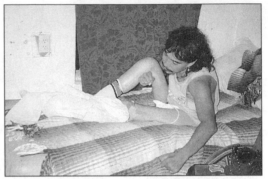

And now he manages to "break the spasticity" and bend the knee.

Using spasticity for dressing. Lying on his back, Julio first bends one knee to his chest, and puts his pants over the foot. Then, he triggers spasticity by tensing his head and shoulder muscles and pushing the leg. His leg straightens stiffly, pushing it into the pants.

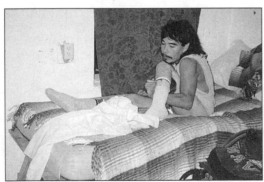

1. Julio bends his knee and positions his open pants in front of his foot.

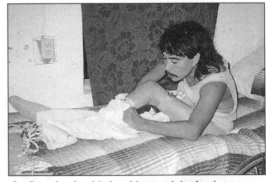

2. On releasing his leg, his spasticity begins to push the leg into his pants.

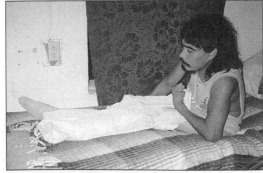

3. As the leg stiffens, Julio does his best to pull up the top of the pants.

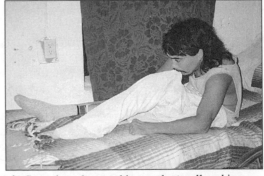

4. Sometimes he uses his mouth to pull up his pants.

USING SPASTICITY TO PREVENT SORES. Julio discovered that he can use his spasticity to help prevent pressure sores. He does this by triggering the spastic straightening of his hips and knees. To do so, he leans backward and pushes with his hands against the hand-rims of the wheel (with the brakes on). As his body stiffens, his backside lifts up off the seat of the chair, relieving the pressure. Julio has found that for him this is the simplest and most effective way of *weight-shifting* to relieve pressure and prevent sores.

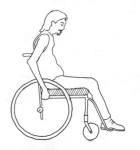 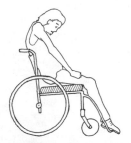 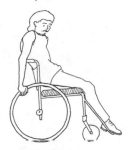

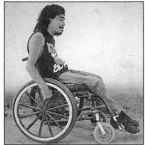

Julio sits normally in his wheelchair.

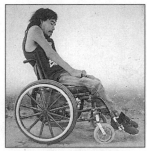

On triggering his spasticity, his buttocks lift off the seat.

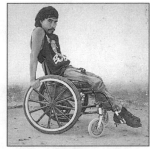

To lift up higher, he uses his shoulders to push himself up.

USING FINGER CONTRACTURES FOR GRIPPING WITH PARALYZED HANDS

As with spasticity, some contractures can occasionally be put to good use. Like many persons with quadriplegia, Julio has learned to use the contractures in his paralyzed fingers to grip things. Persons with a lower neck injury (C-6 or lower) tend to have strong shoulders and some strength in arms and wrists, but complete paralysis of their hands. The fingers tend to develop contractures like this. ⟶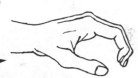

Normally, contractures should be prevented or corrected by range-of-motion exercises. **But with quadriplegia, finger contractures should be allowed to develop to some extent, since the bent-fingered stiffness can be useful for picking things up.**

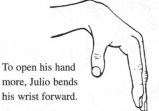 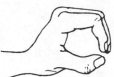 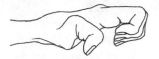

To open his hand more, Julio bends his wrist forward.

To close his hand around an object, Julio bends his wrist back.

CAUTION: Do not let the fingers contract too much!

In this way, Julio can use his paralyzed hands to feed and dress himself independently, and even to propel his wheelchair.

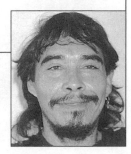

Julio has learned how to make the best use of both his spasticity and his contractures. More important, he has become an excellent teacher and peer counselor, helping other spinal-cord injured persons experiment with new ways of listening to and learning from their bodies. He is especially caring with children who feel lonely and lost.

Julio teaches daily living skills to another quadriplegic youth:

ROMEO was working as an "illegal alien" in the United States to send money to his sick mother back home. Then he became quadriplegic in a car accident. After 3 months in a hospital, he was sent back to Mexico. When he arrived at PROJIMO, Julio soon became his friend, tutor, and role model.

In California, a nurse had given Romeo a "transfer board" for moving from wheelchair to bed. But within 2 days at PROJIMO, Julio showed Romeo to move to and from his wheelchair with no help and without a transfer board. Then Romeo followed Julio's example.

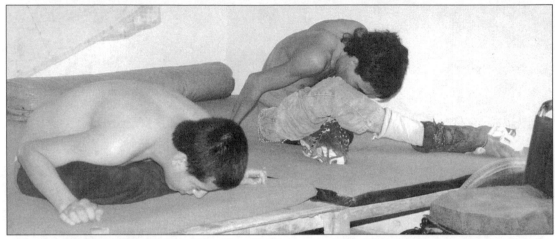

Julio (on right) also taught Romeo to dress himself. First came exercises for bending forward.

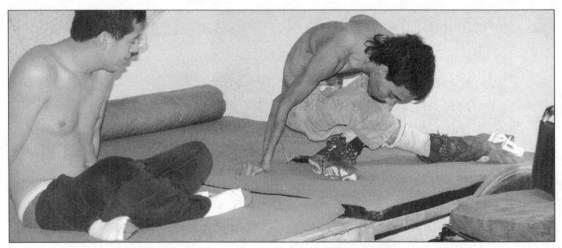

Next, Julio demonstrated different dressing techniques, while Romeo watched.

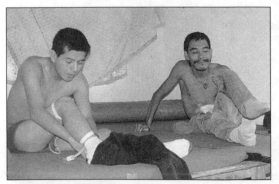
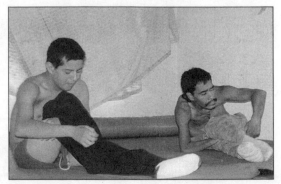

Having a capable person with the same disability as a teacher made learning easier. Both Julio and Romeo benefited greatly.

Part Four

WHEELS TO FREEDOM

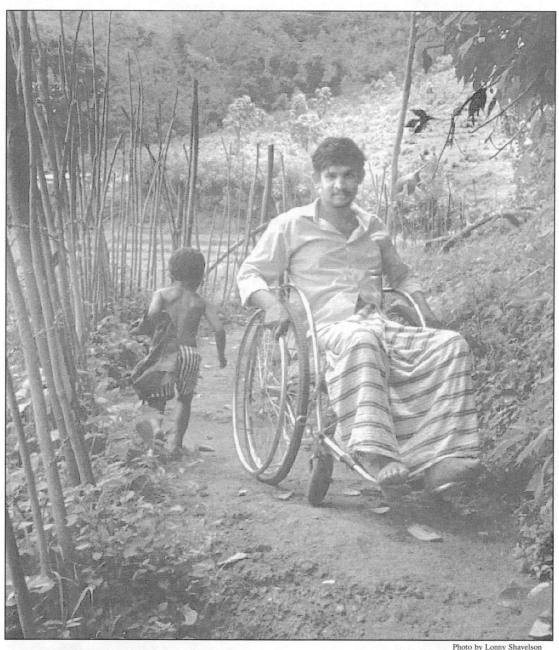

Photo by Lonny Shavelson

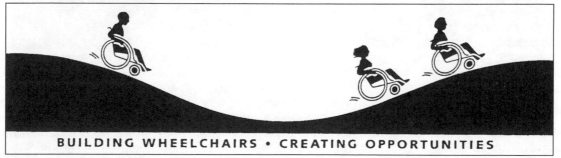

BUILDING WHEELCHAIRS • CREATING OPPORTUNITIES

INTRODUCTION TO PART FOUR

Designing Mobility Aids to Meet Individual Needs

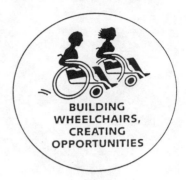

BUILDING WHEELCHAIRS, CREATING OPPORTUNITIES

Wheelchair riders understandably get upset when people say they are "wheelchair confined." Nobody, they say, calls a bike rider "bicycle confined." For someone who cannot walk, a good wheelchair can be a doorway to freedom. It is liberating, not confining.

But if assistive devices—including wheelchairs—are to help disabled persons reach their potential, they must be carefully selected, designed, and adapted to meet each individual's unique combination of needs. In this book's Introduction we saw how standard wheelchairs from the North, donated to 4 women in different countries and circumstances, proved unsatisfactory. This was because the providers did not take into account the particular *needs and wishes of each individual.* Nor did they consider *cultural factors, living conditions, local terrain, available transport, or questions of accessibility.* By contrast, we saw much better results when such factors were taken into account, and when needs and possibilities were discussed with the disabled person and family as part of a creative, problem-solving approach.

Even when persons with the same disability live in the same town, their needs for equipment may vary, depending on their lifestyle, options for schooling or work, and other factors. Cost and convenience must also be considered.

For example, before the wheelchair builders at PROJIMO make a chair for a person, they ask if the chair will need to be transported in a motor vehicle, and if so, what kind. To fit into a passenger car, it helps if the chair can be folded.

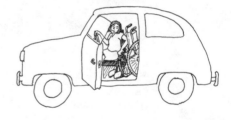

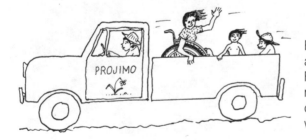

But, if the chair will be carried in the back of a truck, folding may be less important. For many families, keeping the price down may seem more essential. A non-folding chair can be made at lower cost, is lighter weight, and is often more trouble free.

In this part of the book we look at the needs of different persons, not only for **wheelchairs,** but also for other equipment in the realm of "wheeled mobility." This includes **wheeled cots, (gurneys, trollies)** and **hand-powered tricycles.** Our emphasis is on development of a particular mobility aid to meet the specific needs, circumstances, and possibilities of an individual user. For this reason we often describe the situation in story form, and may sometimes include the development of other innovations for the same person.

Wheels work for getting around only when there is access to where you want to go. This means everything from sufficiently smooth, firm **walkways** and **roads,** to **ramps** and in some cases **lifts** or **elevators.** In Chapter 35 we describe a low cost elevator with gravity lift.

In this book we do not include detailed instructions on design and production of standard wheelchairs. Four very different wheelchair designs are in the book, *Disabled Village Children.* Details for building the excellent, low-cost **Whirlwind Wheelchair** are found in *Independence Through Mobility,* by Ralf Hotchkiss (see p. 343). Here we do, however, include some of the most recent breakthroughs in the Whirlwind design (in Chapter 30).

OOPS! THINK AGAIN! — *The Importance of Deciding With, and Not For, the User*

One day, two persons from PROJIMO visited the home of a disabled child in the city of Mazatlán. The child's mother told them about a neighboring family with two children who could not walk. "They're smart little kids," she said, "but their bodies are too weak to walk."

Together, the mother and the PROJIMO workers went to visit these neighbors. They found the two children alone in the house with a baby sitter. The sitter was friendly and invited the visitors to examine the children, who were playing on the floor. It appeared that the children had an inherited muscle weakness, perhaps some form of muscular dystrophy.

MARCOS, the older child, was six years old. He pointed proudly to a big wheelchair in the corner. "Put me in my car!" he insisted. The wheelchair, donated by a government family aid program, was adult size. The small boy sat in it with his feet sticking out over the front edge of the seat. He tried to move the chair by pushing on the wheel rims, but had to stretch his arms far apart to reach them. The chair was so heavy, he could barely move it.

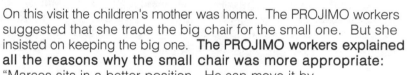

"We have a small, light wheelchair in Ajoya that should fit him much better," said one PROJIMO worker. "We will bring it on our next trip."

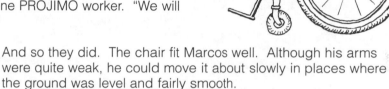

And so they did. The chair fit Marcos well. Although his arms were quite weak, he could move it about slowly in places where the ground was level and fairly smooth.

On this visit the children's mother was home. The PROJIMO workers suggested that she trade the big chair for the small one. But she insisted on keeping the big one. **The PROJIMO workers explained all the reasons why the small chair was more appropriate:** "Marcos sits in a better position. He can move it by himself. It is lighter and takes up less space. And, because the seat is lower, with practice he may learn to climb into and out of it by himself."

The children's mother listened politely, then said, **"But you don't understand! For us, the big chair is best.** You see, I don't have a husband. I sell tacos in the street market. Often I don't have any money to pay a baby sitter. So I have to take both children with me to the market. **In the big chair I can seat both of them together!"**

That was something the PROJIMO workers had not thought of. Given the circumstances, the big chair meets the family's needs better than the small chair.

From this experience, the PROJIMO workers learned the importance of including the family—from the beginning—in the problem-solving process. They yielded to the mother's choice of the over-sized chair.

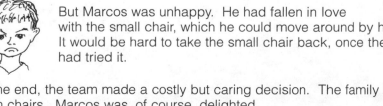

But Marcos was unhappy. He had fallen in love with the small chair, which he could move around by himself. It would be hard to take the small chair back, once the boy had tried it.

In the end, the team made a costly but caring decision. The family kept both chairs. Marcos was, of course, delighted.

Sometimes Simple Solutions Are More Appropriate than Complex Ones

Often a simple device can make as big a difference as a more complex one. And if the device is simple, the user can understand, make, adapt, and control it more easily. Mike Miles, a perceptive observer who worked in community-based rehabilitation in Pakistan for many years, tells a thought-provoking story, which I paraphrase below.

WHICH IS MORE APPROPRIATE? ... WHO IS MORE INDEPENDENT?

One time, in Europe, a man with paralyzed legs wanted to mail a registered letter at the Post Office. He drove his **specially adapted van** to the city center and parked in a disabled-parking spot near the Post Office. Using his van's **motorized lift,** he lowered himself in his wheelchair to the street. In his **battery-powered wheelchair** he zoomed to the front of the Post Office, only to discover that there were three steps he must go up to get inside. Unlike most Post Offices in Europe, there was **no ramp!** Cursing the insensitivity and unfairness of society, he turned his wheelchair around, roared back to his van, hoisted himself and his chair up into it on the lift, and angrily drove home—his letter unmailed.

At the same time, in far-away Pakistan, another man who also had both legs paralyzed wanted to mail a letter at the local Post Office. He hopped on his small **skate-board** and pushed himself quickly along the narrow streets.

He hitched a ride by holding onto the back of a horse-drawn cart. At last he reached the Post Office. To enter it, there were 10 steps and no ramp No worry! He scooted off the skate-board onto the first step. With his arms, he lifted himself on his backside from one step to the next, dragging his skate-board with him. When he reached the top step, he hopped back on his skate-board, rolled to the counter, and handed the letter up to the postal clerk. Thanking him, he turned around, rolled back to the steps, scooted down them on his backside, and rode his skate-board home—his mission fulfilled.

"Which of these 2 men is more independent?" asks Mike. **"Which of the mobility aids is more appropriate? Which society is more at ease with disability? "** ... Clearly, the answers depend on the local situation, cultural factors, and the view point of the persons involved (as well as your own).

COMPLEX AND COSTLY

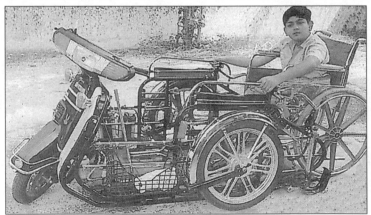

Developed by the Spastics Society of India, Madras.

This motorcycle with two back wheels has been adapted with a ramp at the back so that the wheelchair rider can wheel up into it and drive while seated in his wheelchair.

SIMPLE AND CHEAP

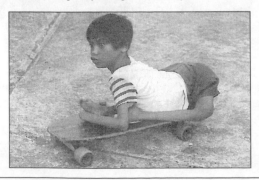

Like this child from India who cannot walk, children (and adults) all over the world use skate-boards, trollies, or make home-made carts to move and play.

Making Wheelchairs from Trash: Innovations in War-Torn Angola

CHAPTER **29**

Disabling Civilians as a Tactic of Low-Intensity Conflict

*As a result of decades of civil war, **ANGOLA**, a country in south-west Africa, has the highest rate in the world of people who have lost legs from land mines. Guerrilla troops, sponsored by the former apartheid (white rule) government of South Africa, have planted millions upon millions of mines. Those injured are mostly civilians, including women and children. Supplied by giant arms manufacturers in the North, **LAND MINES ARE DESIGNED TO CRIPPLE, NOT TO KILL.** This is part of the strategy of "low-intensity conflict." Leaving people seriously disabled puts a greater burden on families and on the nation than does killing people outright.*

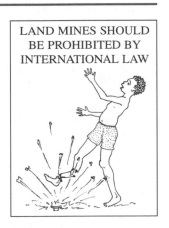
LAND MINES SHOULD BE PROHIBITED BY INTERNATIONAL LAW

National Rehab Centers in Angola—A Chronic Shortage of Materials

To do something for the vast numbers of civilians disabled by war, the government of Angola set up large rehabilitation centers in each province. These were intended to provide disabled persons with rehabilitation, assistive devices, and training in skills such as leather-work and carpentry, so they could soon return to their homes. But at the centers—as in the whole war-torn and economically devastated country—there was a chronic shortage of even basic materials such as leather, wood, nails, and glue. As a result, neither assistive equipment nor skills training were being provided. The rehab centers had become little more than long-term holding camps—sheltered workshops with no work.

To try to find a way out of this situation, in 1990 the Ministry of Social Affairs together with the *Development Workshop* (a Canadian non-profit group) organized a national work-shop. One director and one disabled person from each of 15 provincial centers attended. The author (David Werner) and Kennett Westmacott were among the outside facilitators.

A National Workshop to Develop Equipment and Skills

THE GARBAGE DUMP AS A SOURCE OF SUPPLIES

The purpose of the workshop was to figure out *how to make assistive devices at low cost and with a scarcity of tools and materials.* Rather than simply discuss how to make do with minimal resources, we decided to actually try to make needed aids and equipment for and with the disabled participants. If they themselves could master these skills, they could then not only help meet needs of other disabled persons, but they would have important work.

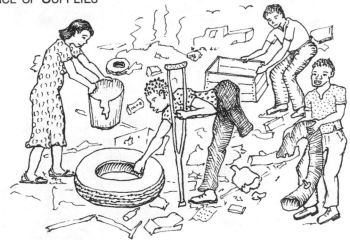
The garbage dump provided a wide variety of useful materials.

To find materials, we first made a trip to the city dump. We collected bits of wire, old plastic buckets, car tires, inner tubes, and bits of metal. About the only wood available was from broken packing crates left over from international aid shipments. Also, there were branches that could be cut from the few remaining ornamental trees.

STARTING WITH BARE HANDS AND SHARP EYES

To start off the workshop, Kennett showed the group how to make a saw by filing teeth into the steel strapping from old packing crates. The blade is stretched between a frame made from sticks, and tightened by twisting a wire. →

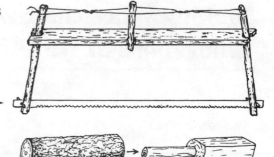

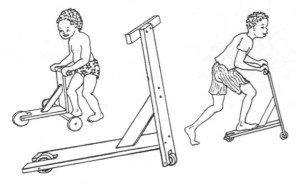

Families and street children are very creative in making equipment for moving from place to place more easily.

To get ideas for building things from scrap, we went into the streets and watched children playing with their homemade scooters, pushcarts, and baby carriages. The wheels of these were made of wood, or with large bearings from junked or bombed trucks. The ingenuity of the street children, inventing playthings out of anything at hand, was an inspiration and challenge to all.

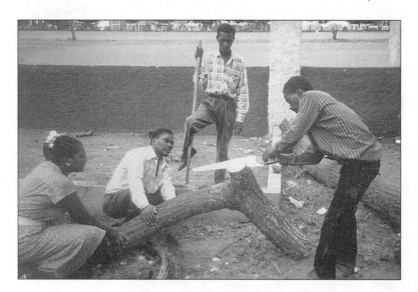

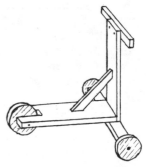

Participants at the Angola workshop cut small wheels from logs. The thicker the wheels, the more weight they are likely to support without breaking.

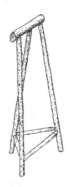

Participants in the workshop make a three-legged walking stick from tree limbs.

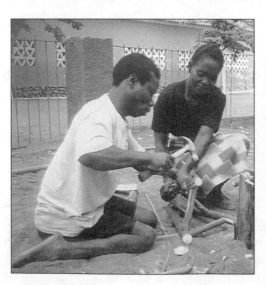

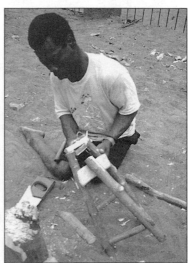

LEARNING TO MAKE ASSISTIVE DEVICES. During the 2-week workshop, the group managed to make a wide variety of assistive devices. These were mostly created to meet the expressed needs of the disabled participants.

For example, one participant, named KOFI, had paralysis in the lower body, with hip and knee contractures. He scooted about on his backside using his hands. He wanted some way to move faster and easier. So the group designed and made for him:

> A log scooter-board with wooden wheels; ———▶
>
> Hand "shoes" with soles made from old tires. ———▶

To meet a wider range of disability needs, the workshop invited disabled adults and children in the local community (on the outskirts of Luanda) to visit. Devices that the workshop participants created to meet the needs of these visitors included:

- A foldable sitting frame for a disabled child

- Artificial legs (both rustic and prefabricated) (see page 180)

- An arm rocker, so that a person with a paralyzed arm can feed herself

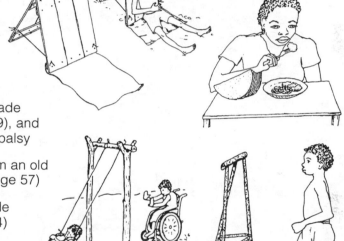

- A special seat with a table made of foam plastic (see page 179), and toys for a child with cerebral palsy

- An enclosed swing made from an old tire, turned inside out (see page 57)

- A 3-legged walking stick made from tree branches (page 174)

- Ramps for wheelchair access and exercise (see page 230)

- An orthopedic lift for a sandal or shoe, made from old foam-rubber "thongs"

- Under-arm and elbow crutches, made from tree branches

- A tray for disabled persons to transport drinks without spilling them (see Chapter 22, page 135)

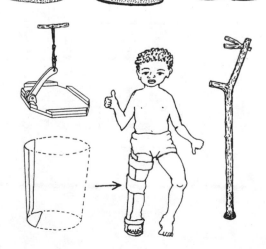

- Wheels, pieced together from old wooden packing crates (see the next two pages)

- A wooden wheelchair, made from packing crates (see page 178)

- Leg braces made from an old plastic bucket, especially designed for a little girl with severe bowing of the knees

How to make a wooden wheel

over 250 mm / 10 in.

Materials:

Wooden planks
Glue
Nails
Old Tire: bicycle or Car.

Basic Tools:

Saw.
Hammer
Book = Square
String = tape measure.

Extra Helpful Tools:

Drill.
Chisel.
Wood file.
Wood plane.
Clamps.

① Select your wooden planks.

The thickness of your planks will equal half the finished width of the wheel.

Cut your planks to length:

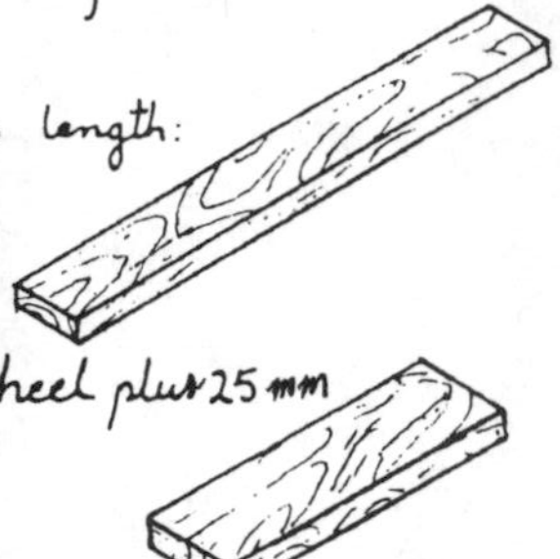

4 × Diameter of the wheel plus 25 mm

8 × Half the Diameter of the wheel plus 25 mm

NB:- It is helpful if these eight pieces are wider than the four.

② Take each of the four long planks.

remove the central square to half the depth of the wood.

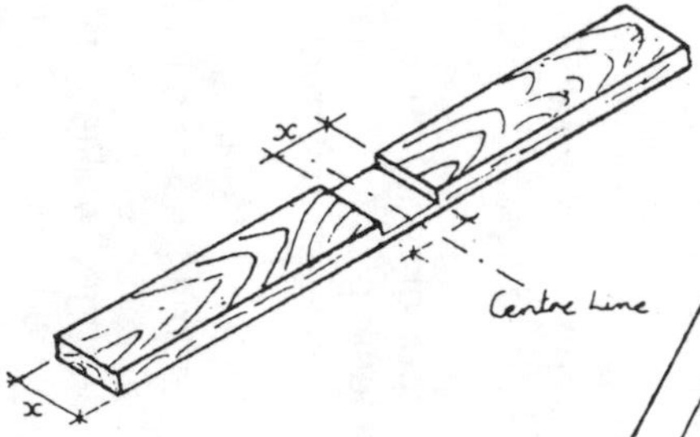

Centre line

③ Place the planks together with glue to form a cross.

Use a book to keep angles at 90°.

If you nail the cross together keep the centre clear you will need to drill a hole for the axle.

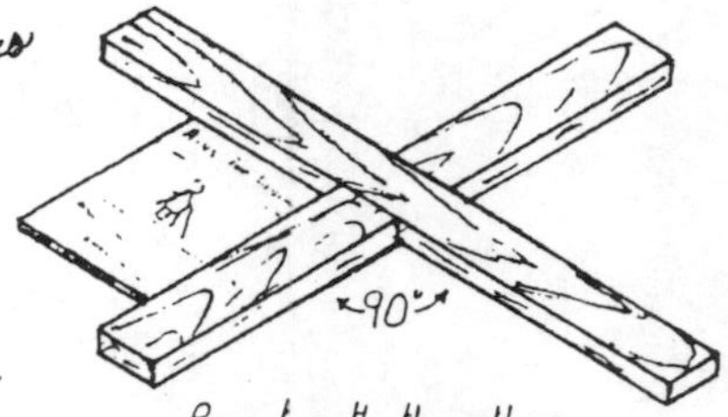

90°

Repeat with the other two planks.

④ Fit the crosses together of the centre.

Drill a small hole in the centre of the crosses.

Put a nail in the drillhole and turn one cross a quarter turn.

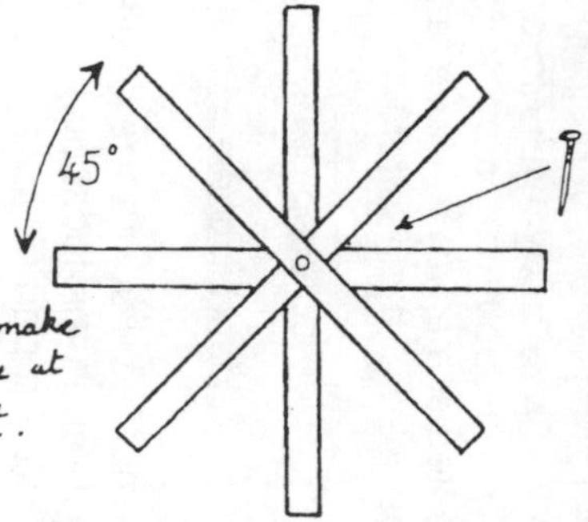

This will make each spoke at 45° apart.

45°

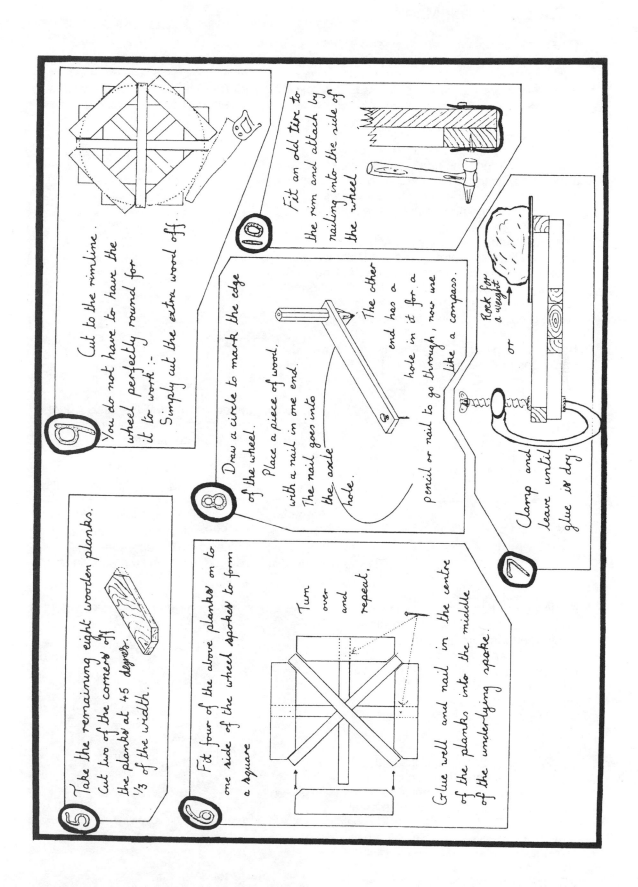

5 Take the remaining eight wooden planks. Cut two of the corners off the planks at 45 degrees. 1/3 of the width.

6 Fit four of the above planks on to one side of the wheel spokes to form a square

Turn over and repeat.

Glue well and nail in the centre of the planks into the middle of the underlying spoke.

7 Clamp and leave until glue is dry.

Rock for a weight or

8 Draw a circle to mark the edge of the wheel.

Place a piece of wood, with a nail in one end. The nail goes into the axle hole.

The other end has a hole in it for a pencil or nail to go through, now use like a compass.

9 Cut to the rimline. You do not have to have the wheel perfectly round for it to work :- Simply cut the extra wood off.

10 Fit an old tire to the rim and attach by nailing into the side of the wheel.

A Wheelchair for Moses

*One of the workshop participants, **MOSES**, had been disabled by a land mine. He walked with great difficulty, supporting his weight with a pole. Moses very much wanted a wheelchair. At first this seemed virtually impossible, given the lack of key materials, especially wheels. But the group was determined to try. The best building material they had was poor-quality, half-inch-thick planks they had scavenged from old packing crates.*

With suggestions from Moses and others, the group drew an initial design for a wooden wheelchair. When the final design was agreed upon, the drawing was enlarged to full size on packing paper, so that the different pieces could be traced onto suitable pieces of wood.

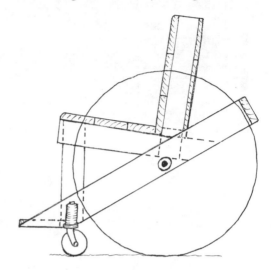

Kennett Westmacott had already taught the participants how to piece together large wooden wheels, using scrap wood from the packing crates. The group put together the wheels and the entire chair using nails pulled out of the packing crates and then hammered straight.

The outer edge of the big wheels were covered with strips of rubber cut from old car tires.

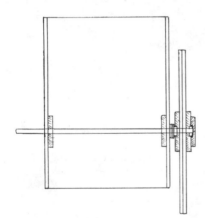

Instruction sheets for making the large wheels were provided by Kennett, and are reproduced (with minor modifications) on the two pages before this one.

With 4 small ball-bearings they had found, they mounted the back wheels on an axle made from a length of 3/4 inch reinforcing rod. The bearings were force-fitted (with a hammer) into inset-holes chiseled into square pieces of Angolan hardwood, found by the scavengers.

For the small front wheels of the chair, participants had hoped to use large truck bearings, similar to those that the street children use for scooters. But the bearings proved difficult to find. At last, someone located a couple of old plastic caster wheels, so these were used. No welding was needed for any part of the wheelchair.

By dividing into small groups that worked at the same time on different parts of the project, the chair was completed in 4 days. It was remarkably sturdy and functional. Moses, who had played a key role in building his chair, loved it. As a last addition, he built a small box on the outer edge of the wooden footrest to hold the front end of his walking stick.

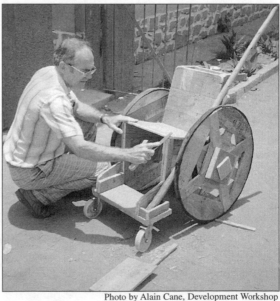

Photo by Alain Cane, Development Workshop

An Outcome: Mutual Respect Gained by Directors and Disabled Participants

Perhaps the most worthwhile part of the workshop was the understanding and respect that grew between the members. At the start, the directors of the rehab centers were hesitant to take part in the manual work. They were reluctant to put themselves on an equal footing with the disabled participants, many of whom were unschooled villagers. The disabled persons, in turn, seemed unsure of themselves and uncomfortable when working alongside the administrators.

However, in the process of working and problem-solving together, everyone began to relax and to appreciate each other's skills. In some areas, such as measuring and interpreting graphic designs, the officials were more able. But in the use of tools and building of devices, many of the people with disabilities were obviously more capable. Each group learned from the other. By the end of the workshop, a strong sense of camaraderie had developed, and everyone seemed more confident.

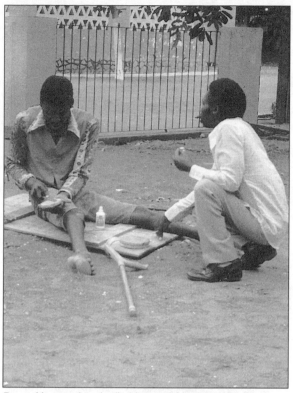

By working together, the disabled participants and the directors of the rehabilitation centers learned to respect each other's different, but equally important, skills.

The Beginning of an Organization of Disabled People in Angola

Another important outcome of the workshop was unplanned. The disabled participants, who came from many parts of the country, recognized that they had a lot of common concerns. They also realized that, by working together to try to solve one another's problems, they could accomplish a lot.

As a result, they began to talk about forming some kind of a network, or organization. This was significant because, at that time, there was no association of disabled people in Angola.

However, there was a major barrier to forming such an organization. At that time, because of all the terrorism and social unrest, the government prohibited all popular organizations, even at the community level. Fortunately, a high official in the Ministry of Social Affairs attended the closing ceremony of the workshop. The disabled participants presented to her their need and desire to form a national organization of disabled people. The official promised to arrange permission for this. We learned later that permission was granted, and an Angolan branch of *Disabled People's International* has now become a reality.

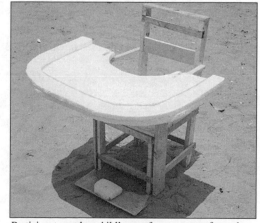

Participants made a child's seat from scraps of wood and foam plastic. They put a raised border on the table to help keep toys from falling off.

Need to Prepare the Stump Before Fitting an Artificial Leg

One of the workshop participants had lost his leg due to a land mine. The group made plans to create a make-shift limb out of bamboo or PVC (plastic pipe) for him. (Designs and instructions for both types of limbs can be found in the book, *Disabled Village Children.*)

However, when a leg-making team from the *Swedish Red Cross* visited the workshop, they brought a **fully adjustable, low-cost prosthesis** (artificial limb) created from local materials. Both the socket and the length of the leg could be quickly modified to fit different persons.

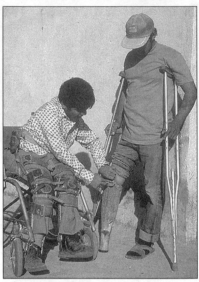

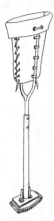

This limb had a laced leather socket attached to a thin steel tube. The length of the tube could be adjusted by a simple telescoping mechanism.

The Red Cross team attempted to fit the limb to the amputee in the workshop. However, they ran into a problem. In the 3 years since his amputation, the man had developed contractures and muscle weakness in the hip. Also, the stump was swollen and flabby. All of this made accurate fitting and safe weight-bearing on the adjustable limb impossible.

A bamboo leg made at PROJIMO, in Mexico (see chapter 18).

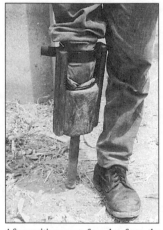

After waiting years for a leg from the government, this man made his own.

From this failed attempt, participants realized that an artificial limb is only a part of the rehabilitative need of an amputee. In the period between losing the limb and getting a prosthesis, it is important that the person:

1. Do exercises to maintain strength and prevent contractures, and
2. Keep the stump bandaged, to prevent swelling and puffiness.

An instruction sheet on stretching and strengthening exercises (partly adapted from the book, *Disabled Village Children)* was developed by the workshop facilitators. It was given to all participants so that they could work with other amputees in the different centers. That way, when there was an opportunity to get an artificial limb, the chances for successful fitting and use would be greater.

The Enormous Need for Artificial Limbs—and an End to Violence

Everyone agreed that there was a **great need for dozens of small, decentralized limb-making workshops** in the provinces, preferably with disabled persons as technicians. Today, Angola has tens of thousands of amputees waiting for limbs. Although the war has more-or-less ended, hundreds of thousands of land mines still cover the landscape. So thousands of men, women, and children will continue to have their legs blown off.

Workshop participants realized that **the only long-term answer is to outlaw land mines by international law.** But that would be just a beginning. Corporate rule, and the power of the multinational arms industry must also be confronted, as well as the unfair distribution of wealth and power that leads to so much poverty, crime, internal strife, and institutionalized violence. **Disabled people need to join with other marginalized and disadvantaged groups in the struggle for a kinder, fairer world.** (See the book, *Questioning the Solution* for more on the politics of health and disability. See page 344.)

Learning From and Admitting Our Mistakes

The illustrated instruction sheet shown below was developed at the Angola workshop. Copies were made for participants to take back to their centers, to help persons who had lost a leg maintain the movement and strength needed to successfully use an artificial leg, if and when they got one. (Another information sheet gave instructions on how to bandage the stump, to prevent the swelling and flabbiness that make it hard to fit a limb.)

Unfortunately, the original exercise sheet, although it was designed by rehabilitation professionals, had some problems. The mistakes were pointed out to me, years later, by Ann Hallum, an outstanding physical therapist who reviewed the manuscript of this book.

Question: *Some of the exercises shown below should usually be done differently, or not be done at all. Do you know which ones? And why?*

Answer: CAUTION with exercises 1, 3, and 4.

Exercises 1, 3, and 4 should be done differently. **They can lead to muscle imbalances and contractures that make walking with an artificial limb much more difficult.**

After the loss of a leg, the person tends to hold his stump lifted up and out, like this.

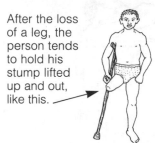

By doing this, he uses and strengthens the muscles that bend the stump up and out, more than those that bend it in and back. This results in a muscle imbalance that can lead to contractures that will interfere with walking.

Therefore, it is best to **do exercises to strengthen the weaker muscles that can help combat contractures. And stretch (but do not strengthen) muscles that contribute to contractures.**

To combat contractures, Exercise 1 should be done to stretch, not strengthen. Exercises 3 and 4 should be done lying down (to reduce flexion contractures of thigh). And if you do exercise 3, avoid opening the thigh to the side past mid-line.

AN INSTRUCTION SHEET WITH *FAULTY ADVICE:*

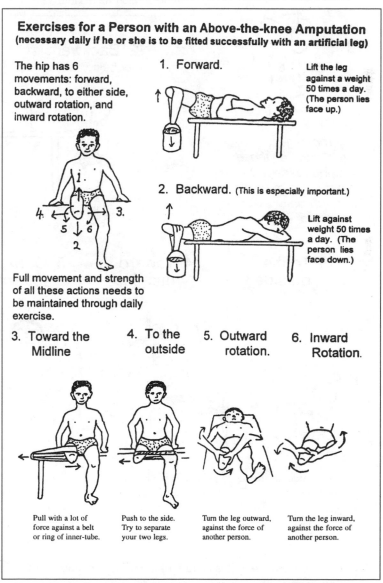

Exercises for a Person with an Above-the-knee Amputation
(necessary daily if he or she is to be fitted successfully with an artificial leg)

The hip has 6 movements: forward, backward, to either side, outward rotation, and inward rotation.

Full movement and strength of all these actions needs to be maintained through daily exercise.

1. Forward.
Lift the leg against a weight 50 times a day. (The person lies face up.)

2. Backward. (This is especially important.)
Lift against weight 50 times a day. (The person lies face down.)

3. Toward the Midline
Pull with a lot of force against a belt or ring of inner-tube.

4. To the outside
Push to the side. Try to separate your two legs.

5. Outward rotation.
Turn the leg outward, against the force of another person.

6. Inward Rotation.
Turn the leg inward, against the force of another person.

A corrected version of this exercise sheet is shown on the next page. . . Live and learn!

This is the **corrected version of the Exercise Sheet** shown on the preceding page.

Exercises for a Person with an Above-the-Knee Amputation
(necessary daily, if he or she is to be fitted successfully with an artificial leg)

The hip has 6 movements:

1) forward
2) backward
3, 4) to either side
5) outward rotation,
6) inward rotation.

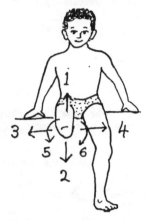

Full movement and strength of all these actions (except the first) need to be maintained through daily exercise.

1. Forward Movement*

CAUTION: Use this exercise to stretch the muscles that flex the thigh, not to strengthen them. Don't lift against the weight; let it pull the thigh backward. Bend the other knee up, to prevent the lower back from bending instead of stretching the hip. It is usually best to avoid exercises that strengthen forward-lifting of the stump (hip flexion).

As a general rule:
DO THIS EXERCISE. ONLY TO STRETCH THE STUMP DOWN. DO NOT LIFT IT UP.

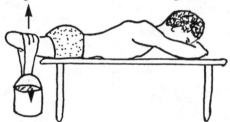

2. Backward (This is especially important for being able to walk with a full range of motion.)

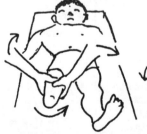

Lift against weight 50 times a day. (The person lies face-down.)

3. To the outside

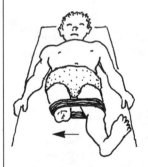

Push to the side, trying to separate your legs.

(But do this so that the stump stays in the mid-line, and does not swing out to the side.)

4. Toward the mid-line

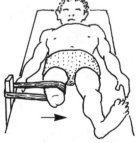

Pull with a lot of force against a belt, or a ring of inner-tube.

5. Outward rotation

Turn the leg outward, against the force of another person.

6. Inward rotation

Turn the leg inward, against the force of another person.

*Note: With Exercise 1, it is important to let the hanging weight stretch the hip down. Do not try **to lift the stump.** This will help avoid hip flexion contractures (inability to straighten the hip) that would make walking more difficult. For a similar reason, **do Exercises 3, 4, 5, and 6 lying down.**

Evolution of the Whirlwind Wheelchair

CHAPTER 30

The Best Wheelchair Designers? Wheelchair Riders!

Everest and Jennings is the brand name of the world's largest wheelchair manufacturer. Many people do not realize that the original designer and founder of this global wheelchair business was disabled and rode a wheelchair himself. **The original "E&J" wheelchair—which was a breakthrough in its day—grew out of a disabled person's creative response to an unmet personal need.**

But as E&J Industries grew, the company became more interested in mass-production than in innovation. Fortunately, however, other disabled persons have continued to advance the state of the art. **Like Herbert Everest, many of the most innovative wheelchair designers in the past 20 years have themselves been wheelchair riders.**

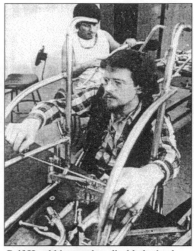

Ralf Hotchkiss teaches disabled wheel-chair builders at PROJIMO.

RALF HOTCHKISS AND THE WHIRLWIND

One of the world's most caring and creative wheelchair designers and builders is Ralf Hotchkiss, who lives in California, USA. Ralf became paraplegic (paralyzed from his chest down) from a motorcycle crash when he was a teenager. Since then, Ralf trained as a mechanical engineer, and has designed and built a wide range of innovative wheelchairs and other equipment.

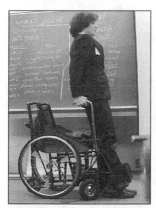

Ralf's early disability-assistive inventions included a **standing wheelchair** that can lift the rider from sitting to standing.

When Ralf first decided to build a **4-wheel drive wheelchair,** he had a hard time figuring a way to transfer power from the large back wheels to the small front wheels. The obvious solution was to use bicycle chains. But for this, the front wheels would need to not swivel (pivot) to make turns, as do caster wheels of most wheelchairs.

Furthermore, caster wheels need to be fairly small to avoid bumping the footrests when they pivot. But, to move easily on rough ground, Ralf's front wheels needed to be relatively large. What to do???

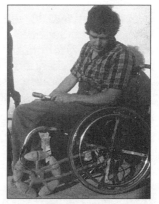

Ralf, in his **all-terrain 4-wheel drive wheelchair.** A bicycle chain transfers power from the back wheel to the front.

The solution, Ralf explains, came from the Bible: the so-called *Ezekiel Wheel, a circle of small wheels that together form a larger wheel.* With this idea, Ralf created a front wheel made of a series of small rubber cones, positioned in a circle around the central hub. Each cone is mounted on its own ball bearings, so it can roll sideways, while the wheel as a whole rolls forward. This combination of several small wheels within a bigger one gives a multi-directional roll similar to that of a caster wheel. However, the forward direction of the main wheel is fixed and it does not pivot. This is what Ralf needed for his 4-wheel drive.

Ralf's "Ezekiel wheel." The small rollers roll sideways. The main wheel rolls forward. This gives a multi-directional caster effect, without swiveling.

Low-Cost, High-Quality Wheelchairs Made by Third World Riders

Although Ralf's 4-wheel drive wheelchair worked well, it never became popular. Building it was too costly and time consuming. Just the front wheels used 24 bearings and 20 individually vulcanized cones.

Ralf's interest turned to developing low-cost wheelchairs for the Third World, using "appropriate technology." His incentive was sparked on a visit to Nicaragua in 1980, shortly after the Sandinistas overthrew the Somoza dictatorship. A group of young Sandinistas who had been spinal-cord injured during the war had formed a grassroots group called *Organization of Disabled Revolutionaries (ORD).* They had so much trouble getting wheelchairs that four of their members were sharing a single wheelchair. Most wheelchairs in Nicaragua were imported from the USA. With the stiffening US embargo, both chairs and spare parts were very hard to find. The ORD members had difficulty reintegrating into society and finding work because they lacked mobility. Some, whose wheelchairs had broken down, had gone back to dragging themselves about in their homes, unable to leave.

For these reasons, the Disabled Revolutionaries set up a small wheelchair repair shop. But they ran into problems. Commercial imported chairs, such as *E&Js,* have poor-quality bearings which wear out quickly in a rough, dusty environment. Because they are not a standard size, they could only be replaced with over-priced bearings purchased from the original manufacturer. The cost was prohibitive. In places like Nicaragua, where bearings of any kind are often not available, wheelchair maintenance becomes extremely difficult.

Clearly, such dependence on expensive, hard-to-maintain, imported chairs increased people's handicaps. Ralf worked with ORD to design a low-cost wheelchair that could be built from local materials by modestly-skilled disabled workers. The result was the *Torbellino,* or Whirlwind Wheelchair. Within a year, ORD was operating a mini-factory in which a team of disabled persons built this home-grown design.

THE WHIRLWIND WHEELCHAIR is relatively easy to build in a modestly-equipped shop. Yet its quality is excellent. As a wheelchair rider himself, Ralf appreciates the need for a light-weight, compact, easy-rolling, trouble-free chair. The design of the Whirlwind is simple and stream-lined, but a great deal of skillful engineering has gone into it.

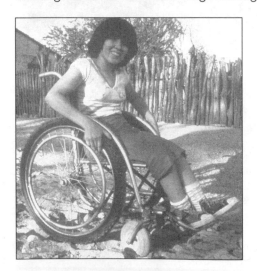

The frame of the chair is made from electric-conduit steel tubing, available in building supply stores around the world. The back wheels are bicycle wheels. The bearings (of the early model) are standard high-speed bearings used in small electric machinery. Used bearings can often be obtained at very low cost in electrical repair shops. These are finely made bearings for high speed use. Even secondhand ones, used in a wheelchair, will long outlast commercial wheelchair bearings.

The beauty of the Whirlwind is that it is made in small community shops by disabled people who recognize the need for a chair that is adapted to the needs of the individual rider.

These wheelchairs tend to be custom-built or adapted. In the process, new design opportunities arise, and the chairs come closer to matching the varied needs of their users.

THE LONG-TERM VISION: WHEELCHAIRS FOR ALL WHO NEED THEM

Since helping ORD in Nicaragua, Ralf has traveled around the world, facilitating workshops and helping groups of disabled persons begin to produce appropriate wheelchairs. One of the first groups he worked with was PROJIMO, in the mountains of Western Mexico. Over the years, Ralf has led workshops and worked with disabled wheelchair builders in 30 countries in Latin America, Africa, Asia, and Russia.

Ralf calculates that, **of the 20 million people in the Third World today who need wheelchairs, fewer than one percent have them.** He dreams of the day when all who need a wheelchair will have a chair fully suited to their needs. To this end, he and his friend, Peter Pfaelzer at San Francisco State University, formed **Wheeled Mobility,** a small non-profit organization which is rapidly turning into an international network of wheelchair builders and designers. **If there are ever to be enough wheelchairs—chairs that are truly liberating to their riders—production must be decentralized and the building process must be demystified, with users leading the process.**

RECENT WHIRLWIND INNOVATIONS

The basic design of the Whirlwind keeps evolving. Not only has Ralf continued to design and test new features himself, but he has gathered new ideas from groups of disabled persons around the world who are building local variations of the Whirlwind.

It should be noted that many of these new features were developed in collaboration with disabled persons who expressed difficulties with the existing design or who wanted some particular modification.

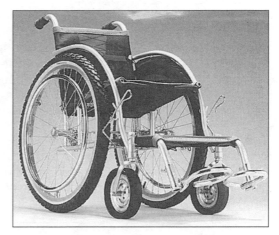

In this book, we do not give detailed instructions for making the Whirlwind wheelchair. A brief description can be found in the book, *Disabled Village Children*. Very detailed instructions—including suggestions for setting up and stocking a shop—are in Ralf's fine handbook, *Independence Through Mobility* (see page 343).

For years, Ralf has been revising and updating this book, but new ideas come so fast that it is a never-ending process. **In this chapter we will give a preview of just a few of the most innovative modifications and improvements of the Whirlwind chair.** While developed primarily for the Whirlwind, most of these innovations can be adapted to other models, or even to commercial wheelchairs.

1. *Front Wheels and Tires*

The front caster wheels and tires of the Whirlwind have presented some big design challenges. Caster wheels are complex and costly. They require two sets of bearings, one vertical and one horizontal, so that the wheels can swivel, as well as rotate. (The swivel is what allows the chair to make turns.)

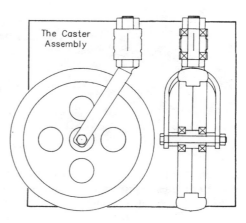

The basic front-caster design and the wheel forks remain much the same as in Ralf's original book (and in *Disabled Village Children*). A new design for bearings is discussed under entry #2. Here, we look at innovations in wheels and tires.

FRONT WHEELS AND TIRES TO SUIT DIFFICULT TERRAIN: A THORNY PROBLEM

Most modern commercial wheelchairs now
come with tiny, hard, rubber or plastic front
wheels. These are good for gliding over
hospital floors or smooth, paved streets. But
they function poorly on the rough, sandy paths
of villages, or on the pitted, irregular roads
of many Third World cities. For difficult
or sandy terrain, front wheels need to be
relatively big (6 to 9 inches in diameter) and
wide (1½ inches or more).

Pneumatic tires (filled with air, under pressure)
are light-weight, and on rough terrain they give
a much smoother ride (which may add to the
life of the wheelchair—and the rider).

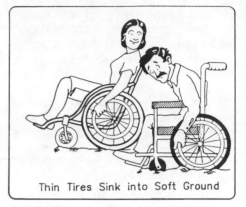

Thin Tires Sink into Soft Ground

Drawing from *Independence Through Mobility*
by Ralf Hotchkiss.

But air-filled tires also have short-comings. On rocky or thorny paths they puncture
easily and often need to be patched and pumped up. Also, pneumatic tires that fit
small caster wheels tend to be outrageously expensive. And, in many countries, they
are simply not available. In the original version of *Independence Through Mobility,*
Ralf gave an address in China where pneumatic tires and tubes can be bought in large
quantities at relatively low cost. But this is hardly an ideal solution for equipment
designed to use local, easily obtained materials.

The wheels have presented another problem. In the early
Whirlwind design, Ralf recommended making front wheels
from two discs of hard wood, glued together, with their grain
crossing (at right angles) to prevent splitting. The photos of
the Whirlwind, below and on p.195, show the wooden wheels.

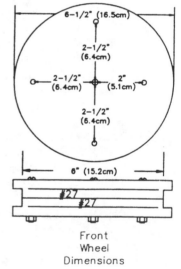

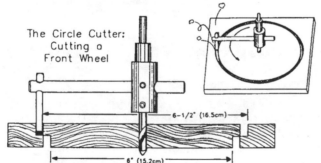

The Circle Cutter:
Cutting a
Front Wheel

6-1/2" (16.5cm)

6" (15.2cm)

Front
Wheel
Dimensions

Designs from *Independence Through Mobility,* for cutting and assembling the wooden front wheels.

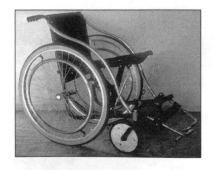

These wooden wheels were tried at PROJIMO in Mexico,
but many users found them unsatisfactory. In spite of
attempts to waterproof them with heavy varnish or
epoxy finish, in the mud and rain they soon rotted and
cracked. Riders in other countries reported similar
problems. Another problem was that some people
who wanted to purchase a wheelchair thought wooden
wheels were primitive and ugly. They insisted on having
"modern" wheels, even if more costly. Whatever the
reasons, such preferences must be taken into account.

Molded aluminum wheels were another alternative considered by Ralf. Workshops in
Brazil and Bangladesh cast and lathe-turn their own aluminum wheels. But for most small
production centers, this is impractical. The set-up costs are prohibitive.

A rubber T tire, clamped between metal plates.

A new design came from RESCU, a production center in Zimbabwe where disabled workers build assistive equipment, including the Whirlwind wheelchair. The front wheels consist of **two round sheet-metal plates which grip a molded rubber tire.**

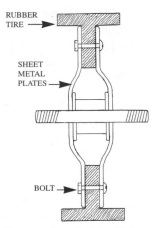

The tire, in cross section, is T-shaped. The center-arm of the T projects inward, and is firmly held with bolts between the 2 metal plates. The tire is vulcanized (heat-molded) in a specially lathe-turned steel mold. Once the mold is made, any shop that retreads car tires can produce these T-tires in small or large quantities at a relatively low cost.

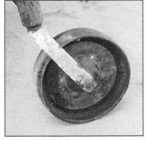

A modified Zimbabwe wheel, made at PROJIMO.

Cross-section of rubber-T tire, bolted between 2 sheet-metal disks that form the wheel.

The wheel is made by cutting two round disks of sheet metal. The disks must be widely separated at the center to hold the hub firmly, and shaped so they can grip the T-tire. A dye of lathe-turned steel is needed to hammer, press or spin the disks into shape.

The advantage of this Zimbabwe wheel is that, after a (fairly costly) initial investment for the molds and dyes, the production cost can be quite low. The tire, made of the same rubber as a car tire, is nearly indestructible. Its broad, T-shaped base has almost the same flexibility and springiness as a pneumatic tire. But it never punctures. Wider tires can be made for sand, to prevent sinking in.

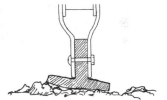

Problem: In Zimbabwe, the wheel was made of fairly thick sheet metal, pressed into shape in a large metal-press delivering tons of weight. In redesigning the wheel for smaller shops without such massive presses, Ralf began to experiment with a thinner grade of sheet-metal that could be hammered into shape when the metal disk was clamped over a dye. The PROJIMO wheel-chair builders tried making these wheels. At first, they appeared to work well. But, after repeated bumps into rocks and curbs, the metal disks bent and finally collapsed. The PROJIMO team tried using thicker sheet-metal, but it was too difficult to hammer into shape. Groups experimenting in other countries ran into similar problems.

Solution: An all-rubber wheel and tire. After exploring many possibilities, Ralf found a simple solution. *Do away with the sheet-metal disks and **mold the entire tire and wheel out of vulcanized rubber, as a single unit.***

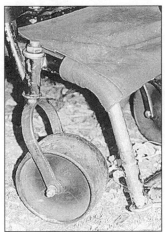

The central part of the wheel is cast thick enough to make it inflexible. The wide outer-edge that rolls against the ground is thin enough to provide a spongy flexibility.

The wide center-part of the wheel is molded to grip the hub. A flange, welded to the hub, is bolted to the wheel.

A big advantage to this all-rubber wheel is that it bends easily, to ride smoothly over irregular terrain. These simplified wheels show great promise. Eventually, they may be used for both front and rear wheels of **all-terrain wheelchairs.**

The all-rubber wheel and tire.

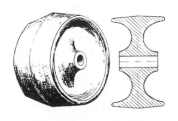

Front view and cross-section of the all-rubber wheel.

2. Bearings

Among the biggest problems with many wheelchairs are the bearings. Commercial chairs use off-size ball bearings of relatively poor quality. They soon wear out, making the wheels wobbly and hard to push. Since the bearings are not a common size, often they cannot be replaced locally, but must be obtained at high cost from the wheelchair supplier or the manufacturer. Where chairs are imported, this may be very difficult or impossible. The Third World is littered with carcasses of fancy imported chairs whose bearings wore out.

For this reason, the original Whirlwind design uses local, widely available bearings. If dust or dirt get into the bearings, it can ruin them. So, sealed bearings are recommended. Though more costly, the user saves money in the long run. **Second-hand high-speed, sealed bearings** of a workable size (5/8 inch inside diameter, 1 3/8 inch outside diameter—or 15 x 35 mm metric equivalent) can often be found in junk yards (in starter motors of old cars) or in small motor or power tool repair shops. (For more details, see *Independence Through Mobility.*)

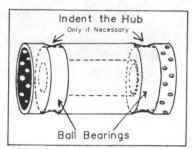

Whirlwind hub design showing fit of bearings. (from *Independence Through Mobility*, p. 82)

Problem: When PROJIMO began making wheelchairs, it could get all the second-hand bearings it needed free or at low cost from friendly repair shop owners in the closest cities. But as the program produced more and more chairs, the repair shops ran out of second-hand bearings. PROJIMO had to buy new bearings, which were very expensive. The 12 sets of bearings needed for a wheelchair cost as much as all the remaining materials! This pushed up the price so much that many poor families could not afford it. Many other wheelchair-making shops have had a similar experience.

Solution: An idea to solve this problem came from India. On a visit there, Ralf Hotchkiss inspected the huge wheels of the traditional ox carts. They used an ancient form of **rod bearings, or "needle bearings."** The wheels rolled on a series of metal rods which fit snugly between the iron hub and the axle.

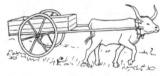

Old Indian ox carts use rod bearings.

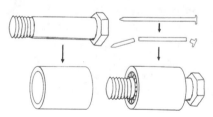

Ralf experimented with hubs that, instead of ball bearings, use metal rods that roll between the axle and the hub tube. But the rods sometimes jammed in the hub.

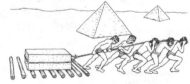

Rod bearings were used to move the rocks to build the pyramids in Egypt.

An old mountain farmer in the eastern USA solved this problem by showing Ralf that thinner rods in a longer hub do not jam. Ralf now uses carpenter's nails with their heads cut off. The nails form a circle of rollers between the axle bolt and metal hub tube.

Ralf has tested the ease with which the wheels turn compared to ball bearings, and finds them equal. The cost of materials for rod bearings is a fraction of that of commercial ball bearings. Rod bearings require more work, but durability tests indicate that they last many times longer. (Whereas ball bearings bear the weight of chair and rider on a tiny point on each tiny ball, with rods, the weight—and wear—is spread over the full length of the rods.)

These new (though ancient) bearings show great promise. Hopefully they will contribute toward providing high-quality, long-lasting wheelchairs to many of the millions of people who need them, at a cost more within their reach.

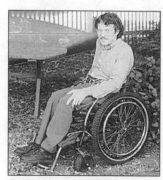

Ralf in his wheelchair with rod (nail) bearings.

3. Folding Mechanism, with Adjustable Chair Width

Different adjustments on wheelchairs. People who ride wheelchairs come in all shapes and sizes. So should wheelchairs. Many commercial chairs—although the basic models are standardized—come with adjustable footrests, armrests, and alternative positions for the rear hubs.

Hub position. By changing the up-and-down position of the hubs in relation to the chair, the height and tilt of the seat can be changed. By changing the front-to-back position of the hubs, the balance of the chair can be changed. For example, a person without legs may need the rear hubs mounted farther back to avoid falling over backwards when going up-hill.

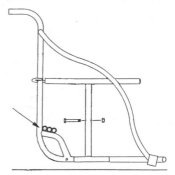

A series of axle tubes on the frame of the Whirlwind permits the hub position to be adjusted. (Hotchkiss)

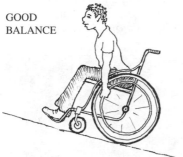
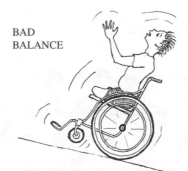
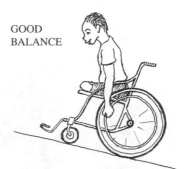

GOOD BALANCE

BAD BALANCE

GOOD BALANCE

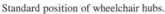

Standard position of wheelchair hubs.　　Legless rider tips backwards on hill.　　Hubs farther back for legless rider.

An advantage to producing wheelchairs in small, community-based shops is that often they can be custom-made. Rather than adding a lot of mechanisms for adjustments to meet different user's needs (which add to both weight and cost), each chair can be personalized from the start, to meet the specific needs of the intended user. If the wheelchair makers are also wheelchair riders, they are likely to be more aware of and responsive to those needs, and to include the user in the planning and design process.

Nevertheless, even in a small community shop, some amount of standardization can make production quicker, easier, and cheaper. It helps to have a selection of ready-made chairs available when they are needed. That way the person can try different chairs and pick the one that comes closest to meeting her or his needs. Last minute adjustments (or even more substantial changes) can then be made according to the individual's requirements.

Goodness of fit—in terms of size, width, seat angle, angle and height of back, need for armrests, position of footrests, etc.—is essential. Decisions need to be made *with* the user, *not for* her, allowing enough time to test different alternatives and make well-informed decisions.

ADJUSTABLE FEATURES OF THE WHIRLWIND. Although the Whirlwind has a basic (if evolving) design, it can be built and modified in different ways for different users. The **height of the footrests** can be easily adjusted by the user. Also, in response to his own need and that of others with spastic ankles, a PROJIMO wheelchair builder, Martín Pérez (see Chapters 37 and 39), has designed a simple way to **adjust the sideways angle of the footrests.**

One of the greatest needs for adjustability in wheelchairs is the **width of the seat,** and thereby the **width of the whole chair.** Correct width is important for the stability and comfort of the rider, and for her ease in pushing the chair. A new design for easy adjustment of chair width has been developed, together with a new mechanism for folding the chair.

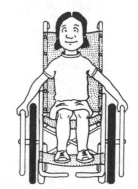

A chair that is too wide is hard to push. (From *Independence Through Mobility,* page 26)

Folding is important. For many wheelchair riders, it is essential that their chair can fold, to fit into a narrow space. This is especially important for those who need to travel in a bus, carry their chair in the back of a car, or pack it on a donkey.

Problem: The original Whirlwind design included an upright X-brace that folded like scissors, as do most commercial chairs. But to fold well, the measurements, welds, and alignment must be exact. In PROJIMO, as in many small shops run by disabled persons, many workers are still learning their skills. There are few highly skilled craftspersons. The resulting wheelchairs were often very difficult to fold. Users expressed their frustration.

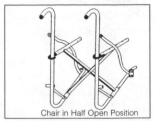

Chair in Half Open Position

The X-brace folds like scissors.

Solution: a horizontal folding device. To solve this common problem, Ralf and friends experimented with alternative folding devices until they came up with one that was more fool-proof. The new design folds horizontally, rather than vertically. Although it has more pieces and uses more welds than the X-brace, it requires less skill and precision to build, and gives consistently good results. PROJIMO now uses this new folding device in all its Whirlwind chairs, and has had fewer complaints.

The horizontal folding brace is attached to the side frames of the chair: at the back, with short, strongly-welded vertical hinges, and at the front, with vertical bolts that allow the cross bars to pivot.

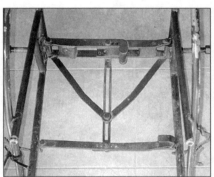 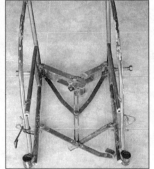 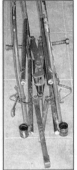

Narrowing the chair to get through doorways.

On experimenting with the new folding mechanism, users discovered that they could easily narrow the width of the chair while sitting in it. They pull the handle under the seat forward, and then pull the wheels in, closer to their body. This offered a solution to another big problem of wheelchair riders in many countries: getting through narrow doorways. (See Luz's story on page 17.)

A short handle below the front of the cloth seat can be pulled forward or pushed back to fold or open the chair.

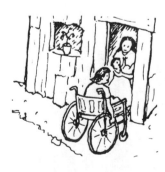

With the new design, to go through a narrow door the user simply pulls the sides of the chair in against her hips, and rolls through. (With an X-brace, narrowing the chair is much harder, because it folds against gravity and the person's own weight holds it wide open.)

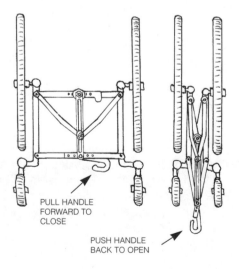

PULL HANDLE FORWARD TO CLOSE

PUSH HANDLE BACK TO OPEN

Adjustable chair and seat width. The horizontal folding mechanism also lends itself to adjusting the seat width to match the hip-width of the user. Small holes can be drilled in the cross bars of the adjustment device, so that the chair width can be adjusted, depending on which set of holes the center bolt is passed through.

Upholstery. To avoid having to make new upholstery with different measurements for different seat adjustments, Ralf has devised wrap-around seat and back-rest cloths that can be laced up at different widths.

The patterns for the back-rest and seat are similar. They consists of one square just a little bigger than the desired size of the back-rest or seat, and another square, 4 times as big.

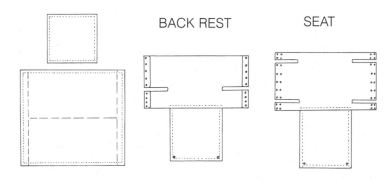

BACK REST   SEAT

Hem the edges of both squares to prevent fraying. Then, fold the big square in half, and cut grooves as shown here. Sew together at all edges, except where the small square will be attached. Turn the resulting sack inside out, and sew on the small square. Make holes for lacing as shown.

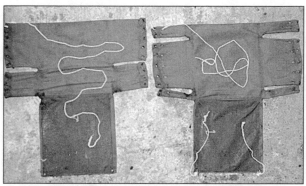

Completed back-rest and seat, ready to be laced into place. The small square folds over and protects the lacing.

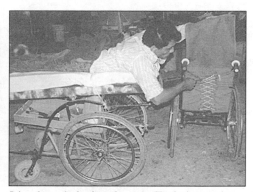

Jaime laces the back to the seat. The lacing can be loosened or tightened for different wheelchair widths.

How appropriate is the new folding mechanism and adjustable seat? The answer depends on who you ask. Wheelchair riders and users (including Ralf) have mixed feelings. One of the beauties of the early Whirlwind design (with the vertical X-frame) is its simplicity, streamlined look, relatively few parts, and few welded joints (all of which contributed to the chair's low weight and low cost).

The new folding mechanism with its adjustable seat width solves a number of problems but sacrifices some of the Whirlwind's graceful look and adds a bit of weight. Some users like being able to adjust the chair to their own body width, and to narrow it easily to pass through narrow doorways. Other users think it "looks funny" and prefer the more conventional X-brace. (For some people, appearance is more important than function.)

The PROJIMO wheelchair builders are delighted because—although the new folding mechanism takes more welds and looks more complex—for them, it is easier to build successfully. That is important. **Designs must be appropriate for builders as well as users.**

The search for better designs continues. Ralf's team is now experimenting with a folding mechanism developed by blacksmiths in Nyabondo, Kenya. This uses a vertical X-brace that is easier to build than is Ralf's original design.

There is always room for improvement. And improvements are always possible when builders and users work together creatively.

4. A Jump Step and Toilet Seat for a Wheelchair

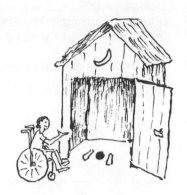

Two problems: In many Third World countries (as also in France), toilets and latrines are made for squatting over, rather than for sitting on. Basically they consist of a hole in the floor. This can be a big challenge for the wheelchair rider.

Also, in some countries, people traditionally work and eat at floor level. In the Introduction of this book (page 15), we saw the difficulty that Mira had with her standard wheelchair. Its height kept her from joining in kitchen work and family meals, where everyone squats or sits on the floor.

Finding Solutions: Solutions to each of these difficulties have been found by wheelchair riders and travelers. A simple solution to both problems has been devised by Ralf Hotchkiss. The device started as an improvisation to meet his personal needs, as well as those of other adventurers who travel in off-road situations and sometimes fall out of their wheelchairs.

For Ralf and others whose spinal-cord injury is at a relatively high level, getting back into the wheelchair without help can be difficult. Wheelchair users, as part of their rehabilitation, are often taught to get back up from the floor using a stool or a box of an intermediate height. But on a country road or desert trail, a stool or box may not be available.

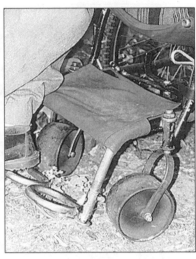

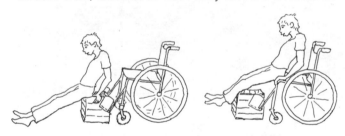

Some people get up into their wheelchair using a low box or stool . . .   but Ralf uses a built-in jump seat.

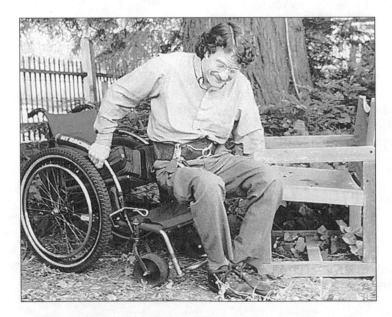

JUMP SEAT. To get back into his wheelchair from the ground in such circumstances, Ralf designed a small cloth step, or "jump seat" (transfer seat), halfway between his wheelchair seat and the ground.

This way, he can first lift himself onto the low-level seat, and from there, into the wheelchair seat. (The front edge of the jump seat also functions as an ankle-band, to keep his feet from slipping backward off the footrests.)

TOILET SEAT. While traveling in Kenya, Ralf faced the difficulty of trying to use pit latrines that had no seat. A Kenyan wheelchair rider suggested that he cut a round hole in the jump seat of his chair, and perch on that. Ralf did so, and it worked.

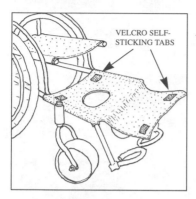

VELCRO SELF-STICKING TABS

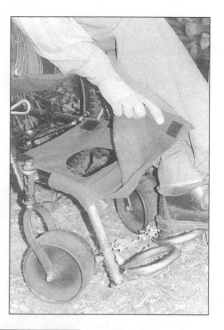

In the revised design of the jump seat and toilet seat, a flap is included which is kept in place for transfers, and is folded up out of the way for toileting or bathing.

The flap fastens into place with Velcro tabs.

(Velcro is a self-adhesive plastic tape, where tiny hooks on one surface catch on loops of the other.)

Note: Where Velcro is not available or is too costly, the flap can be held with buttons or ties.

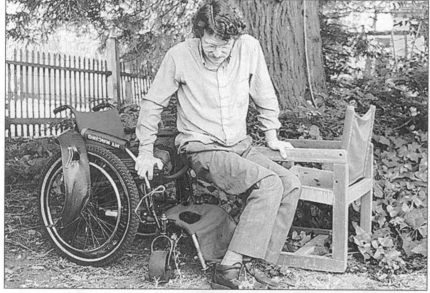

The new jump-seat design lends itself to many circumstances.

Consider again the example of Mira, mentioned above and in the Introduction. In order to work in the kitchen and eat with the family at ground level, she obtained a low-riding wheelchair, or trolley. But a jump seat on her standard wheelchair also might have helped her to easily move to the floor for meals and other activities.

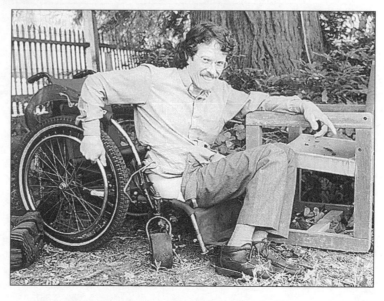

TROLLEY AND WHEELCHAIR TOILETS IN BANGLADESH

Trolley. At the *Center for Rehabilitation of the Paralyzed (CRP)* in Dhaka, Bangladesh, low-riding trolleys are often used instead of wheelchairs because people traditionally eat and cook at ground level (see page 15). The trolley rider sits on a soft coconut-fiber mat on top of an air-filled inner-tube (from a motor-scooter). To convert the tube to a toilet seat, the person just removes the mat.

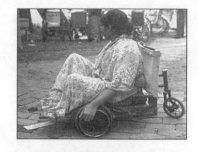

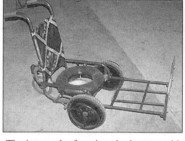

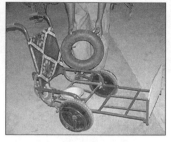

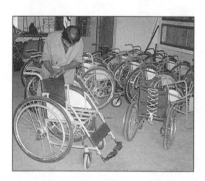

The inner tube functions both as a cushion and as a toilet seat. Centered under the hole, in the tube, a small removable aluminum removable pot fits into the metal frame of the trolley.

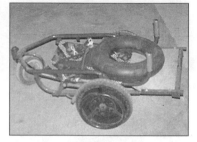

For travel on crowded buses, the trolley is collapsible. The back folds down. The projecting leg-rest slides in.

Wheelchair. The center in Dhaka (CRP) makes wheelchairs with a frame similar to Ralf Hotchkiss' Whirlwind. As with the trolley, however, a motor-scooter inner-tube is used as an air cushion, and also serves as a toilet. ——▶

◀—— Notice that the CRP wheelchairs have several of the same innovative features as does the new Whirlwind design. These include the laced back-rest which allows adjustment of the chair width.

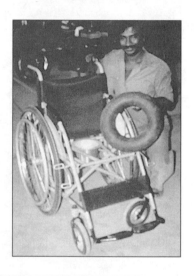

> ### The goal of a wheelchair is to increase the person's possibilities.

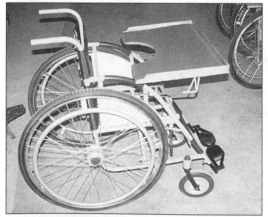

A nice feature of the CRP chair is a removable table that easily slips into small tubes welded to the arm-rests.

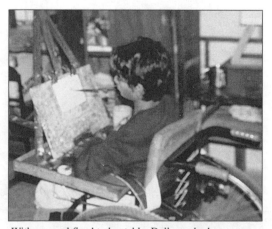

With an easel fixed to her table, Dolly—who has cerebral palsy—paints greeting cards with her mouth.

THE BEST OF BOTH WORLDS

Some of the best innovations come about through bridging conventional barriers and sharing widely varied experiences and skills. Remarkable designs have been developed when—by working together as equals—the gap has been closed between the First and Third Worlds, between professional and lay-persons, between the provider and recipient. Wonderful things happen when persons from different backgrounds pool their abilities and their dreams and learn from each other. According to Ralf Hotchkiss, this has been the secret to the evolution, and the many breakthroughs of the Whirlwind wheelchair.

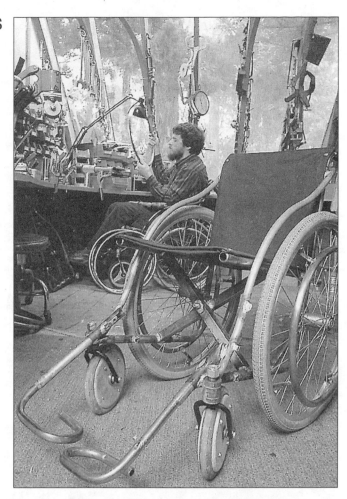

In the workshop in his California home, which has been imaginatively adapted for doing work from a wheelchair, Ralf experiments on and improves new designs and inventions by disabled wheelchair builders from many parts of the world.

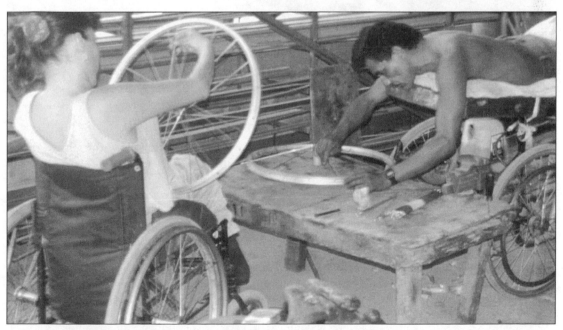

Jaime, one of Ralf's students and co-workers at PROJIMO, joins his girlfriend, Irma, in spoking the wheels of an improved model of the Whirlwind wheelchair. By sharing ideas and working together, Ralf and the PROJIMO team make design improvements that neither may have realized alone.

SAFETY FIRST in Wheelchair Design

For many wheelchair riders, **the biggest danger of all is pressure sores** (see Chapter 27). Good cushions help. But the design of the chair can also make a difference. If the rider has a spinal-cord injury fairly low down his back, he may prefer **a low back-rest like this.** Every few minutes he can lean far back to lift his backside off the seat, thus helping to prevent sores. (But if his injury is higher-up, he may want a higher back-rest for more support.) **Each individual's needs differ and may change over time.**

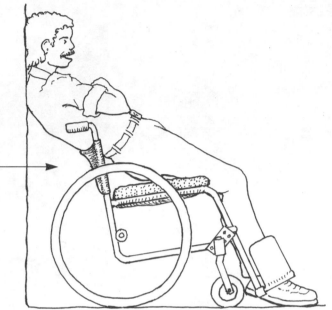

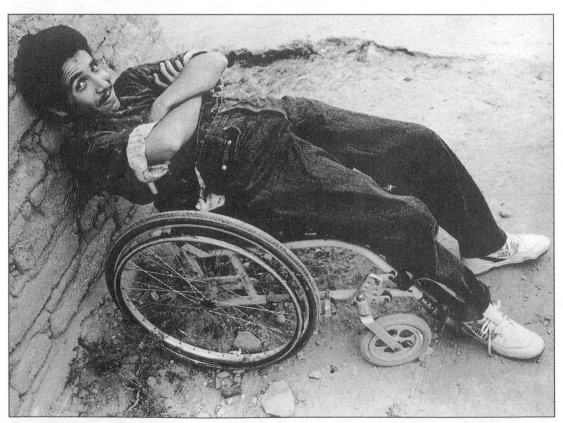

Wheelchairs serve many purposes. Here, Raymundo, a brace maker and wheelchair builder at PROJIMO, has found an effortless way to relieve the pressure on his backside and prevent sores.

For Long Runs on Lousy Roads: A Hand-Pumped Tricycle

ALEJANDRO'S CHANGING MOBILITY NEEDS

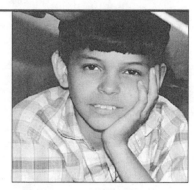

ALEJANDRO was 12 years old when he was shot through the spine by a policeman. The events surrounding this brutal incident will be briefly described in Chapter 40, page 261, under the heading, "Defense of Human Rights." Here, we will focus on Alejandro's changing mobility needs, and the equipment designed at PROJIMO to help him move about at the different stages of his rehabilitation and re-entry into community life.

*Alejandro first arrived at PROJIMO two months after his injury. For a child who was completely paralyzed from the mid-back down, he was in good spirits. Although he had been told he might never walk again, he was eager to get back into action. He progressed through using 3 forms of locomotion: **a gurney, a wheelchair,** and **a tricycle**.*

A GURNEY to Recover from Pressure Sores and Prevent Urinary Infections

Like so many spinal-cord injured young people who come to PROJIMO, Alejandro already had deep pressure sores when he arrived. The sores had begun to form while he was in the hospital. Therefore, his first mobility aid was a wheeled cot, or gurney (see Chapter 37). This allowed him to lie on his stomach, taking pressure off the sores on his butt. In the wheelchair shop, the gurney was built to the boy's size.

At Alejandro's request, **a simple rack to hold a container with drinking water** was made from a plastic gallon bottle and attached to the front of the gurney. Handy access to drinking water is essential, especially in a hot climate, because *one of the best ways to prevent bladder and kidney infection is to drink lots and lots of water.* For Alejandro to have his own water container (with its attached plastic straw) within easy reach wherever he went, was an important (and possibly life-saving) measure.

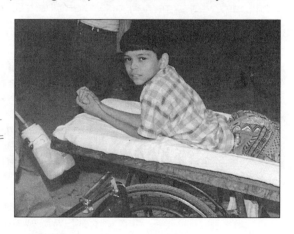

The gurney had another feature to help prevent urinary infections: **a built in free-flow urinal** (see next page).

With spinal-cord injury, the person usually loses bladder (and bowel) control. To get the urine out and prevent wetting the clothing, a catheter (thin tube) is often used. Whenever possible, however, it is important that spinal-cord injured persons avoid using a permanent (Foley) catheter (see box). If the catheter is left in continuously, it is likely to cause urinary infections (see page 147).

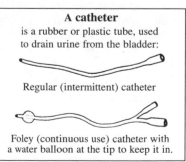

A catheter
is a rubber or plastic tube, used
to drain urine from the bladder:

Regular (intermittent) catheter

Foley (continuous use) catheter with
a water balloon at the tip to keep it in.

WARNING: For persons with a spinal-cord injury (or spina bifida),
pressure sores and urinary infections are the most common causes of death.

To help Alejandro keep dry, and yet avoid the need for a permanent catheter, his gurney had a hole cut out of it in the position of his genitals. This way, he could urinate into a container hanging under the gurney, without needing a permanent catheter. (The hole also prevents injuring the genitals, which, because they lack feeling, can be easily injured.) Gurneys can be built with a potty or other removable container attached under the hole in the gurney. Or, a large funnel can be mounted under the hole, with a plastic tube that drains into a urine bag.

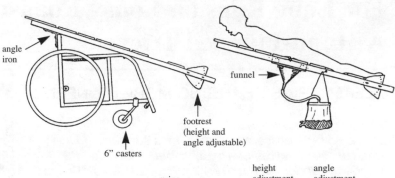

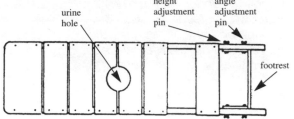

A Wheelchair to Take Part in Village Life

Partly because he was so active on his gurney, Alejandro's large pressure sores healed quickly. Within 2 months, he was ready for a wheelchair. He experimented with different models at PROJIMO until he had an idea of what would work best for him. The wheelchair builders then took his measurements and built a version of the **Whirlwind wheelchair** (see Chapter 30). In his new chair, Alejandro was extremely active, and he took part in a wide variety of adventures with other youth in the village, including swimming in the river.

At first, Alejandro used an air-filled cushion on his wheelchair to prevent pressure sores. But even with the cushion (and in spite of repeated advice from Mari and others to often lift his butt off the seat) Alejandro began to develop new sores.

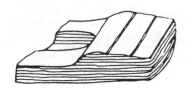

When well-made, tests show cardboard cushions prevent pressure sores as well as costly air-balloon cushions do.

His younger brother, Neto, with guidance from the PROJIMO team, helped him make **a personalized cushion out of layers of cardboard** glued together with white glue (see Chapter 27). Before the glue was dry, they sprinkled the cardboard with water to make it softer. Then, Alejandro sat on the cushion so that it would take the shape of his backside. Finally, they cut an oval out of the back part of the cushion to further reduce pressure over the butt-bones where the pressure sores often form. To make the cushion softer, they covered it with a layer of fairly dense foam rubber. The whole thing slipped into a protective cloth pillowcase.

With his cardboard cushion—plus daily treatment of the sores with honey and sugar, and remembering to shift his weight regularly— Alejandro's sores healed rapidly.

Time passed . . . When Alejandro first came to PROJIMO, the team had realized that the treatment of his pressure sores would take months. Because proper management of his sores at home was unlikely, they arranged for him to stay in Ajoya (where PROJIMO is based) and to attend the village school. For a time he did well, but eventually he dropped out and got married to a girl of his own age (14 years old). He took his young wife to his parents home, but life was difficult. His parents drank a lot and neither was employed. Often the family went hungry. Alejandro began to think of how he and his young wife could have a better future.

A TRICYCLE to Continue Schooling

Fortunately for Alejandro and his family, PROJIMO has relations with *Liliane Fonds*, a non-government charity in Holland that assists individual disabled children and their families. Liliane knows that a family's economic survival is basic to a disabled child's survival and well-being. A little "seed money" from Liliane helped the family begin to earn a living through the informal economy. Marcelo, at PROJIMO, built **a metal cart for frying and selling tacos,** which the family could put on a street corner in the evening and earn a modest income.

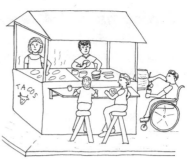

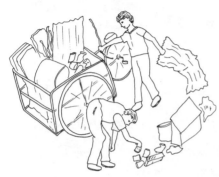

Later, Liliane financed a strong, **pedal-powered tricycle with a big carriage area.** With this, Alejandro's brothers (who could find no formal employment) rode through the city streets collecting old cardboard, aluminum cans, and scrap metal. They could sell these for enough to put a bit of food on the family table.

Even so, sometimes there was not enough to eat. In Mexico, as in so many countries, unemployment increases and wages decline as the gap between rich and poor continues to widen. Unable to do many forms of physical "unskilled" labor, Alejandro began to think about returning to school.

Dolores Mesina—a big-hearted social worker who had polio as a child and has close ties with PROJIMO (see page 261)—arranged for Alejandro (at age 16) to get a **scholarship to a technical school.** Alejandro could study practical skills there, ranging from small-motor repair to secretarial and computers skills. He was eager to attend.

However, there was a major difficulty: how to get there. The school was on the far side of the city, 5 kilometers away. Buses were not equipped to take wheelchairs, and they were terribly crowded. Taxis were too costly. The roads were too rough and the traffic too heavy for travel in his wheelchair to be safe.

Alejandro thought of a solution for getting to the distant school: **a hand-powered tricycle.** Geoff Thomsby, a wheelchair builder with experience in Africa, had volunteered at PROJIMO for over a year. He had taught the PROJIMO workers to build a hand-pumped tricycle that he had developed from models used in Cameroon, Africa. While at PROJIMO, Alejandro had tried out a tricycle, and loved it. With its large size and big front wheel, it zoomed safely over uneven terrain. For long distance travel, the rider could keep up a relatively high speed without tiring nearly as much as with a regular wheelchair, even a "Whirlwind."

Again Liliane Fonds assisted with the costs. Alejandro went back to PROJIMO and helped to repair a used tricycle, which the team agreed to let him have at a reduced price. The fact that Alejandro himself helped repair the tricycle gave him both the knowledge and the responsibility for its upkeep. Alejandro now cruises all over the city of Mazatlán, visiting friends and attending social gatherings. The tricycle has been Alejandro's ticket to a new level of freedom.

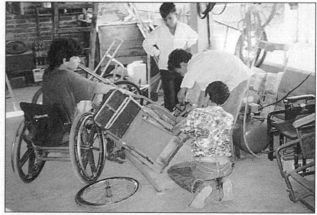

Village children help Alejandro repair his hand-powered tricycle.

HAND-POWERED TRICYCLES

Strengths and Weaknesses

Although hand-powered tricycles are widely used in Asia and Africa, they are little-known in most of Latin America. But there is certainly a need for them.

The main advantages of the tricycle are that its large front wheel, large size, and hand-power mechanism (whether by crank or pump) permit **easier, faster safer travel over rough terrain.**

The tricycle is most useful for disabled people with specific needs, such as:

* Persons, like Alejandro, who **travel long distances** to school or work on rough roads or in heavy traffic.

* Persons with **only one hand** strong enough to push a wheelchair—such as those with one-sided paralysis.

* People who **can walk short distances**, with or without crutches, but need wheels for going longer distances.

Disadvantages. The tricycle is not ideal for every rider's needs. Its **large size** (length and width) makes it unfit for indoor use (or for bus travel).

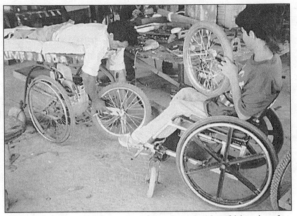
Jaime teaches Alejandro to spoke the wheels of his tricycle.

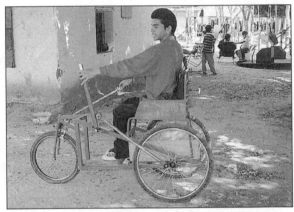
Alejandro with his tricycle (when he was 16 year old).

At PROJIMO the two workers who at once fell in love with the tricycle were Armando and Inez. Both use crutches. Although Armando walks with crutches in the wheel-chair shop, he enjoys using the tricycle to move about in the village. It is easier for him than a wheelchair, because one arm (as well as both legs) is weak from polio. He powers the tricycle with his stronger arm, and steers it with his weaker one.

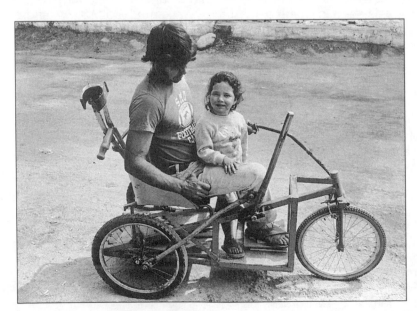

Inez's arms are both strong. But he lives at the far end of the village, a long distance away on crutches. The tricycle gets him there quickly. It is big and strong enough so he can give his two young daughters a ride on it, which they love.

Inez gives one of his daughters a ride on his tricycle wheelchair.

A Tricycle and Dignity for Don Miguel

A person who found the tricycle wheelchair especially enabling was DON MIGUEL. Don Miguel (who recently died) was an elderly man who had come to PROJIMO with a huge, open sore (ulcer) on one leg. The lack of feeling and scars from burns on his hands and feet gave the clue that he had Hansen's disease (leprosy). At first he denied this. But, later, he admitted that he had undergone treatment for the disease.

The ulcer needed long-term treatment, and the leg needed to be kept elevated (higher than the level of his heart) when he was not physically active. So, Don Miguel was invited to spend an extended period of time at PROJIMO, for treatment and rehabilitation.

In truth, Don Miguel's biggest need was to feel respected and needed. Because of people's fear and lack of correct information about leprosy, he had been rejected wherever he went. His relatives occasionally helped him with a little money, but preferred that he keep his distance. He had a kindness and wry sense of humor about him, born of loneliness. A good man, but misunderstood.

In PROJIMO, Don Miguel found a new family: people who welcomed and accepted him. Why a group of disabled persons should be more accepting of someone with leprosy than most other people, is hard to say. Perhaps it was because they, too, have felt rejected, slighted—or worst of all, pitied—for their various disabilities. Stigma is stigma.

In PROJIMO, Don Miguel discovered not only that he was welcome, but needed! Though he had arthritic pain secondary to his disease, he was more able-bodied than many PROJIMO workers. He began helping in any way he could. He moved and bathed persons in need of assistance. And he took over the maintenance of the grounds and playground.

There was always a lot of garbage to clean up. This Don Miguel would do religiously every morning. But moving about was difficult for him. One day, he asked if he could use a tricycle. Everyone said yes. To help him with the clean-up, **the wheelchair builders made a large cart which could be attached to the back of the tricycle, like a trailer.** Don Miguel would ride around the grounds, getting out here and there to put trash into the cart.

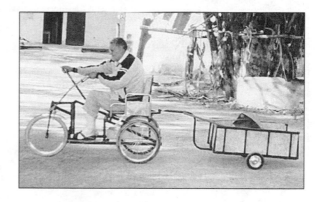

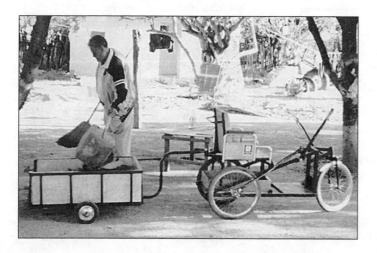

Don Miguel stayed at PROJIMO for nearly two years . . . the last two of his life. He was a good influence on the team, a peacemaker in times of strife. Everyone liked him. One day he said he was leaving, and a few weeks later the team learned from his family that he was dead. He had been a warm and stabilizing influence on the program.

We miss him.

Design and Construction of A Lever-Powered PROJIMO Tricycle

The PROJIMO tricycle is one of many different designs in different parts of the world. One feature of the PROJIMO tricycle that differs from many is its **lever-powered drive.** Most tricycles are powered by hand-rotated pedals (often modified bicycle pedals), and the power is transferred to either the front wheel or one of the back wheels by means of a bicycle chain. The problem with chains is that they can break fairly easily. The lever-powered drive mechanism is more resilient and requires less maintenance. Also, rear-wheel (rather than front-wheel) drive provides better traction on sand and steep slopes.

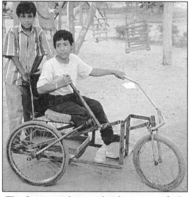

The front steering mechanism uses a fork made with strong metal tubes. The front wheel is a 24-inch bicycle wheel.

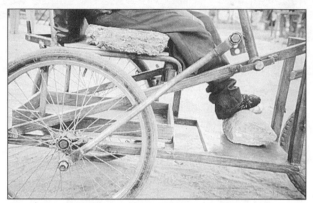

The hand-powered lever is attached to an arm welded to the hub and a bracket welded to the frame. It works like the drive mechanism of a railroad train.

Examples of Different Tricycle Designs from Different Lands

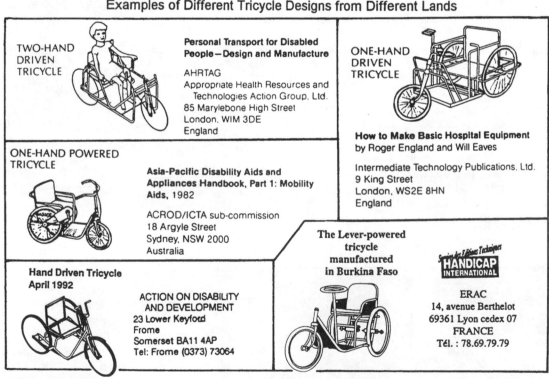

TWO-HAND DRIVEN TRICYCLE

Personal Transport for Disabled People — Design and Manufacture

AHRTAG
Appropriate Health Resources and Technologies Action Group, Ltd.
85 Marylebone High Street
London. W1M 3DE
England

ONE-HAND DRIVEN TRICYCLE

How to Make Basic Hospital Equipment
by Roger England and Will Eaves

Intermediate Technology Publications. Ltd.
9 King Street
London, WS2E 8HN
England

ONE-HAND POWERED TRICYCLE

Asia-Pacific Disability Aids and Appliances Handbook, Part 1: Mobility Aids, 1982

ACROD/ICTA sub-commission
18 Argyle Street
Sydney. NSW 2000
Australia

Hand Driven Tricycle
April 1992

ACTION ON DISABILITY AND DEVELOPMENT
23 Lower Keyford
Frome
Somerset BA11 4AP
Tel: Frome (0373) 73064

The Lever-powered tricycle manufactured in Burkina Faso

HANDICAP INTERNATIONAL

ERAC
14, avenue Berthelot
69361 Lyon cedex 07
FRANCE
Tél. : 78.69.79.79

Note: Some tricycles are powered with only one hand. Others are powered with both hands (in which case the steering mechanism and drive mechanism are usually on the same bar, attached to the front fork). Some have hand-powered drive pedals (handles) on both sides of the tricycle, so that when one of the rider's arms tires she can use the other. It is important to pick the design that best meets the needs of the particular user. Booklets exist on different designs of tricycle wheelchairs. Some examples are shown here. (Also see Resource List #2 at the end of this book, page 343.)

Worldwide Sharing of Tricycle Know-How, Coordinated by
APPROPRIATE MOBILITY INTERNATIONAL

Great progress is under way in terms of the sharing of knowledge about different designs of hand-powered tricycles. A world-wide information sharing network has been launched by a group called *Appropriate Mobility International (AMI),* based at Delft University of Technology, in Holland. Joep Verweij of AMI has collected information and photos on scores of tricycle designs from rich countries and poor, world-wide. He has assembled these in an Overview Report titled *Inventory of Tricycle Models* (see page 344). The wide diversity of design is a testimony to the creativity of disabled people and local craftspersons. Here are a few examples of this diversity, taken from the *Inventory of Tricycle Models,* and elsewhere:

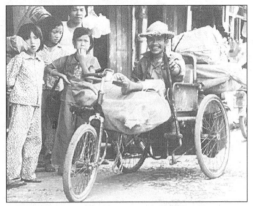

Thailand. A hand-pump powers one rear wheel. Steers with foot. Heavy duty for hauling cargo.

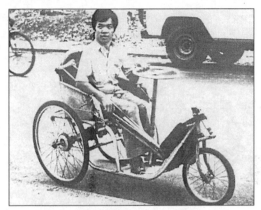

Vietnam. Designed in **France**. Steering column pumps back and forth to give dual rear-wheel drive.

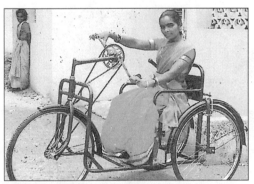

India. Hand-crank powers the front wheel. Good for flat paved roads; poor traction on hills and sand.

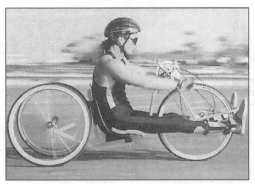

Racing trike. Sold commercially in **USA**. Front-wheel drive. Rider's forward position increases traction.

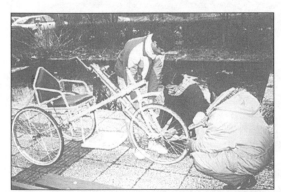

Workshop managers from **India** and **Sri Lanka** discuss an experimental model for a new design of wheelchair, developed in partnership with *Appropriate Mobility International (AMI),* in **Holland**.

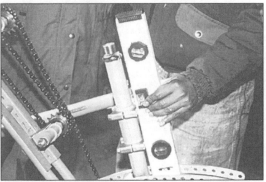

Most features of the AMI experimental model (shown on the left) are adjustable, so it can be tested by different riders with the wheels, hand-crank, and other parts at different angles and positions.

High-Tech Communications for Grass-Roots Shop Workers:
"Tricycle Production Manual," by the *Folks at Appropriate Mobility International*

Based on their research and the design perspectives of tricycle users and designers from all over the world, folks at AMI and the *Center for International Cooperation and Appropriate Technology* have put together a remarkable instruction manual. With **hundreds of line drawings and very few words,** the manual guides the reader through the steps of building an improved model of a hand-operated tricycle.

The Table of Contents of the Manual uses the pictures shown below to indicate headings:

1. TRICYCLE
2. PRODUCTION
3. ADDITIONS
4. MATERIALS
5. INFORMATION

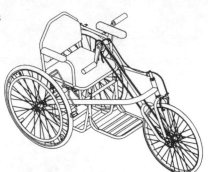

Research in preparation of the manual included a study of people's ability to interpret pictures. As a result, many of the drawings—which have been done with great precision with a computerized graphics program—are 3-dimensional, as shown below.

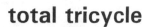

total tricycle

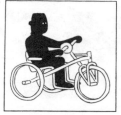

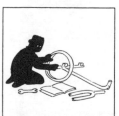

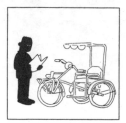

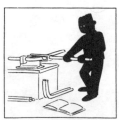

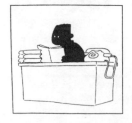

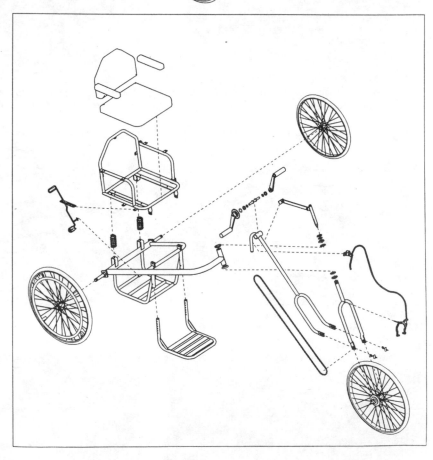

This innovative manual deserves careful study, not only by wheelchair builders, but by anyone interested in exploring new ways of communicating clearly. Through the use of step-by-step series' of computerized drawings, it attempts to bridge the gap between sophisticated technology and the traditional skills of local craftspersons, whose understanding tends to be based on real (or at least realistically drawn) objects rather than written words. (See Resource List #2, on page 344.)

A CONVERTIBLE TRICYCLE-WHEELCHAIR FOR ALEJANDRO

At the time this book went to press, Alejandro had been offered a scholarship to study English at the *Academia de Inglés Golden Gate,* in his home city of Mazatlán. (The Academy is run by a disabled youth, José Angel Tirado, whom PROJIMO assisted in his childhood. See page 315.) To get to the Academy on the rough, heavily trafficked roads, Alejandro could use the sturdy tricycle made for him at PROJIMO. But this outdoor vehicle was much too big to move about inside the Academy or to enter a classroom.

Therefore the PROJIMO team decided they should make a tricycle that Alejandro could quickly convert into an ordinary wheelchair for indoor use. Armando remembered seeing a design for such a tricycle in a booklet called *Making Health Care Equipment* (see page 343). It consisted of a standard wheelchair to which a tricycle front-end (including a large front wheel, hand pedals, and a steering mechanism) could be easily attached or removed.

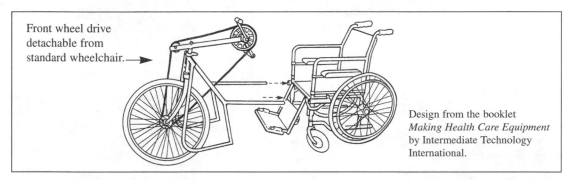

Front wheel drive detachable from standard wheelchair.

Design from the booklet *Making Health Care Equipment* by Intermediate Technology International.

Alejandro thought that such a trike would meet his needs. For long distance rides on rough roads, he could use the full tricycle. On arrival at the Academy (or at home) he could unplug the front section and enter the building in the compact wheelchair.

For this experimental model, Armando and Marcelo adapted a standard donated wheelchair. They used a 24-inch bicycle wheel at the front. They welded together a tube frame, with rods that could slip into the side tubes of the chair seat.

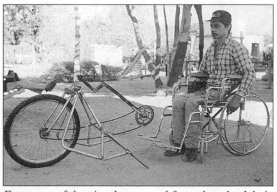

Front part of the tricycle removed from the wheelchair.

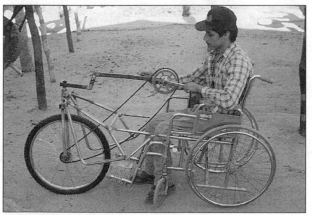

Marcelo experiments with the new design.

Need for improvements:

At the time of this writing, the experimental design had been built and tested, but still had problems. The chain that linked the hand crank to the front wheel occasionally jumped off the sprockets (which needed better alignment). Also, some sort of device or blocks were needed to hold the chair's caster wheels a couple of centimeters off the ground—so that Alejandro can plug in or remove the tricycle unit while sitting in the chair.

Tricycle designs must be adapted to local needs. In urban Mexico, a standard tricycle is too long to fit into buildings and classrooms. In rural Africa, a standard tricycle is too wide to ride on narrow dirt trails. An African boy's innovative solution is shown on the next page.

PAFUPI BUILDS HIS OWN TRICYCLE FOR NARROW TRIALS

PAFUPI lived in a remote village in Malawi, Africa. Because his legs were paralyzed by polio, he had started school later than most children. The school was too far away to walk to on his braces and crutches. He dreamed of having a hand-powered tricycle. But the trails where he lived were much too narrow for the big, wide tricycles made in the cities.

Pafupi was good with his hands and had an inventive streak. As a child he had made a guitar from old tin cans and scraps of leather. And he had learned to play it fairly well.

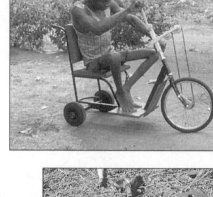

When he was 17, Pafupi decided to make a small tricycle that was narrow enough to ride on local trails. He used parts of 3 old bicycles, an old flywheel, and bits of scrap metal. He had no welding equipment. So he hammered the ends of the pieces together precisely, like interlocking fingers. Although the joints were slightly flexible, they were remarkably strong.

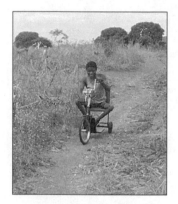

On his way home from school, Pafupi rides his improved "narrow gauge" tricycle, designed for the narrow trails.

The tools Pafupi used to make his tricycle were very basic: a small block of iron which he used as an anvil, 2 hammers, and a piece of an old hack-saw blade held in a curved metal pipe.

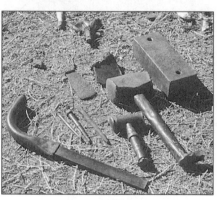

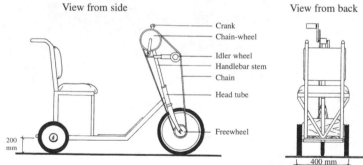

View from side

Crank
Chain-wheel
Idler wheel
Handlebar stem
Chain
Head tube
Freewheel

200 mm

View from back

400 mm

View from above

Hand grip   Fork

People Potential
PLUM COTTAGE
HATTINGLEY
ALTON
HAMPSHIRE GU34 5NQ U.K.

On a trip to Malawi, Kennett Westmacott, an innovator of disability aids, saw Pafupi on his home-made tricycle. (In England, Kennett and his wife, Jean, run *People Potential,* where they teach ordinary people to design and make simple assistive devices. See pages 72 and 74). Fascinated by the appropriateness of Pafupi's home-made tricycle, Kennett and his students tried to build one like it in a training workshop. But their modified version had problems. To get it to work well, the group had to rebuild the tricycle, closely following Pafupi's design. Then they modified it with a bigger front wheel and other helpful changes.

An outstanding feature of Pafupi's tricycle was that he could pedal it in reverse (make it back up), something Kennett had not seen before in small, chain-driven tricycles.

The group was amazed that Pafupi—a village boy in primary school—was able to create such a well-adapted and functional vehicle, all done with very simple tools and without welding. Their respect for the skill and creativity of disabled villagers increased greatly.

CHAPTER 32

Mobility Aids, a Walking Toilet, and a Seeing-Eye Person for Carlos

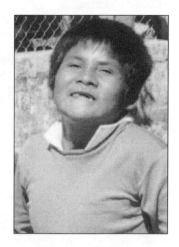

CARLOS is the son of migrant farm workers from Oaxaca, one of the poorest states of Mexico. During harvesting season, his family used to come north to Sinaloa (the state where PROJIMO is located) to pick tomatoes. When he was 8 years old, Carlos already worked with his parents in the fields. Sadly, when he was 10, the boy was hit by a truck and his brain was severely damaged. He remained mentally and physically disabled, and also visually impaired.

Months after his accident, Carlos was taken to PROJIMO by state social workers. While he was still in the hospital, his parents had abandoned him. Apparently they had gone back to Oaxaca, without leaving an address. The social workers asked if PROJIMO could provide rehabilitation for the boy. In effect, PROJIMO became Carlos' new family.

On arrival, Carlos already had secondary physical and emotional problems. His spastic body had become very stiff, and he had contractures of his hips and knees. He was almost totally blind, and his mind did not function well. He had very little short-term memory and difficulty learning even simple things. The few words he spoke were mostly abusive swear words. He got angry easily, and often cursed and spit at persons trying to help him. He would repeatedly plead "I want water!" or "I want food!" even when he had just had plenty to eat and drink. He constantly wet and pooped his clothing and bed.

Carlitos (as he was affectionately called) needed a lot of personal assistance, plus a huge amount of understanding and patience. Fortunately, an older woman named Rosa, who has worked at PROJIMO for years, became like a mother to him. Rosa lovingly bathed him and washed his soiled clothes 2 or 3 times a day.

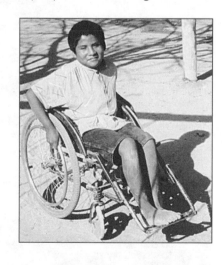

Mobility. To help Carlitos move himself about, one of the first things the shop-workers did was to build a wheelchair adapted to his size and needs. At first he could not move his wheelchair at all. But, little by little, he learned to roll it about. In time, he could more or less find his way on the pathways between buildings.

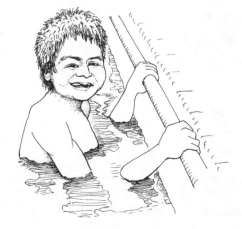

Water Play as Therapy. In preparation for standing and walking, the team helped Carlitos with range-of-motion and stretching exercises. These helped to correct contractures and reduce the spasticity of his hips and knees. At first, he angrily resisted the exercises. But when the team tried working—and playing—with him in water, he loved it. The water supported his weight and let him move without the fear of falling. His pleasure and activity in the water seemed to help his stiff body to loosen up.

Standing. Although Carlitos' knees still bent stiffly when he tried to stand, the team felt he had the potential for learning how to stand and walk. At first he was non-cooperative, and understandably so. After nearly a year without weight-bearing, standing hurt his feet. But with daily practice his feet toughened.

The team found that the best way to get Carlos to try to stand was to put him with another child who was learning to stand.

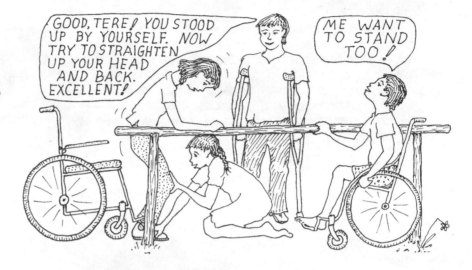

Carlitos watched Tere trying to stand at the parallel bars.

When Tere's helpers praised her enthusiastically for her efforts, Carlitos suddenly said, "Me want to stand!"

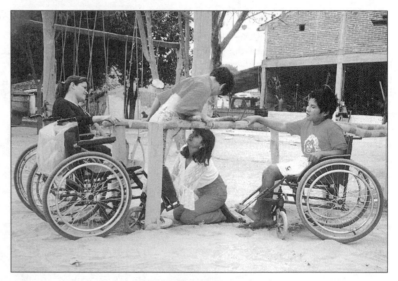

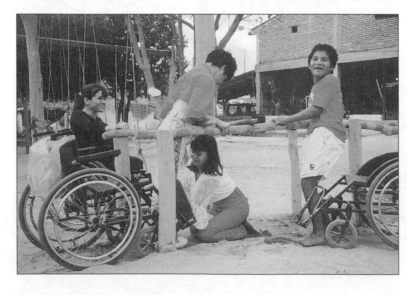

He made an effort to do so . . . and finally succeeded in pulling himself up to stand.

Walking. When Carlitos first tried to stand at the parallel bars he had very poor balance. He practiced daily. Little by little, his balance improved until he could take a few steps, holding onto the bars.

After months of practice, he learned to walk back and forth between the bars with fair stability. When Carlos began to say "I want walker!" the team asked Jaime to design a walker that would meet the boy's needs.

Mari and Inez tested him with walkers of different sizes and heights. At last they found a combination of features that allowed him to stand straighter and more firmly. Jaime, a paraplegic wheelchair builder who works lying on a gurney (wheeled cot), built the walker out of steel tubing. He used thin-wall electric conduit tubing, the same material used to make the wheelchairs.

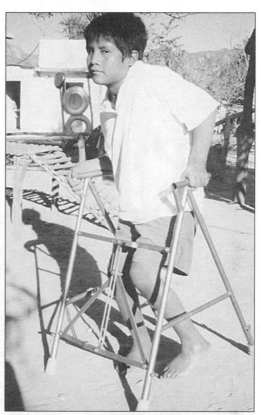

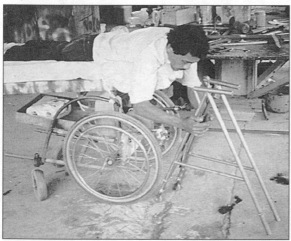

To make the folding mechanism, Jaime used the same recent innovation that the shop workers use on an improved design of the Whirlwind wheelchair (see p. 190).

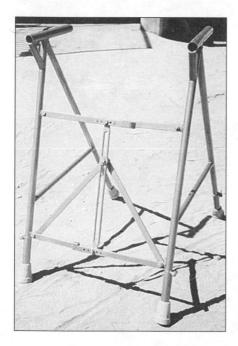

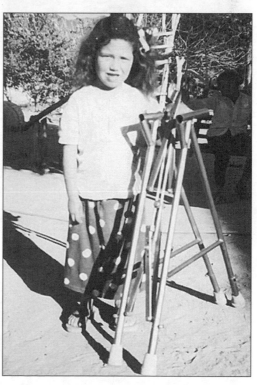

The folding mechanism worked well, providing a stable walker that was easy to fold.

A Wooden Walker with a Seat

Carlitos enjoyed walking with his new metal walker. But his attention span was brief and he tired quickly. After a few minutes, he would want to sit in his wheelchair. And a few minutes later, he would want to walk again. Because he was blind and had difficulty remembering, it was hard for him to find things. All day long he would call out to people to bring him his walker or his wheelchair. When everyone was busy there was sometimes a delay, and he would get angry and frustrated. "Carlos want walk NOW!" he would wail.

One day, Juán, a disabled carpenter and brace-maker, asked Carlos, "Carlitos, would you like a walker with a seat on it, so that you can sit down and rest when you're tired of walking?"

"Yes" said Carlos eagerly. "Carlos want walker with seat." So Juán made him a unique wooden walker with a seat.

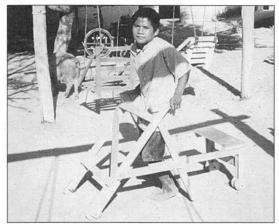

Carlos walks with his wooden walker.

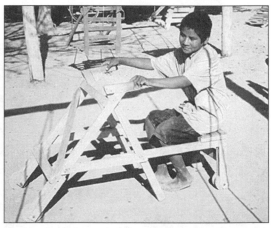

Carlos sits and rests in his walker.

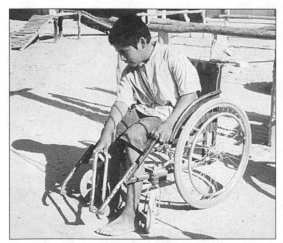

To move from wheelchair to walker, Carlos first lifts aside the footrest. (A single footrest for both feet, hinged on one side, makes this easier for him.)

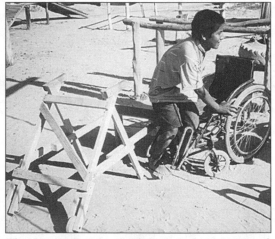

Then he stands and turns his body to sit on the seat of the walker. Next, he will lift his feet over the wooden bar.

Although transferring from his wheelchair to the wooden walker required stepping over the wooden bar that supported the seat, Carlos soon learned to transfer without help.

With his new walker, Carlos became more independent. He no longer needed to always ask people for help, and he began to take pride in doing things for himself. His self-help skills in walking helped prepare him for a better response to toilet training (see p. 212).

A "Seeing-Eye Person" for Carlos.
With his walkers, Carlos' walking improved. But being blind, he had a hard time finding his way. Someone suggested a seeing-eye dog. But it was easier to provide a "seeing-eye person."

At PROJIMO there are always young wheel-chair users who have trouble moving about by themselves. These include Tere and Lupita, who have spastic arms and legs. One day, Tere was practicing standing at the parallel bars. At the same time, Carlos was walking in circles around the outside of the bars, holding on with only one hand. To do this, Carlos had to circle around Tere's wheel-chair. Once when he took hold of the handles of her wheelchair, he laughed and tried to push it, like a walker. That gave Rosa an idea.

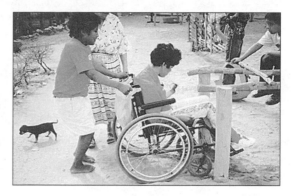

A Wheelchair as a Walker.
When Tere finished her standing session at the bars, she said she wanted to go to the laundry area to wash her clothes. Because she has difficulty moving her wheelchair on the uneven ground, she asked Rosa to push her. Half-joking, she said, "Carlitos, why don't you push Tere to the laundry area?"

Carlos grinned with excitement. "Yes! Carlitos want push Teresita!"

At first Tere was reluctant. Although she and Carlos were friends, she feared he would wheel her into a pit or tree. But Rosa explained to Tere that, by letting Carlos push her, she would be helping him with his therapy, his independence, and his self-esteem. So Tere agreed to give it a try.

Rosa guided Carlos' hands to the handles of Tere's wheelchair. Carlos pushed it eagerly. To keep on course, Tere told the blind boy where to go. At first he was confused. But after a while he learned to tell "Left!" from "Right!" and steer accordingly. Carlos had never seemed so happy, nor Tere more scared.

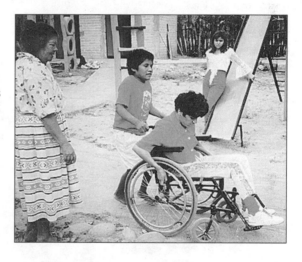

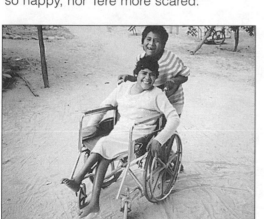

Carlos as a wheelchair-rider's attendant.

By that afternoon, Carlitos proudly also began to help Lupita move from one area of the play-ground to the other. He was walking more and better than he had ever walked before. And he was able to find his way, thanks to his "seeing eye persons." This mutual self-help by persons with different disabilities helped to build self-confidence in all who were involved. Carlos took great pride in his new role as a "wheelchair attendant."

Peer therapy. Tere, likewise, took pleasure in knowing that she was helping Carlos both develop his walking skills and gain a sense of being useful and appreciated. Lupita, whose mental handicap is as great as that of Carlos, was all smiles with the enthusiastic services of her newly found driver. In this way, multiply disabled young people have learned to help one another.

Toilet Training as Preparation for Standing, Balance, and Manual Skills

Carlos' toilet training advanced slowly, with modest gains. At first, he always pooped in his cot at night. Then he began occasionally to crawl off his cot and poop on the floor. To reinforce this response and take it further, Juán—with the help of two village school children—made a simple wooden toilet seat that could be placed over a bucket next to Carlos' cot.

To involve Carlos more with **making his toilet,** the group asked him if he wanted to help sand the wooden seat. Carlos, always eager to "work," responded, "Yes, Carlos want sand toilet." Perhaps because he had already tried sitting on the toilet and identified it as *his,* he did the sanding with more energy and persistence than usual.

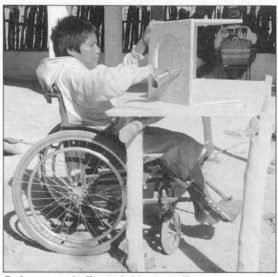

The next step was practice **using his toilet.** This involved sitting on the edge of the bed, standing up (while holding a metal bed frame turned on its side at the head of the bed), unbuttoning and loosening his pants, lowering his pants enough to avoid soiling them (while leaning against the bed frame), and sitting on the toilet. After using the toilet, he learned to repeat the same steps in reverse.

Carlos energetically sands his own toilet seat.

Steps in Carlos' toileting practice:

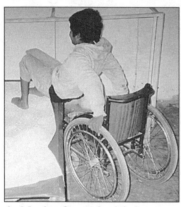

1. Moving from wheelchair to cot.

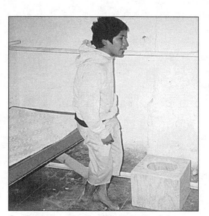

2. Standing up holding the bed frame.

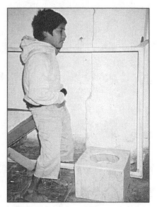

3. Loosening his pants.

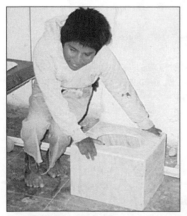

4. Shifting to the toilet.

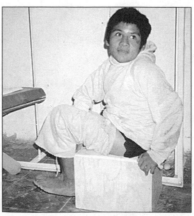

5. Sitting on the toilet.

Carlitos still has a long way to go until he has no accidents in his bed. But his bedside potty not only helps him with toilet training, it also helps with standing, balance, dressing and undressing skills, body coordination, and manual dexterity. He is eager to learn new skills, and takes pride in having helped make the toilet he is learning to use.

A WALKING TOILET FOR CARLOS

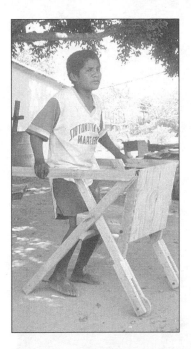

Problem. Carlos' new *walker-with-a-seat* (described on page 210) allowed him to sit down when and where he wanted. But the design had one big problem. Because the seat was mounted behind the space where he stood to push the walker, the whole device was over a meter long. This made moving in close quarters very cumbersome. If Carlos was to learn to walk to the dining room, he needed a walker that was more compact.

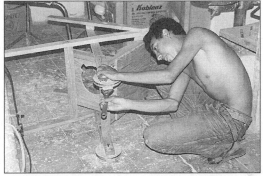

Martín, a village youth with severe chronic asthma, puts bigger wheels on Carlos' toilet walker so that it will roll more easily on rough ground.

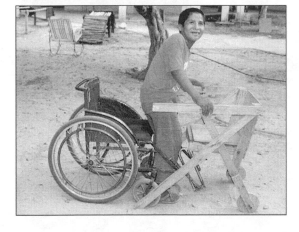

To solve this problem, PROJIMO designed a compact walker with the seat in front of him, not behind. Although he had to turn around to sit down, this walker had the advantage that it had *no poles to step over.*

Also, it *simplified transfers from the wheelchair.* Carlos could wheel his wheelchair between the rear legs of the walker, take hold of the walker's handle-bars and easily stand up.

Adaptation for urinating. One complication to having the seat of his walker in front of him was hygiene. Now that Carlos was partly toilet-trained, to urinate he would simply stand up and lower his pants. With his old walker (with the seat behind) that was all right. But to avoid wetting the forward-positioned seat of the new walker, the seat needed to be hinged so that Carlos could lift it out of the way before urinating.

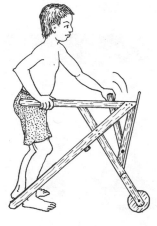

After a few days of coaching, Carlos took pride in lifting the seat before urinating.

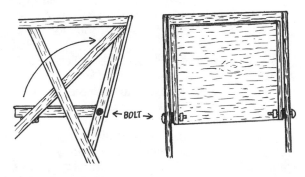

← BOLT →

The hinges for lifting the seat consist of a bolt slipped through holes in the walker frame and the seat frame.

Adding a potty. The idea to adapt the walker as a portable toilet came from necessity. It was springtime. The plum trees at PROJIMO hung heavy with fruit. The ripest plums fell to the ground. Carlos would park his walker in the shade of the trees, sit on the seat, and lean over to feel with his hands for the fallen fruit. In a short time, he would stuff his belly to bursting.

But this feast had a nasty side effect: *diarrhea.* Because Carlitos was blind and forgetful, he had not learned to take himself to the outhouse. Sometimes, when he had to go in a hurry, he called someone to take him. And sometimes he would poop in his pants. Rosa, who had to bath him and wash his clothes, was at her wits end.

To solve this problem, Polo helped to convert Carlos' walker into **a mobile toilet.** He cut a hole in the seat to hold a plastic bowl. Supported by its rim, the bowl could be lifted out to empty it. To use as an ordinary seat, a square board, hinged at the back, could be lowered over the bowl. To urinate, Carlos could swing the whole toilet up out of the way.

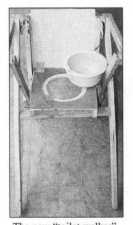
The new "toilet walker" with the potty removed from the toilet seat.

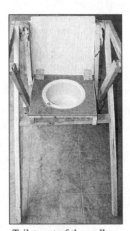
Toilet seat of the walker with the lid lifted out of the way.

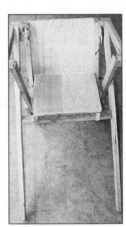
Toilet seat with the cover closed over it to form an ordinary seat.

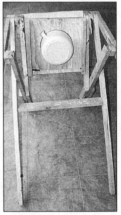
Walker with the entire seat, toilet, and cover tilted out of the way.

The invention saved the day. From one day to the next, Carlos became more independent in his toileting. The stimulation caused by his high-plum diet gave him plenty of practice, and he quickly learned to lift the lid and lower his pants.

What he never learned to do was to empty his potty. We all learned—the hard way— about the need to empty Carlos' potty often enough, especially during plum season.

One day, when he had filled his potty to the brim, he lost his bearings and fell over with his walker. He and the walker were covered with the potty's rank contents. Cecilia and the author helped with the clean up. It was no fun!

But, despite the occasional mishaps, Carlos loved his new walker. It not only gave him new freedom to move about, but helped him become more fully self-sufficient with his toilet.

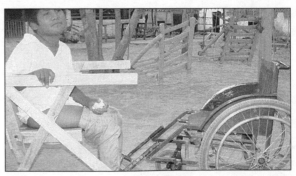
Carlos proudly uses his new mobile toilet.

Improvement

Bit by bit, in the 3 years that Carlos has been at PROJIMO, both his physical and mental abilities have improved. He has remembered songs from early childhood, and has learned new ones. He now talks more cleverly, remembers people's names, gets angry less often, and laughs gladly in response to friendliness or assistance. His common phrases now include "I want to walk" and "I want to work." He takes pride in using his toilet, and in staying dry and clean (sometimes).

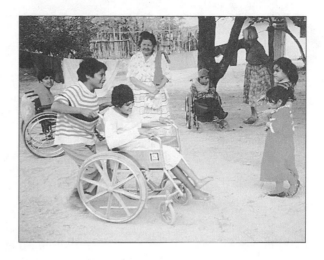

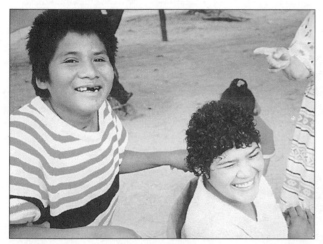

His attention span is still brief, but for several moments at a time, he helps with activities in the toy shop. All in all—through a team effort in which disabled persons help each other—Carlos has come a long way.

Most important of all, Carlos has made friends and learned how to enjoy life and people.

In addition to better balance, he now has more self-confidence in his abilities. **It was a day for celebration when, at last, Carlos began to stand without any support or assistance.**

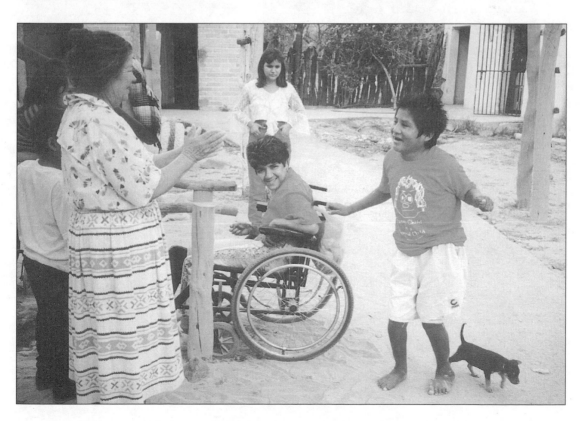

CARLOS HELPS ALONZO LEARN TO WALK

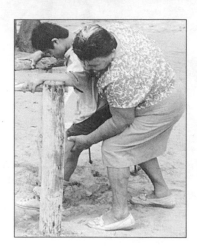

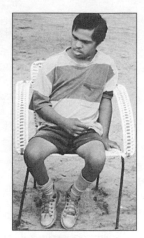

ALONZO is a 17-year-old youth with a condition called Cretinism, which he was born with because his mother lacked foods with enough iodine during pregnancy. Alonzo is developmentally delayed and small for his age. He speaks only a few words. He frowns a lot. To nearly every request he snaps "No!" Physically, he is strong and should have been able to walk, but he did not. To move him, his mother half-carried and half-dragged him. When she tried to help him stand or walk, he would sink to his knees.

The PROJIMO team invited Alonzo and his mother to stay at the center for a few days, to help him start walking. But Alonzo refused to cooperate. His mother did her best to stand him at the parallel bars, but he stubbornly resisted.

Inez, who helps with physical therapy, had an idea. He asked Carlitos to help teach Alonzo. Carlos (who, like Alonzo, had resisted beginning to walk when first at PROJIMO) loved the idea. Carlos started by demonstrating how he could walk between the bars.

"Look!" he cried. "Carlos can walk. So can you!" Alonzo watched with wonder.

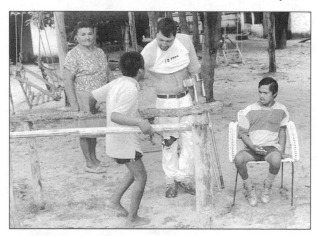

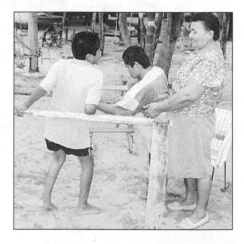

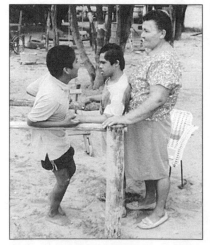

Now, when his mother lifted Alonzo to the bars, he resisted less. Carlos guided his friend's hands to the bars. To his mother's surprise, her son stood on his own.

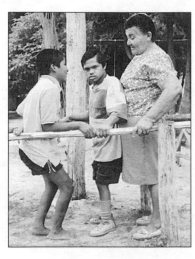

With Carlos encouraging him, Alonzo began to take a few steps. By the next day, he could walk between the bars by himself—and he almost smiled.

Alonzo Discovers the Advantage of Carlos' Walker

By the second day, Alonzo was more confident and willing to walk at the bars. His mother wanted him to try a walker. Inez chose a big blue wooden walker with front wheels. At first Alonzo refused. So Carlos paraded back and forth on his own walker. Alonzo decided to try.

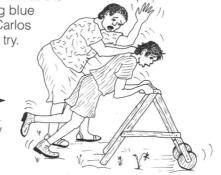

But a problem arose. Alonzo would push his walker and take small steps. But his feet did not keep up with his body. He leaned farther and farther forward until he almost fell. ⟶ His frightened mother would jump to catch him. After a few near-falls, Alonzo and his mother grew discouraged. Suddenly Alonzo, scowling, pointed at Carlos who was parading back and forth on his long wooden *walker-with-a-seat.*

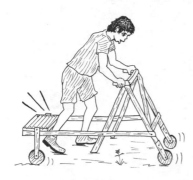

"Do you want to try Carlos' walker, Alonzo?" asked Inez intuitively. Alonzo frowned …but he did not say "No!" "That means Yes!" his mother interpreted. ("Yes" was not part of Alonzo's vocabulary.)

Carlos willingly moved to his wheelchair. Inez helped Alonzo step into his friend's walker. Without prompting, Alonzo began to walk. As before, he started to lean forward precariously. But before he fell, his legs bumped into the seat behind him, acting like a brake. With this braking action, Alonzo felt safer. By evening he was running all around the playground, his nervous mother close on his heels. Bruised stripes formed on the back of his calves from the many bumps against the seat edge. But Alonzo was so excited about his new skill that he did not mind.

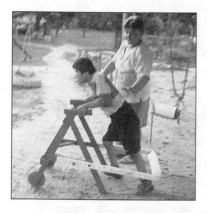

Building on Alonzo's discovery, the next day Polo modified the big blue walker.

⟶

He attached some adjustable side-bars that extended backward to support a padded cross-bar, to function as a leg-brake.

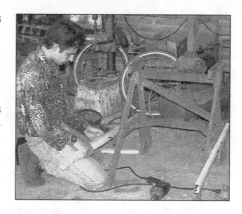

On testing, the new leg-brake worked fairly well. But Alonzo still leaned forward a lot. His mother still hovered over him, fearing he would fall. So Polo adjusted the rear brake-bar closer to the walker. ↓

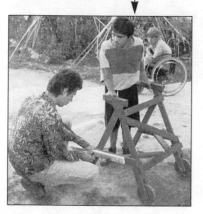

Now, with less leg room, it stopped Alonzo from leaning forward as much. He could walk more upright, and with greater control. ⟶

At last his mother was willing to stand back and let him walk alone.

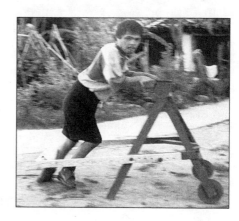

Carlos Helps Alonzo To Walk By Holding a Rope

To help Alonzo improve his balance so that eventually he could walk without any assistive device, the PROJIMO team suggested that his mother encourage him to walk while holding onto a rope stretched between two trees. The rope, being less stable than parallel bars or a walker, requires more balance. **Rope walking** can therefore be another step toward independent walking. At first the rope can be stretched tight, then gradually loosened as the child's balance and control increase.

As with the parallel bars and the walker, at first Alonzo was afraid to try to stand or walk holding the rope. Once again, Carlos came to the rescue. He walked back and forth holding the rope while Alonzo sat watching him. →

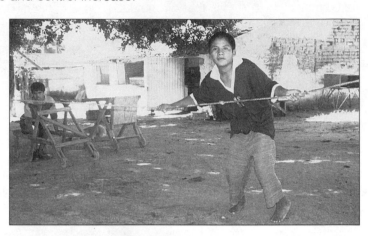

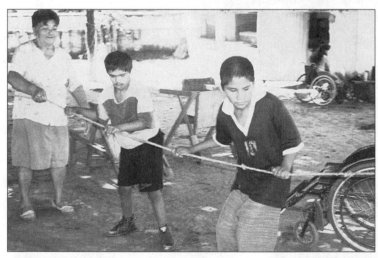

At last Alonzo was willing to try. First he hung fearfully onto the rope without moving. Then Carlos coaxed him into a "follow the leader" game, back and forth along the rope. In the end, they both had a good time.

In 4 days at PROJIMO Alonzo made great progress learning to walk—and with trying new things. His mother learned to be less over-protective and to let Alonzo do more on his own, even if it meant taking some risks. For Carlos, being asked to assist another child with problems similar to his own was a marvelous experience. He took joy and pride in helping. Folks at PROJIMO remembered how unreachable Carlos had been when he first came, and realized how far he had come.

Like many of us, Carlos discovered that one of the greatest joys in life comes from reaching out to others in need.

For more about Carlos, see Chapter 34.

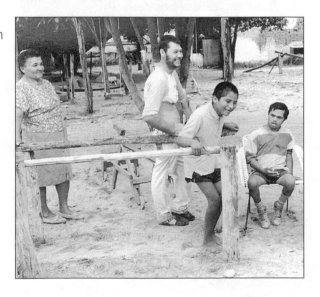

CHAPTER 33

Bars for Beno, and a Walker that Turns into Crutches for Lino

This chapter looks at walking aids, harmful and helpful, for two children with spina bifida: Beno and Lino.

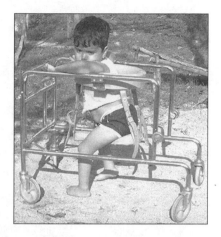

A Costly Walker for Beno that Did More Harm Than Good

BENO was four-years-old when he proudly showed the PROJIMO team how well he could walk with his big new chrome-plated walker. A month before his family (from a fishing village near the coastal city of Mazatlán) had taken him to a rehabilitation hospital where a doctor had prescribed the giant walker. It had cost the family a third of its year's earnings. But was it good for Beno?

Mari and Conchita had their doubts. The big square walker had a sling seat. To push it, the boy sat leaning forward with his hips bent almost at a right angle to his back. This was not a desirable position for a child with *spina bifida,* like Beno.

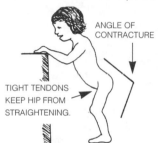

ANGLE OF CONTRACTURE

TIGHT TENDONS KEEP HIP FROM STRAIGHTENING.

A child with spina bifida (page 131) often has weak muscles in the lower back and hips. This weakness is likely to lead to hip contractures that prevent the hips from straightening. As a result, many of these children have trouble standing up straight (or even lying down straight). Their butt tends to stick out backwards. If they will ever be able to walk upright and independently, they need exercises, activities, and assistive equipment that help stretch and straighten the hips.

Beno's big metal walker did just the opposite. Taking steps while seated in it, he was crouched in a position that would add to hip contractures, not prevent them! Also, walking in a sitting position prevented Beno from bearing weight on his legs, which is important for bone growth and muscle development.

Mari and Conchita explained all this to Beno's parents, and advised them not to let Beno continue using the walker.

Parallel bars. As an alternative, Conchita adjusted the parallel bars in the playground high enough so that when Beno walked between them, they helped him to stretch his hips and to stand as straight up as possible. The parallel bars, which were made out of poles from the forest, had the advantage that the family could build their own at home at almost no cost.

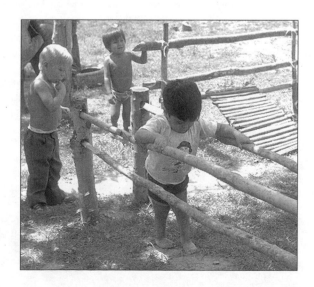

Later, PROJIMO workers designed a wooden walker for Beno to help him stand as upright as possible and stretch his hip-flexor muscles. (An unusual walker for another child with spina bifida is illustrated on the next page.)

A Low-Cost Crutch-Walker for Lino

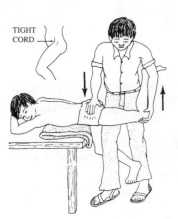

TIGHT CORD

Hip-stretching exercise to correct or prevent hip-flexion contractures.

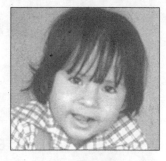

LINO, like Beno, was born with spina bifida. The defect in his spinal cord was sufficiently low on his back (near his butt) that he had fair upper leg strength. This meant he had a good chance of learning to walk, first perhaps with a standing board (parapodium) and then with a walker and perhaps crutches.

If a child with spina bifida is to be able to walk with crutches, or possibly without them, it is important that, from early childhood, every effort be made to prevent hip-flexion contractures. Care should be taken to keep the hip joints extended as straight as possible by means of exercises, positioning, and appropriate assistive devices.

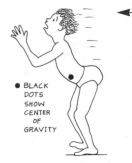

● BLACK DOTS SHOW CENTER OF GRAVITY

With hip contractures the child finds it hard to stand.

Because of weak lower back and hip muscles, the child with spina bifida is likely to find it hard to stand independently.

Some of these children learn to stand by thrusting their hips forward and their upper body backwards, so that their center of gravity is behind the hips. ⟶ But to stand this way, it is essential that hip-flexion contractures be prevented (or corrected). In fact, **it helps if the hip joints over-extend,** or bend farther back than a simply straight position.

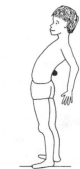

Thrusting his hips forward, this child can stand alone.

Lino was fortunate because, since early childhood, his family helped with exercises and positioning to keep his hips fully flexible. When he was three, PROJIMO helped him start to use a walker, with confidence that he would soon "graduate" to walking with crutches.

In designing a walker for Lino, Marcelo—an innovative shop-worker at PROJIMO—recalled his own childhood as a boy with both legs paralyzed by polio. Many disabled children who are learning to walk first use a walker and then, when they become a little more stable, change to crutches. For many children, the transition from walker to crutches is a fearful and traumatic experience. The walker gives them substantial stability. Crutches, at first, tend to wobble all over. In learning to use them, the terrified child often loses his balance and takes some nasty falls.

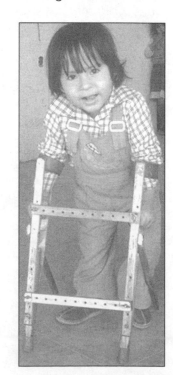

For this reason, Marcelo designed for Lino a **walker that could gradually be converted into crutches, with no sudden and frightening transition.** The walker consisted of 2 forearm crutches, which were connected with cross struts held in place with bolts and butterfly nuts. This way, the bolts could be gradually loosened to make the walker more wobbly and less stable. Then one after another of the cross-pieces and back-supports could be removed, until only the crutches were left.

This kind of innovation, which takes into consideration the child's worries and fears, is much more likely to take place when the technicians themselves are disabled.

CHAPTER 34

A Front-Wheel-Drive Wheelchair for Aidé:
Lessons Learned from an Experiment that Failed

AIDÉ is a 14 year old girl who is multiply disabled as a result of brain damage at birth. Her mind works at about the level of a 6- or 8-month-old child. She cannot speak, but she does communicate, in a limited way, through grunts and facial expressions. Physically, she has good head and trunk control. But she has a lot of spasticity, especially in the lower part of her body. On her first visit to PROJIMO, she was unable to move herself about or feed herself. She had little sense of the potential usefulness of her hands. But she would occasionally take hold of different objects and hold them for a moment, then drop them.

Aidé's family is very poor. Her parents put most of their energy into obtaining food and other resources to meet the family's basic needs. They did not know what to do with Aidé. As a result, they did little more than feed, bathe and clothe her.

Unmet Potential. Even at PROJIMO, no one expects that Aidé will ever be able to do much for herself. She responded little to early stimulation activities or play-things that were tried with her.

The team thought that if Aidé could begin to move herself about a bit in a wheelchair, this self-created movement might increase her awareness of her body's position and the usefulness of her arms and hands. They provided a wheelchair. Inez held her hands on the hand-rims and rolled the chair back and forth, hoping she would begin to make the connection between the movement of her hands and that of the chair. ──────▶

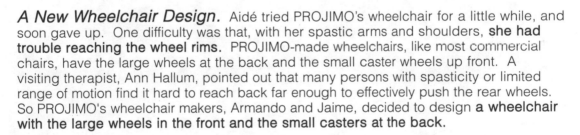

A New Wheelchair Design. Aidé tried PROJIMO's wheelchair for a little while, and soon gave up. One difficulty was that, with her spastic arms and shoulders, **she had trouble reaching the wheel rims.** PROJIMO-made wheelchairs, like most commercial chairs, have the large wheels at the back and the small caster wheels up front. A visiting therapist, Ann Hallum, pointed out that many persons with spasticity or limited range of motion find it hard to reach back far enough to effectively push the rear wheels. So PROJIMO's wheelchair makers, Armando and Jaime, decided to design **a wheelchair with the large wheels in the front and the small casters at the back.**

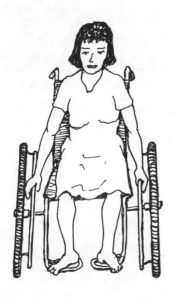

Another reason why persons like Aidé have trouble moving their wheelchairs is that the hand-rims, which are mounted on the outside of the large wheels, are so widely separated. So, Armando decided to try **mounting the hand-rims on the inner side of the wheels.** Closer to the rider's body, they would hopefully be easier for her to reach and to push.

A possible advantage of the inward position of the hand-rims is that the wheels are further apart. This wide wheel-base should provide stability and less likelihood of tipping over. The chair could be safer for persons with strong uncontrolled movements.

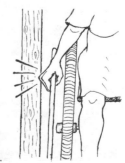

Also, for a person with limited control, hand-rims on the inner side of the wheels protect the knuckles from banging into doorways and other objects.

The newly designed chair, with front-wheel-drive and internal hand-rims, was built in 4 days. It was tested, not only by Aidé, but also by Tere, Lupita, and Carlos, all of whom have spasticity that makes it hard for them to push rear-wheel-drive wheelchairs.

Although the new chair did help to resolve some of the difficulties that some users had, **none were happy with it.**

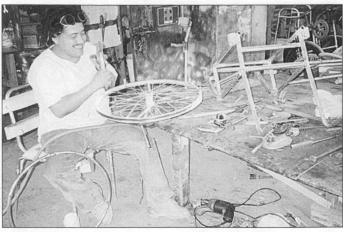

Armando builds a front-wheel-drive wheelchair for Aidé.

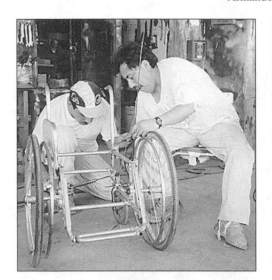

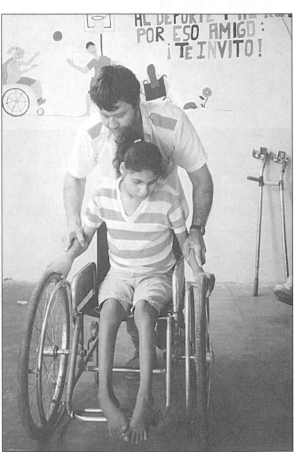

Inez worked a lot with Aidé in her new chair. He found it easier to position her spastic hands on the wheels, now that they were mounted further forward. She seemed more comfortable that way and, in time, began to close her hands on the wheels.

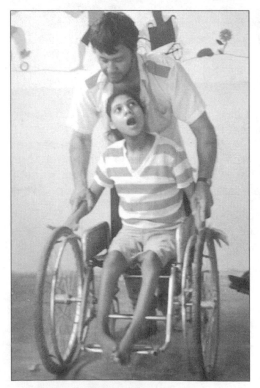

Inez would hold her wrists and push them forward, helping Aidé to move the chair.

However, Aidé was unable to grip the hand-rims that were mounted to the inside of the wheels. Her spastic fingers would bump into the wheels.

SHORTCOMINGS OF THE NEW DESIGN

It is still too early to know if the new wheelchair will benefit Aidé. So far, she still has not made much effort to push it by herself. However, she has begun to occasionally take hold of the large front wheels. This she had not done when the wheels were mounted further back.

Inez continues to work with Aidé daily. He hopes that, at some point, she will discover the joy of moving herself by pushing on the wheels.

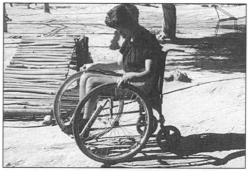

Tere did not like the new design because she could not grip the inwardly mounted hand rims. Also, the poor traction of the large front wheels caused her to get stuck on soft loose soil.

Tere, Lupita, and Carlos also tried the front-wheel-drive wheelchair. Both Tere and Lupita could reach the front-mounted wheels more easily. But, when they tried to grip the inward-mounted hand-rims, like Aidé, they had trouble fitting their spastic fingers between the rims and wheels. So Armando widened the space between wheels and the rims.

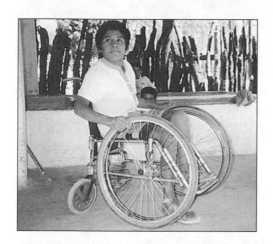

But still the girls had trouble. The team decided that **putting the hand rims on the inner side of the wheels was simply not practical.** Neither girl found the new design acceptable.

Carlos, on the other hand, did not care where the hand-rims were. He always grips the tire, not the rim. However, the chair's unusually wide wheel-base gave the blind boy more stability when he tilted off a curb with one wheel, and in other spots where he might have tipped over in a narrow chair. **For Carlos, the wider wheel-base was helpful.** (To avoid accidents, Carlos also learned to "see" with his foot. See next page.)

Poor traction was the biggest problem with the front-mounted large wheels. On a smooth, level cement surface, Carlos, Lupita, and Tere could move the chair about fairly easily. But, on an upward slope, or on sandy or uneven ground, the front wheels slipped. This happens because the rider's weight is mostly over the small, back caster-wheels, which dig into sand and stop short on a pitted surface. There is simply not enough weight over the large front wheels for them to firmly grip the ground.

With the front-wheel-drive chair, the only way to get good traction on a sloping or irregular surface is for the rider to lean far forward, shifting her weight over the front wheels. This, of course, can be difficult, especially for persons with spasticity. The team concluded that **front-wheel-drive wheelchairs are of limited usefulness, particularly in rough, sandy, or uneven terrain.**

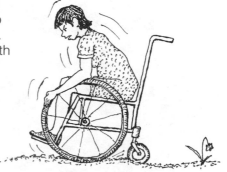

Learning from our mistakes. Not all innovations are successful. But we can learn a lot, even from efforts that fail. One lesson is extremely important:

> **Adequate trials of new designs are essential, and must include the intended users, within the local environment where they live.**

Carlos and his "Seeing-Eye Foot"

Because Carlos is almost completely blind, he sometimes has a hard time finding his way in his wheelchair. However, he has figured out different ways to stay on paths and to avoid bumping into things.

In Chapter 32 we saw how Carlos recruited a "seeing-eye person" to guide him while he pushes her wheelchair.

Since Carlos needs both his hands to drive his wheelchair, he cannot use a cane to feel his way, as many blind persons do. **Instead of a cane, he has learned to use his right foot.** He takes his foot off the foot-rest and puts it lightly on the ground in front of him. As he rolls forward, with his foot he can feel when he begins to go off a pathway or curb.

That way, he can often correct his direction before he has a mishap.

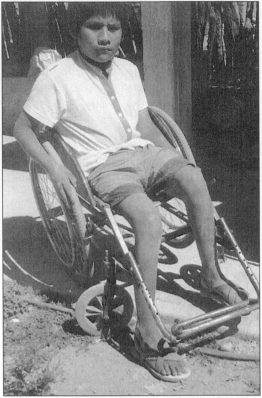

Feeling his way with his foot, Carlos rolls his wheelchair off the cement path onto the soil. But sometimes he misjudges and tips over.

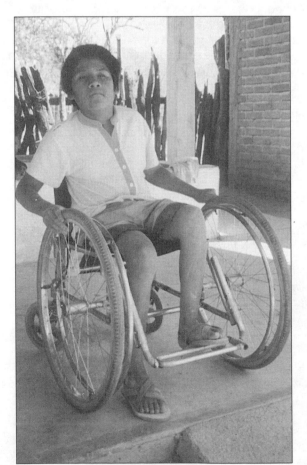

Although Carlos' seeing-eye foot serves him well, sometimes he forgets to use it. Or, at times, he tries to maneuver his wheelchair over curbs or rough terrain, and the chair tips over. He has had a few nasty falls.

For this reason, **the front-wheel-drive wheelchair, with its widely separated front wheels, is safer for Carlos than is a narrow chair.** The wide chair tips over sideways less easily. **Having the large wheels in front also appears to give more stability.**

Nevertheless, on loose or sandy soil, the front-wheel-drive chair has poor traction. Often, Carlos found himself trapped in pockets of loose soil where the front wheels would slip, and where he could not wheel himself out without help. As a result, **Carlos prefers his narrower, rear-wheel-drive wheelchair—even though he tips over more often.**

The wide wheel-base of the front-wheel drive wheelchair gives Carlos extra stability. Here, he avoids falling off the curb by feeling his way with his foot.

WARNING: Don't Assume That All the Designs You See in Pamphlets or Books on "Appropriate Technology" Are Appropriate.

Many booklets on "appropriate technology" for disabled people show designs of wheelchairs and hand-powered tricycles with front-wheel-drive. Such chairs are often given to disabled persons, especially in Asia and Africa. They may work fairly well in exhibition halls, and on level hard-surfaced roads. But **on rough terrain they are likely to further handicap the user.** The rider may need an assistant to push her in circumstances where a better designed wheelchair or tricycle could provide more independent mobility.

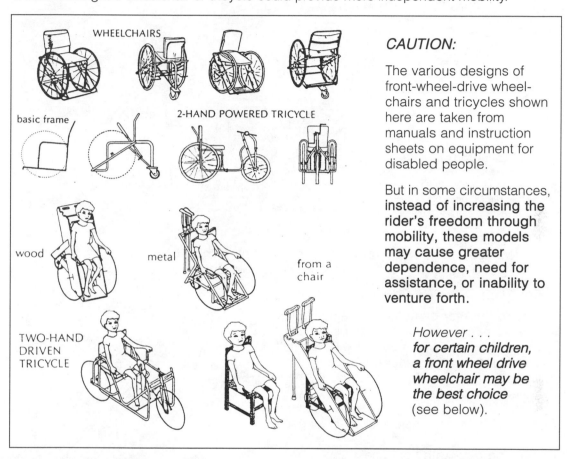

WHEELCHAIRS

basic frame

2-HAND POWERED TRICYCLE

wood

metal

from a chair

TWO-HAND DRIVEN TRICYCLE

CAUTION:

The various designs of front-wheel-drive wheelchairs and tricycles shown here are taken from manuals and instruction sheets on equipment for disabled people.

But in some circumstances, **instead of increasing the rider's freedom through mobility, these models may cause greater dependence, need for assistance, or inability to venture forth.**

However . . .
for certain children, a front wheel drive wheelchair may be the best choice (see below).

SOME CHILDREN WITH CEREBRAL PALSY FIND BIG FRONT WHEELS EASIER TO REACH AND PUSH

As with most rules, there are exceptions. Front-wheel-drive chairs are often inappropriate. But some children with spasticity, like Aidé, may find large front wheels easier to handle. Trollies and wheeled cots (see page 235) often work better with the big wheels up front.

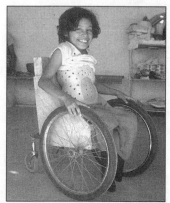

A scooter board for certain children with cerebral palsy has been designed with the **large wheels positioned right under the child,** and with **small wheels both at the back and front.** For travel on rough ground, the child can learn to balance on the center wheels and barely touch the ground with the others.

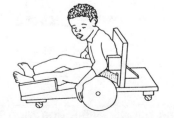
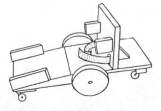

This girl with spastic cerebral palsy finds front-wheel-drive easier.

This scooter slopes forward, so that a child with hips that thrust him backward, or that do not bend to 90 degrees, can sit up straight. (See positive seating, Chapter 4.)

REMEMBER: Some of the best design improvements come from the ideas and suggestions of the persons who try them out and will use them. This is true even for children. The child may not always be right. But doctors, therapists, and technicians are not always right either, especially if they do not live in the same situation and experience the same barriers and desires. By respecting each other's special knowledge and looking for solutions together, we can more nearly meet the disabled person's needs.

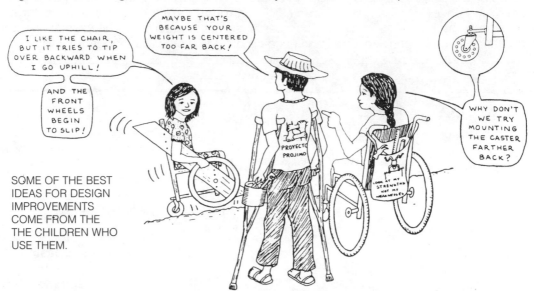

SOME OF THE BEST IDEAS FOR DESIGN IMPROVEMENTS COME FROM THE THE CHILDREN WHO USE THEM.

Note: The above front-wheel-drive chair not only risks tipping backward, it will lose traction going uphill. The front wheels do not support enough of the child's weight to grip well, so they will slip.

Mounting the rear caster wheel farther back will help prevent the chair from tipping over backwards on an uphill slope. It will also shift more weight over the front wheels and give them better traction. For these reasons, this modified design is included in the book, *Disabled Village Children*. But even when the rear caster is farther back, traction is not good.

Another problem with front-wheel-drive wheelchairs is that **the rider can not do "wheelies."**

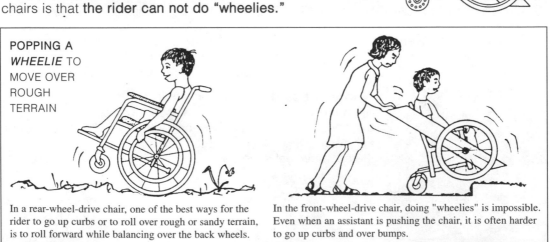

POPPING A *WHEELIE* TO MOVE OVER ROUGH TERRAIN

In a rear-wheel-drive chair, one of the best ways for the rider to go up curbs or to roll over rough or sandy terrain, is to roll forward while balancing over the back wheels.

In the front-wheel-drive chair, doing "wheelies" is impossible. Even when an assistant is pushing the chair, it is often harder to go up curbs and over bumps.

A rule to consider:

> **Never follow instructions blindly. Use common sense and creativity.**

A Gravity-Powered Elevator for Wheelchair Accessibility

Lack of Accessibility

Getting to the upper floors of buildings with more than one level is, in many countries, a major obstacle for disabled persons, especially wheelchair riders. I (the author) am an advisor to PROJIMO in the village of Ajoya, Mexico, and live on the second floor of a small, two-story cement-block building there. My friends at PROJIMO rightly criticized me for living in inaccessible quarters.

But how could the upper-level of my home be made more accessible to wheelchair riders? The entry is via a steep wooden stairway: little more than a solid step-ladder that leans against a rectangular opening in the upstairs floor. A ramp would be out of the question in the small room with so many steep stairs. The only possibility would be some sort of elevator. But a commercial motorized elevator, or lift—even a small one, designed to glide up a stairway—would be far too expensive. Besides, the supply of electricity to the village is too unreliable. What to do?

A Simple, Home-Made Elevator

To make the upstairs accessible to wheelchair riders, a visiting inventor from Holland, Reinder van Tijen, together with two disabled craftspersons at PROJIMO, Martín Pérez and Marcelo Acevedo, helped to design and build **a simple elevator lifted by gravity.** The elevator consists of a plywood platform mounted on a frame of steel tubing. Welded to the frame are sets of ball bearings that roll along a diagonal pipe attached to the stairway.

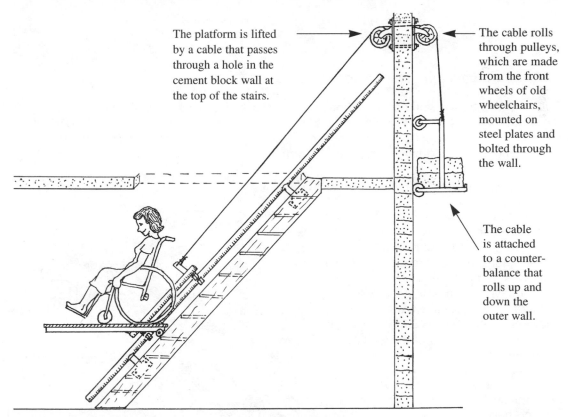

The platform is lifted by a cable that passes through a hole in the cement block wall at the top of the stairs.

The cable rolls through pulleys, which are made from the front wheels of old wheelchairs, mounted on steel plates and bolted through the wall.

The cable is attached to a counter-balance that rolls up and down the outer wall.

The counter-balance is weighted with cement blocks, the number of which can be varied so as to match the weight of the particular wheelchair rider. When properly counter-balanced, the elevator glides effortlessly up and down the stairwell.

Details of the elevator

A short diagonal pipe welded to the metal frame of the elevator is equipped at either end with 4 sets of ball bearings. These bearings fit snugly around the diagonal pipe next to the stairs.

Another set of ball bearings, attached to the other side of the elevator frame, rolls up and down the edge of the wood plank on the right side of the stairs.

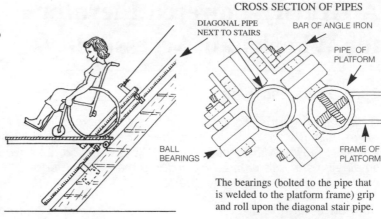

CROSS SECTION OF PIPES

DIAGONAL PIPE NEXT TO STAIRS

BAR OF ANGLE IRON

PIPE OF PLATFORM

BALL BEARINGS

FRAME OF PLATFORM

The bearings (bolted to the pipe that is welded to the platform frame) grip and roll upon the diagonal stair pipe.

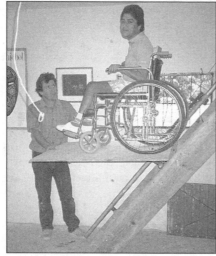

In her wheelchair, Tere rides up the elevator.

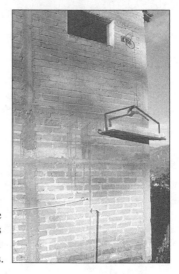

The counter-balance on the outside wall is weighted with cement blocks.

Safety problems that needed solving

The simple elevator worked well. It has now been used by wheelchair-riding visitors for more than 4 years. Since the time it was built, however, visiting engineers warned that the elevator was unsafe. The biggest risk factor, they insisted, was the lack of an automatic locking mechanism to safely hold the platform in place when it reached ground level.

As designed, the platform had to be locked by the rider on reaching ground level. A bolt was slipped through two holes: one in the elevator frame, and one in the diagonal pipe on which the elevator rolled. As long as this bolt was in place before the rider rolled off the platform, there was no problem. But, if he forgot and rolled off without inserting the bolt, the elevator would rocket skyward. This happened once, when a small boy was standing on the edge of the elevator. The platform took off like a rocket. The surprised boy shot upward and fell off into a water tank below. Fortunately, he was unhurt. But if anyone had been on the stairs when the elevator rocketed upward, heaven help them.

An automatic parking brake for the gravity-run elevator. Although visiting engineers insisted that the elevator needed an automatic locking mechanism, none offered a design. Finally, it was Marcelo, the disabled PROJIMO craftsperson, who designed and built a fail-safe automatic locking mechanism for the elevator. He made it out of scraps of iron bar, a spring, and a few bolts.

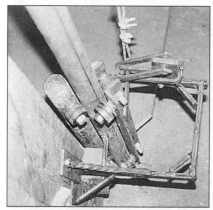

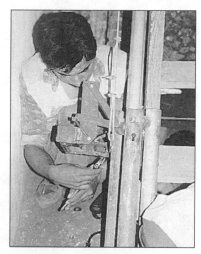

Marcelo modified the design of a latch he built for PROJIMO's main gate, which locks automatically when it swings closed. (He made it after the gate was left open at night and cows ate the banana plants.)

Marcelo installs the safety latch.

This photo, taken from behind the stairs, looks down at the U-shaped bracket, to which is attached the automatic latch.

The device is simple. A U-shaped iron bracket is bolted to the side beam of the stairs. To this is attached a V-shaped latch, made by welding flat iron bars. The latch, which pivots on a bolt, is pulled forward by a spring. This latch hooks onto an upright post, welded to the platform frame (the post to which the elevator lift-cable is attached). When the elevator comes down, the post pushes the latch out of the way. Having passed, the latch springs back, hooking onto the post and locking the platform at ground level.

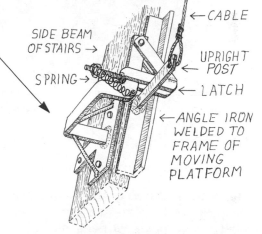

SIDE BEAM OF STAIRS →

SPRING →

← CABLE

UPRIGHT POST →

← LATCH

← ANGLE IRON WELDED TO FRAME OF MOVING PLATFORM

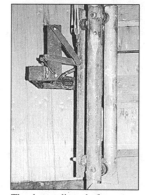

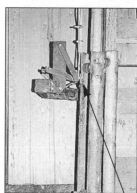

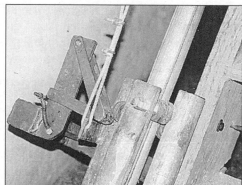

The descending platform approaches the latch.

The post pushes the latch to the side and slides past it.

The latch springs back over the post, locking it in place.

The device was tested 100 times and appears fool-proof. The only way to unlock the latch is to put enough weight on the platform so that it lowers a bit more, then push the latch out of the way. As an added safety mechanism, the original bolt-lock can still be used when the elevator is not in use—giving double protection.

In conclusion: Thanks to the warnings of visiting engineers, plus the creative design and building skill of Marcelo, the gravity-run elevator is now much safer.

Stairs Need Not Be So Big an Obstacle When There are Willing Friends

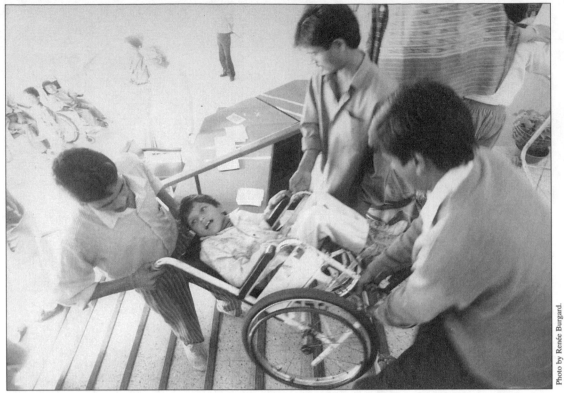

Photo by Renée Burgard.

Sometimes a barrier can become a chance for camaraderie. Here friends of a boy in India help him up a long flight of steps. (A lot depends on our culture and point of view. See the story by Mike Miles on page 172.)

Ramps

In many circumstances, ramps are far cheaper and more practical than elevators.

The recommended grade (steepness) of a ramp depends on the strength of its users, and whether they have, or need, assistance. Ramps for public use should have a very gentle slope, so that persons with weak arms can go up them without assistance. But in limited space, a steep ramp may be better than none.

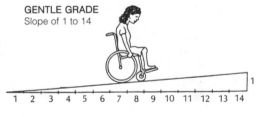

GENTLE GRADE
Slope of 1 to 14

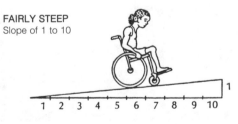

FAIRLY STEEP
Slope of 1 to 10

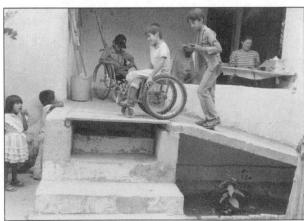

This ramp in a Mexican village clinic was built in a very limited space. The board over the steps lifts out of the way, so that people can use the steps when the ramp is not needed.

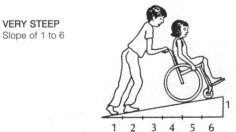

VERY STEEP
Slope of 1 to 6

Paraplegics Who Walk Where Wheelchairs Won't Enter (India)

CHAPTER 36

Innovations For, By and With Spinal-Cord Injured Persons in India

Centers for rehabilitation in the United States and many other countries encourage most spinal-cord injured persons to use wheelchairs as their primary way of moving about. Except for a few persons with low-level or incomplete injuries, walking is considered too difficult.

This emphasis on *wheelchair riding with ease* rather than *walking with difficulty* reflects the current trend in rehabilitation. The goal of *maximum function* is placed before *normalization*—even if this means doing some things "abnormally" (differently from how most people do them). Today, many spinal-cord injury self-help groups strongly encourage members to "*Accept yourself as a wheelchair rider and get on with your life.*" Individuals are gently discouraged from putting a lot of hope or energy into *"learning to walk again."* Instead, they are urged to **"join in the fight for accessibility and social acceptance of wheelchair riders."**

I was, therefore, surprised by the approach of the rehabilitation center linked with the *Christian Medical College* in Vellore, India, which I visited in 1995 during a UN workshop on "Indigenous Assistive Devices for Disabled Persons." **At the center, many paraplegic persons were being vigorously trained to walk with leg braces and elbow crutches.**

Started in 1934 by a visionary woman doctor who was paralyzed in a car accident, the Vellore Center is recognized as the country's best, most comprehensive spinal-cord injury program. I was impressed, not only by the quality of services and innovativeness of activities, but by its human warmth and convivial spirit. The center's outstanding staff made a point of including disabled persons in the problem-solving process: as friends, co-workers, and equals.

Innovations at the center included a **traditional village,** complete with thatched huts and vegetable gardens. Here, disabled villagers lived and relearned the skills and the **activities of daily living in a typical rural environment.** We saw persons working and moving about there on crutches, or sometimes, crawling with knee-pads—but few used wheelchairs.

At first, I was concerned by the emphasis on walking rather than on wheelchair use. In recent years, India's government has launched a major program of wheelchair production. In cities, at least, increased attention is placed on wheelchair access (though there continues to be a huge unmet need).

I asked the Director: "Why such a strong emphasis on walking? Wouldn't it be more realistic to teach most paraplegic persons to use primarily wheelchairs?"

"Not at all!" he said. "Most spinal-cord injured persons who pass through our center come from remote villages, where wheelchair use is almost impossible.

"You will see for yourselves when we go to a village this afternoon."

He was so right!

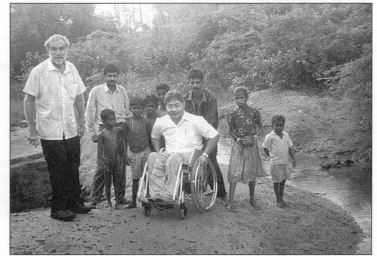

To reach the village of a paraplegic man in rural India, a wheelchair-riding United Nations coordinator of our group had to be helped across streams and through sand, mud, and high grass. (David Werner is on the left.)

Visit to an Independent Sugar-Cane Farmer Who is Paraplegic

We visited a paraplegic man on the outskirts of a small village. To reach his homestead, we drove the last 2 or 3 miles over a narrow, muddy, rutted country road, difficult to travel even in a Jeep. For the last 200 yards, we had to travel by foot. We quickly realized the limitations of a wheelchair in such places.

On arrival, we made our way through a muddy field behind a large mud house. There we saw a man standing next to a small, rustic gasoline-motor-run sugar-cane mill. He was skillfully pushing armfuls of green cane into the rolling jaws of the machine. Helping him was a boy who, we learned, was his son. We had to look twice to realize that the man was disabled. He wore full-leg braces and arched his body backwards to stand and work with both hands, without having to support himself with his crutches.

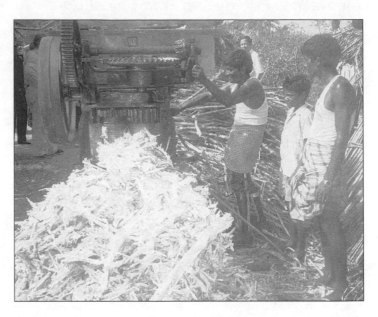

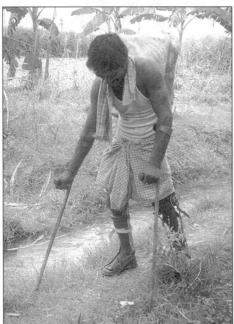

RAM, the man at the mill, saw us approaching. He bounded over a pile of milled cane and greeted us warmly. He was dark, muscular, and had a look of uncrushable self-assurance. He appeared to be in excellent health (better than many people in India's hunger-ridden rural areas).

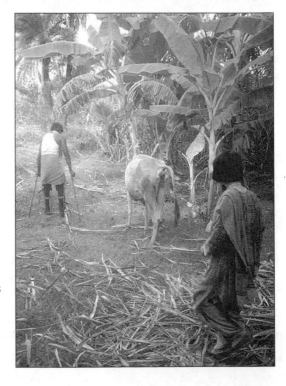

We observed Ram doing a variety of daily chores, ranging from clearing pathways to leading his cow to pasture across the narrow dikes of a rice field. Totally self-sufficient, he provided for his wife and children through his own hard physical labor. He had the innovativeness of one who, since childhood, has lived in a difficult environment where dexterity and creative ingenuity are essential skills for staving off hunger and for survival.

A pit latrine. Ram's innovations included a pit latrine with a wooden toilet seat (unusual for rural India, where the custom is simply to squat). He had built it next to a cement-covered mud-brick water trough. (The pit was over 2 meters deep, in order to avoid contamination of the surface water that fed the trough, which ran through a shallow ditch from a spring, 200 yards away.)

Home-grown castor-oil catheter lubricant. Ram had also found a way to catheterize himself at low cost. Like most spinal-cord injured persons who lack normal bladder control, to drain out urine he needed to pass a catheter (clean rubber tube) through his penis into his bladder every few hours.

Rubber catheters can be cleaned and reused hundreds of times (see Chapter 25, on catheterization). But for each use, they need to be lubricated (oiled). And commercial medical lubricants—such as *KY Jelly*—are expensive.

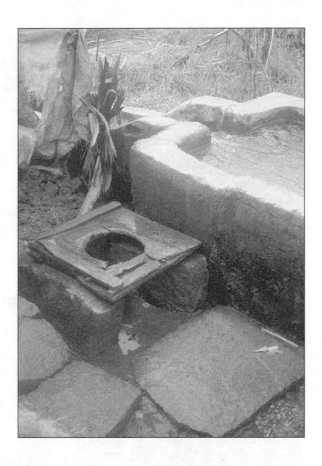

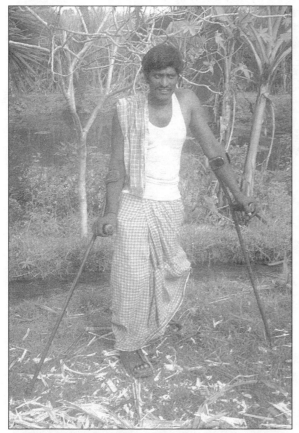

Ram stands in front of castor trees he planted to make castor oil for lubricating his catheters.

To save money, Ram had stopped using costly medical lubricants and had begun to use castor oil. But he soon learned that commercial castor oil was contaminated, causing repeated urinary infections. So he planted his own castor trees, harvested the beans, and pressed them carefully under clean conditions to extract the oil. With this clean home-made oil, he explained, he now had almost no problems with urinary infections.

A two-rear-wheel-drive tricycle. For most of his farm work, Ram moved about with full-leg orthopedic braces and crutches made at the rehab center in Vellore. But for travel into town, he used an "all terrain tricycle" that he had designed and built with help from a local welder.

Most hand-powered tricycles made in India have front-wheel-drive, and they are therefore useless in mud and sand. The front wheel has little traction and tends to slip because the person's weight is mostly over the back wheels.

But Ram's tricycle was different.

Ram's tricycle has 2 hand cranks (adapted bicycle pedals), one on either side. With bicycle chains and sprockets, they power both back wheels. ⟶

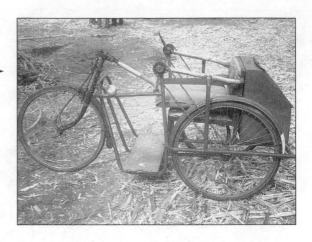

The steering mechanism consists of a bar extending back from a bicycle fork that holds the single front wheel. When traveling on a fairly hard, flat roadway, Ram can steer with one hand and pedal the chair with the other (one wheel drive). For two-wheel-traction in mud or sand, he can pedal with both hands. But that means he must let go of the steering rod.

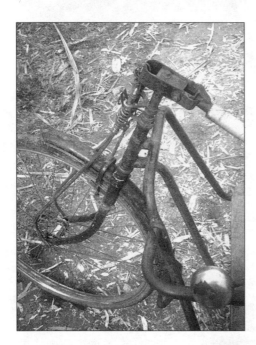

In order to keep the chair moving ahead in a straight line when he is not holding the steering rod, Ram improvised a spring device on the steering shaft of the front wheel fork. (See photo on left.)

The 2 springs persistently push the front wheel into a straight position. When Ram comes to a curve in the path, he lets go of one pedal just long enough to get around the curve. When he lets go of the steering rod, the front wheel automatically straightens.

Another advantage of this two-hand rear-wheel-drive tricycle (compared to one-hand-drive ones) is that for long distances it is less tiring to use. The rider can provide power with both arms at once, or use only one arm while resting the other.

(For more ideas on hand-powered tricycles, see Chapter 31. For a "4-wheel drive" all-terrain tricycle, see the drawing at the bottom of page 343.)

Observing the innovative problem-solving skills of rural disabled persons like Ram made a deep impression on the visiting rehabilitation specialists and technicians. By the end of the 10 day workshop; many declared they would work more as "partners in problem solving" with disabled clients, and encourage them to design or improve upon their own devices and solutions.

The visiting professionals gained greater respect for the creativity and abilities, not only of disabled people, but of *poor, unschooled, disabled people.* And that was a big step forward.

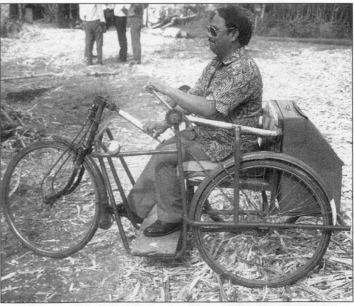

One of the participants in the UN workshop tries out Ram's tricycle. Hand-pedals that power both rear wheels make it an "all terrain vehicle."

CHAPTER 37

Martín Builds a Jointed Gurney to Keep His Hips from Stiffening

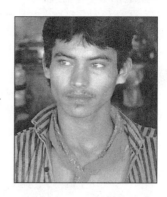

MARTÍN Pérez, since he was 10 years old, lived on the streets in Culiacan, the capital city of the state of Sinaloa, Mexico. He survived by stealing, doing odd jobs, and trafficking drugs. At age 15, as a result of a gang dispute, he was shot through the spine and became paraplegic (paralyzed from the middle of the back down). Upon his release from the hospital, he was sent to PROJIMO.

On his arrival, Martín was near death from a urinary infection and pressure sores that had developed in the hospital. He was angry and depressed, but had the will and spirit of a survivor.

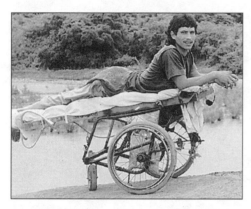

As is usual in PROJIMO, other spinal-cord injured persons took over the management of Martín's urinary problem and pressure sores. In the wheelchair shop, they built a wheeled cot, or gurney, so that he could be active while lying on his stomach, and so his sores (on his backside) would heal.

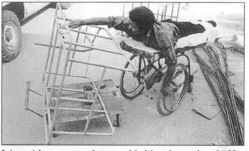

Frozen hips. Martín recovered his health, and his sores healed in record time. But a new problem was developing. His hip joints were beginning to *ossify*—in other words, the flesh around the hip joints was beginning to turn into bone.

Jaime rides a gurney because his hips do not bend. Here he paints the frame of a tricycle trailer (see page 201).

This problem, called *myositis ossificans,* occurs occasionally in spinal-cord injured persons. It happened to Jaime, a worker in PROJIMO's wheelchair shop. Because his hips are solidly fused into a straight position, Jaime works while lying on a gurney (see photos on pages 195, 200 and 247).

There is a debate among specialists as to what to do when *myositis ossificans* starts to develop. Some recommend very limited motion of the hips, in the belief that movement causes irritation and speeds the deposit of bone. Others argue in favor of aggressive range-of-motion exercises, to try to stop the joints from freezing up. Martín learned that Jaime had not exercised during the time when his hips became ossified. Therefore—at a stage when Martín's hips had almost no movement left—he set about **exercising to bring back flexibility.** Every morning his hips were so stiff he could barely move them. But he would diligently exercise for an hour or more to recover lost range of motion.

First, Martín would brace his feet against the wall and pull on a rope for several minutes, until his hips started to bend.

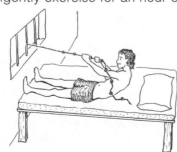

Then, he would sit on the edge of his cot, grasp first one knee and then the other, and steadily pull them toward his body.

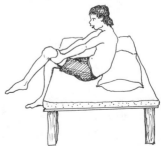

With his persistent exercise program, Martín managed, in time, to regain complete range of motion of his hips. Nevertheless, every morning his hips would partially "freeze up." For years, he had to keep up his morning exercise routine to maintain flexibility.

Martín's great strengths and weaknesses. In PROJIMO, Martín's presence was a mixed blessing. On the negative side, he had a violent temper which sometimes led to acts of physical violence. He also used drugs (mainly marijuana) on the PROJIMO grounds, even though drug use was prohibited by group decision. He was also openly critical of weaknesses in the organization and its leadership, which caused his own errors to be less tolerated. (Eventually he was expelled.)

On the positive side, Martín developed into an extremely innovative and creative wheelchair builder. He solved design problems in the Whirlwind wheelchair that disability engineer Ralf Hotchkiss had struggled with for years (such as a very simple mechanism to adjust the angle of the footrests).

Ralf was so impressed with Martín's abilities that he invited him to live in his home and to work in his shop for a number of months. Martín even became a teaching assistant in Ralf's course in rehabilitation design and engineering at San Francisco State University, in California.

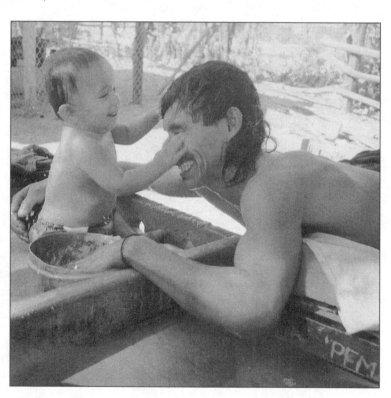

Also on the positive side, Martín was very friendly and helpful to some of the neediest disabled children at PROJIMO. Whenever they needed help with their aids or equipment, they went to Martín, who would always help them in a warm, personal, and effective way.

A Jointed Gurney for Post-Surgery Recovery

Martín was sometimes too active and hard working for his own good. He had begun to use a wheelchair before the last pressure sore on his backside had healed. As a result, the sore—although it had healed except for a small opening on the surface—had formed a large and stubborn cavity underneath. Periodically this cavity became infected. Surgeons from *Interplast* (International Plastic Surgery) who examined Martín decided he needed surgery to repair the deep sore. They offered to do the operation free of charge, in Stanford, California.

Martín's biggest worry was the post-operative period. The surgeons told him he would need to lie on a special "air bed" for 6 weeks, to allow healing. But Martín—who knows his own body well—feared his hips would freeze up forever if he lay flat for so long and could not do his daily bending exercises. In order to maintain flexibility, he felt that **during the post-surgery period he needed to be positioned at different and changing hip angles.** He told the surgeons he could make a jointed gurney with adjustable hip and knee angles to use post-operatively. But the surgeons were skeptical.

The surgeons doubted that Martín could make a satisfactory gurney. And if he did, they doubted that he would be able to lie on it face down all day long.

But Martín was persistent. The doctors decided to test him. They insisted that he spend three days and nights continuously on the gurney, to prove that he could do it without complications. Martín did this successfully, and the doctors at last agreed to let him use the gurney following surgery, instead of being on the special hospital bed.

Excellent results. To the doctors' amazement, on his jointed gurney Martín's post-operative recovery went remarkably quickly and well. They observed that Martín was very active on the gurney. They agreed that such activity increased blood circulation, which probably speeded surgical healing. (This finding is consistent with other observations by the PROJIMO team on the healing of pressure sores, after surgery and otherwise. See "Medical Treatment of Osvaldo's Pressure Sores," page 252.)

THE GURNEY

The flexible gurney that Martín made for his post-surgical recovery period was built on top of a standard donated wheelchair. The hip and knee angles could be easily adjusted by hand. He upholstered each section of the gurney with water-resistant vinyl (plastic cloth).

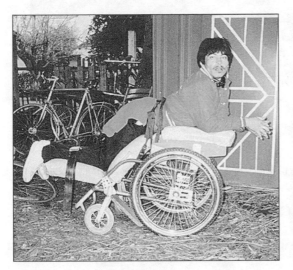 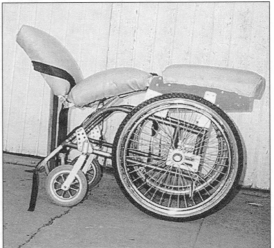

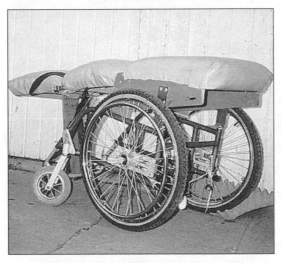 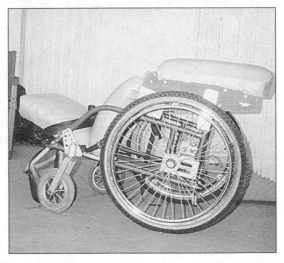

The above photos show Martín trying out his new gurney, and the gurney alone in 3 of the many different positions to which it can be adjusted.

Different Kinds of Jointed Gurneys

Other jointed gurneys have been custom-built at PROJIMO and used by persons
with a variety of needs. Here is a gurney for a boy, DANIEL, who is paraplegic due to
tuberculosis of his spine. When Daniel came to PROJIMO, his body, hips and knees
were contracted in a sitting position, and he had severe pressure sores. Therefore, the
team built for him an adjustable, jointed gurney that could gradually straighten him out.

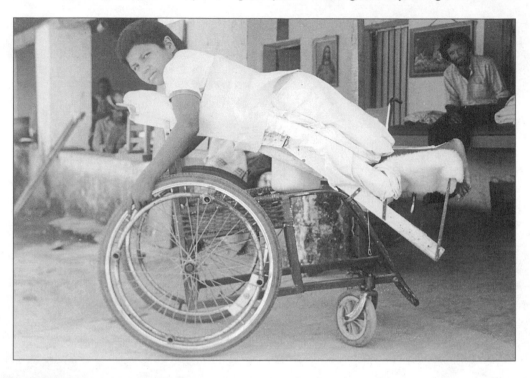

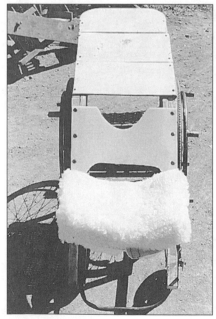

The gurney has a hole in it through which the boy
can pass urine—with or without a catheter—into a
bag or bottle. (Spinal-cord injured persons usually
lack urine control. See page 147.)

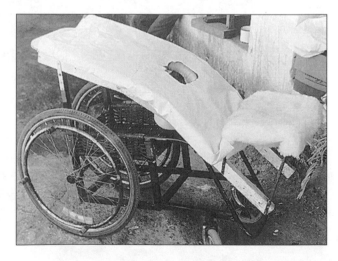

In contrast, the next chapter describes a jointed gurney that was built for a boy (Osvaldo) to
gradually bend his hips and knees, which had stiffened in an extended (straight) position.

Additional information on designs for wheeled cots or gurneys can be found in the book,
Disabled Village Children. Also see the next chapter, pages 246-248.

Osvaldo: A Triplegic Boy with Many Challenging Needs

OSVALDO'S childhood was like that of many boys in a poor urban community. He lived with his ailing mother on a hill on the outskirts of Culiacan, the state capital of Sinaloa, Mexico. His father had abandoned the family years before. His mother worked in a factory, for wages so low that sometimes there was little to eat. Osvaldo went to school, but he often skipped classes to do odd jobs or to play.

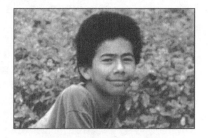

When he was 13 years old, an event happened that drastically changed Osvaldo's life. He was playing with friends on the roadside outside the family hut, when a truck parked at the top of the hill, and the driver got out. Then the hand-brake failed, and the truck rolled down the steep dirt road toward the children at play. It suddenly pitched off the narrow road, straight into the children. One child was killed, four were injured. Because the driver had not been in the truck (and had slipped the police a bribe) he was not held responsible.

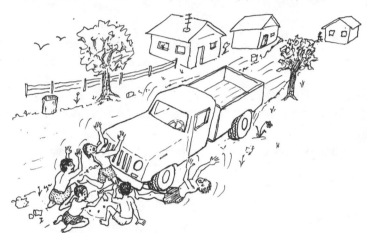

After he was hit, Osvaldo—dazed and bleeding—tried to stand up. But he could not move his legs or his right arm. Neighbors took him to the hospital. The doctors found **his spinal cord was crushed at mid-back level** (T6). He had a double fracture of his right leg, above and below the knee. His right shoulder was broken and dislocated, with nerve damage that left his **right hand and arm paralyzed.**

So it was that, at age 13, Osvaldo became *triplegic* (paralyzed in 3 of 4 limbs). He had **lost all movement and feeling in his lower body** and had **no urine or bowel control.** In the hospital his broken spine was stabilized surgically with metal rods. (Fortunately, Osvaldo's mother had social security insurance which covered most of the medical expenses.)

On his release from the hospital, Osvaldo was taken by ambulance to his home. Unfortunately, neither he nor his mother had been given instructions about prevention of pressure sores and urinary infections. So, day after day, Osvaldo lay on his back on a burlap cot without moving. A month later, when a nurse made a home visit, she found that his back, buttocks, and heels were covered with **pressure sores.** The hospital then provided an "egg crate" foam mattress, and a nurse instructed the boy's mother to "Turn him frequently from side to side."

But this was easier said than done, as his mother soon discovered. Osvaldo had sunk into **severe depression which expressed itself as anger,** directed mostly at his mother. His paralyzed right hand was extremely sensitive: it gave him unbearable, burning pain, especially when it was moved. He rested it over his chest without moving it for weeks and months. In time, his right arm became stiffly fixed in front of him. **He was so afraid of having his painful hand touched or moved that he refused to let his mother get near it.** Whenever she tried to move him he would weep and protest. Using his good left arm, he fiercely fought off her attempts to turn him on his side. Because of his lack of urine and bowel control, she had a hard time keeping him clean.

PROJIMO TO THE RESCUE

In November, 1991, on a visit to the capital city, two disabled workers from PROJIMO learned about Osvaldo and visited his home. Five months after his accident, the boy was near death. Emaciated, anemic, and very depressed, he had deep pressure sores, a urinary infection and chronic fever. His doctors had not stressed the importance of drinking lots of water to reduce the risk of urinary infection. Adding to the danger, they had not changed him from a permanent catheter (urine-draining tube) to intermittent catheterization (see page 147). His dark urine had so much crud in it that the catheter often clogged. His pressure sores, which his mother did her best to clean and bandage, were infected and had black necrotic (dead) areas.

The worst sores were on the back of his ankles. They formed after the visiting nurse—worried about the sores on his heels—told his mother, "Keep a rolled-up towel under his ankles." His mother had carefully followed the nurse's orders. Four months later (when the PROJIMO workers visited the home) deep sores had formed where the towel was still obediently positioned. The sore under the left ankle was so deep that it bared the Achilles tendon.

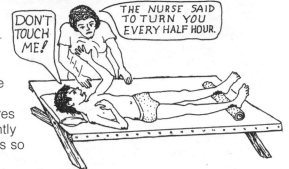

This was a powerful lesson for the PROJIMO workers. They saw the danger of simply giving cookbook-like instructions without explanations. On the contrary, it is important to:

> Help people to **fully understand the reasons** for doing things, so that they are able to **make well-informed decisions,** based on their own observations and changing needs.

Further complicating Osvaldo's condition was his delicate, often angry mood, his fear of pain or injury, and the excruciating sensitivity of his paralyzed right hand. Yielding to his tearful protests, his mother had given up attempting to turn him onto his side or belly. So, for five months he had lain on his back, his pressure sores getting larger and deeper, and his body growing as stiff as a board.

On seeing Osvaldo, the PROJIMO workers felt that—due to the difficult combination of physical and emotional needs—more might be accomplished in their small community rehabilitation center than in the home. They invited him and his mother to spend a while at PROJIMO. At first, Osvaldo was afraid to leave home … or even to be moved from his cot. But the warmth and concern of the PROJIMO workers gave him a new sense of hope. Gathering courage, he accepted their offer. The next morning, with Osvaldo lying on a foam mattress in the back of a station wagon, the group made the 4-hour trip to PROJIMO.

The Need for a Creative and Loving Approach

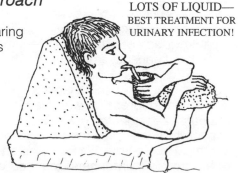

LOTS OF LIQUID—
BEST TREATMENT FOR
URINARY INFECTION!

The complexity of Osvaldo's needs called for very caring rehabilitation and innovative assistive equipment. His urinary infection and sores required urgent attention. For the former, the team gave him antibiotics and encouraged him to drink **lots of fluids.** However, he often refused to drink, even when we explained its importance. Since Osvaldo's favorite drinks were orange juice and hot chocolate, we pampered him with all of these he could drink. As his urinary infection got better, so did his mood and appetite.

The team put Osvaldo on a **high calorie, high protein, high iron diet.** Improving his nutritional status and blood level would help to heal his pressure sores, and fight off the urinary infection.

Managing Osvaldo's Pressure Sores—and Lifting His Spirits

The next job was to find a way of taking the pressure off of Osvaldo's pressure sores. To manage the sores on the back and buttocks, PROJIMO usually builds a gurney, or trolley (narrow wheeled bed), on which the person can lie face down. That way he can wheel himself around, and energetically work and play. Keeping active not only makes lying face down for long periods more tolerable, but it also stimulates circulation, which speeds healing.

With Osvaldo, however, lying face down was not an easy matter. From having lain flat on his back for months, his entire body had become as stiff as a board. Also, his paralyzed right arm was almost "frozen," with his forearm over his chest. Both the shoulder and hand were so super-sensitive that he would howl even before someone touched them.

The first job was to win Osvaldo's trust and to involve him in the problem-solving process. The team tried to give him a sense of control that would help him overcome his fear. Often, it seemed that **his fear of the pain was worse than the pain itself.** Certainly it made the pain worse.

On discussing Osvaldo's wishes and needs with him and his mother, it became clear that the management of his sores needed **an integrated plan to lift both his body and his spirit.** His various physical and emotional needs needed to be answered in a "whole-person," or holistic, way. The group agreed that the major short-term objectives with Osvaldo were:

- to figure out ways to get the pressure off Osvaldo's sores for prolonged periods and, as soon as possible, to find a way for him to lie face down without lying on top of his stiff, hypersensitive right arm and hand;

- to help him regain flexibility of his hips and knees, so that he could begin to sit: first in bed, and later (after his pressure sores healed) in a wheelchair;

- to correct the foot-drop (contracture of the heel cords) that had begun to form;

- to help him increase the strength and ability of his useful (left) arm—a greater challenge because he had been right-handed;

- to design mobility aids that Osvaldo could move and steer with only one arm;

- to provide a range of enjoyable and useful activities so as to encourage self-care, self confidence, and more independence;

- while doing all of the above, to provide a friendly, understanding, stimulating, entertaining, and adventurous environment—to help Osvaldo pull out of his depression and rediscover joy in life, the will to live, and ability to love.

Talking with Osvaldo was not easy. It took time for him to gain enough confidence in himself and in others to speak seriously. What seemed to distress him most was his sense of powerlessness and total immobility. He feared remaining dependent, not being able to do anything for himself, to move, or to go anywhere without help.

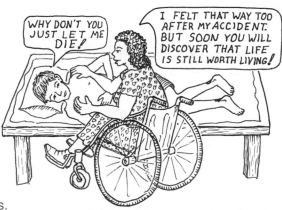

Therefore, **helping Osvaldo learn to do more for himself, manage his personal body functions, and move under his own power** were seen as urgent goals which could contribute to his healing in many ways.

In these pages, we will not describe all the aspects of Osvaldo's rehabilitation—rather we will focus on several of the most innovative aids and activities.

Innovations For and With Osvaldo

To help meet the various objectives of Osvaldo's rehabilitation—or revitalization—the PROJIMO team designed a number of innovative devices. They will be described here in the order in which they were created and used.

It is important to note that **most of these innovations were developed with the active participation of Osvaldo himself.** In the process, this 13-year-old boy acquired a much clearer understanding of his body, its unusual needs, and how to meet them. He began to rediscover and become friendly with his own mysterious body, and to increasingly take charge of his own rehabilitation and care. Soon he was reminding and guiding his attendants (especially his mother) about how to position him and where to place padding to prevent pressure sores. His testing, criticism, and suggestions for improvements of devices became a valuable part of the innovative process. As he became an active participant in the design of his own equipment, he gained new confidence, lost much of his fear of trying new things, was less fretful, and gradually became again a friendly, playful boy—although strangely perceptive and wise for his age. (He avidly read *Disabled Village Children* and gave suggestions for the rehabilitation of other children.)

AN ADJUSTABLE BED—TO HELP REDUCE PRESSURE OVER SORES, BEND HIS STIFF BODY, AND PREPARE HIM FOR SITTING

Complexity of the problem: Clearly, for rapid healing of his pressure sores, Osvaldo needed to stop lying on his back and start lying on his belly or side. However, the team realized the need to move toward this slowly, at a pace the boy could tolerate and control. Osvaldo was terrified of being shifted to a new position that might trigger the pain in his hypersensitive shoulder and hand. It had taken his last bit of courage just to come to PROJIMO, and the team did not want to push him too hard or fast. In the first days, especially, it was essential that his experience at PROJIMO be as reassuring and uplifting as possible. Therefore the team, together with Osvaldo and his mother, tried to think of ways to reduce the pressure on the sores on his back and buttocks—and to help him regain some flexibility in his hips and knees—while still lying face up.

Partial solution: To reduce pressure over the bony areas with sores, Osvaldo was laid on a **double foam mattress,** the lower one thick and fairly firm, the upper one quite soft. To help speed healing, the sores were packed daily with a paste made of **bees' honey and sugar** (see page 156).

From lying flat on his back for so long, Osvaldo's hips and knees had grown so stiff (with extension contractures) that they almost would not bend at all. Bending exercises were introduced. What was needed, however, was prolonged, very gentle stretching. It would have helped to have a hospital bed that could be gradually cranked up into a sitting position, slowly bending the hips and knees. But such a costly item was out of the question.

Partial solution: an adjustable, hinged plywood bed board.

Materials: 1 sheet plywood; 2 strips old cloth (about 6 inches wide); white glue.

Construction: A piece of plywood the size of the cot was cut in three pieces based on Osvaldo's body measurements (A=feet to knees, B=knees to hips, C=hips to head). The plywood sections were then joined together with cloth hinges made with strips of old towel and white glue.

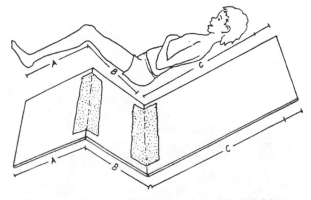

Three sections of plywood joined together with cloth hinges.

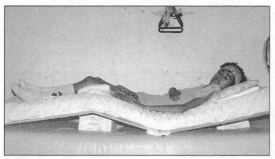

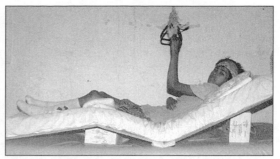

Osvaldo, beginning to bend at the hips.

Osvaldo, with a little more bend at the hips.

1. A metal triangle, hanging from a rope over Osvaldo's bed, allowed him to lift himself up periodically with his good arm. This took pressure off his back, and also helped strengthen his arm.

2. By putting padding under Osvaldo's knees, some of the weight could be taken off his backside.

3. This padding reduced the pressure on his buttocks and lower back, where he had some of his worst sores.

4. Padding was also placed under his lower legs, to take pressure off his heels and ankles.

5. By putting boxes of different sizes under the bed-boards, the angle of his hips and knees could gradually be increased.

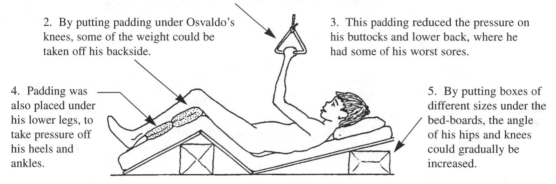

Results: Flexibility of Osvaldo's body returned surprisingly quickly. Within a few weeks, both his hips and knees flexed to almost to 90 degrees. Also, being able to move into a partly sitting position allowed the boy to do more things more easily (eat, read, draw pictures, and take part in what was going on around him). His disposition improved accordingly. And his pressure sores began to heal.

Technical problem: With repeated removal and replacement of the hinged plywood bed-board between the two foam mattresses, the cloth hinges began to tear loose.

Solution: hinges made of thin cord.
As an experimental alternative, hinges were made using cord (thick string). The cord passes through small holes in the edges of the plywood sections.

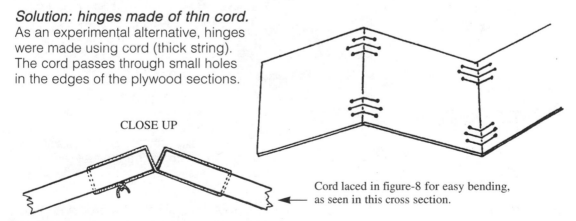

CLOSE UP

Cord laced in figure-8 for easy bending, as seen in this cross section.

Results of cord hinges: These hinges were as quick and easy to make as the cloth hinges, and they could be used at once (whereas several hours of drying time were needed before the cloth-and-glue hinges could be used). The cord hinges are stronger and hold up longer than the cloth hinges (although this clearly depends on the relative strength of the cord, the cloth, and the glue).

A Simple Aid For Active Correction And Prevention of Foot-Drop, In Bed

The problem: From lying in bed so long, Osvaldo had begun to develop contractures of his heel cords (Achilles tendons). This made it difficult to bring his feet up to 90 degrees. He wanted to do this with the dream of someday standing or even walking— or at least so his feet would be in a good position and he could wear shoes.

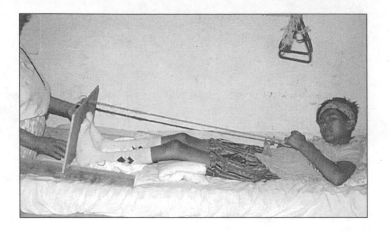

Osvaldo wondered if there was some way he could do the exercises by himself to regain the flexibility of his ankles.

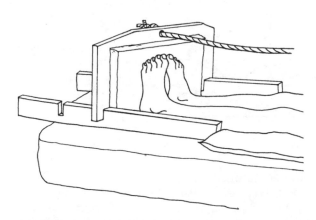

The solution: a flexible footboard pulled by a rope.

Materials: a short piece of thin wood plank; 2 narrow boards about 2 cm. by 6 cm. by 60 cm. long; a piece of rope (about 1 meter); a piece of dense rubber foam (to cushion the feet).

Construction: Notch wood, drill hole, and assemble as shown.

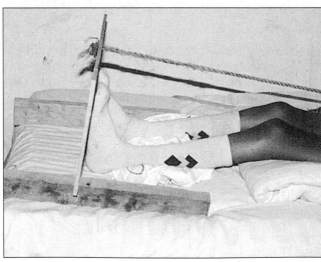

How it works: The footboard is placed to keep the feet upright (as near to 90 degrees as possible). For his heel-cord stretching exercises, Osvaldo pulled the rope himself.

As Osvaldo pulls the rope, the front ends of the side boards sink into the foam mattress, angling the footboard forward and stretching the feet (and heel-cords).

Results: The device worked fairly well. The hinge-like action, which allowed the footboard to angle forward more when pulled, was unplanned and recognized only when tried. The device actively involved Osvaldo in exercises to correct and prevent further contractures of his ankles. Moreover, to do the exercises, he had to move his upper body and shoulders somewhat, which he had resisted doing because of his hypersensitive right arm. So the foot exercises were also good therapy for his painful shoulder and arm.

AN ADJUSTABLE BED TABLE

The problem: Osvaldo, who before his accident had been right-handed, needed to develop confidence and skill in using his left hand. He also needed activities to keep him interested and busy during the long periods of lying in a flat or semi-sitting position. For this, he needed a table which could easily be rolled over his bed, and which could adjust both in slant and in height. The group decided that a wooden design, which any village carpenter could make, would be ideal.

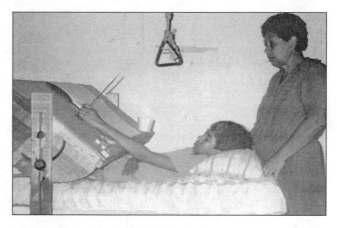

Solution: Two of the workers in the carpentry shop (Mario, who is paraplegic, and Rafa, who is quadriplegic) designed and built the wooden table shown below.

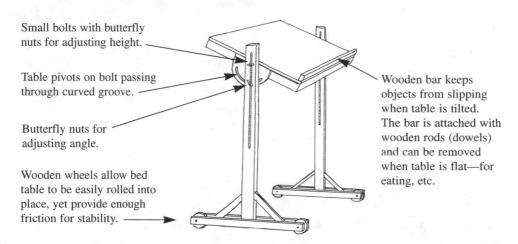

Small bolts with butterfly nuts for adjusting height.

Table pivots on bolt passing through curved groove.

Butterfly nuts for adjusting angle.

Wooden wheels allow bed table to be easily rolled into place, yet provide enough friction for stability.

Wooden bar keeps objects from slipping when table is tilted. The bar is attached with wooden rods (dowels) and can be removed when table is flat—for eating, etc.

Results: The table was handsome, strong, and it worked well. It was large and solid enough to double as a drafting table. It could also be used as a typing or work table by someone in a wheelchair. This model can be easily made or adapted by a local carpenter. Wooden wheels help keep the cost down. The only welding necessary was to fasten the "wings" on the butterfly nuts. (Ordinary nuts and bolts would work as well, but require a wrench.) For transport, the wing nuts can be removed and the whole table packed flat.

The adjustable bed table made it easier for Osvaldo to do many activities in bed. He took particular pleasure in drawing. He began to confront the challenge of learning to draw and write with his left hand.

Games. Some of the school children who came to visit Osvaldo made a **checker board** for him. While playing such games with other children, often the sign of a smile would creep over Osvaldo's face.

The main disadvantage of the table was its heavy weight and bulky size (as compared to the welded commercial hospital bed-tables that roll in from one side of the bed).

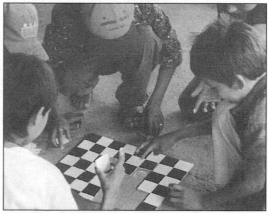

Village children make a checker board to play the game with Osvaldo.

GURNEY (NARROW WHEELED BED) WITH ONE-HAND DRIVE

Problem: To heal his pressure sores, Osvaldo needed to lie face-down for long periods. However, his paralyzed right arm was stiffly contracted over his chest. The arm was so hyper-sensitive that it would take a long time with therapy to regain enough flexibility to place it out of the way so that he could lie face down.

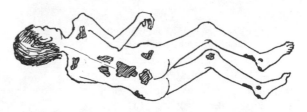

Another problem was how to help Osvaldo regain flexibility (bending ability) of his hips and knees while lying face down. A special gurney could be built for him with adjustable angles at the hips and knees. Actively moving about on the gurney would also stimulate circulation and thereby speed healing of the pressure sores.

But the biggest problem was: How could Osvaldo wheel and steer a gurney with one hand?

Solution: A one-hand-drive gurney with adjustable hip and knee angles, and with a cut-out section and lower-level table for his paralyzed arm.

A rectangle was cut out of the bed of the gurney at the level of Osvaldo's right shoulder, so his stiff arm could rest on a small, cushioned table underneath.

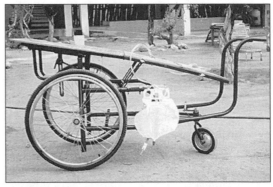

Gurney in straight position.

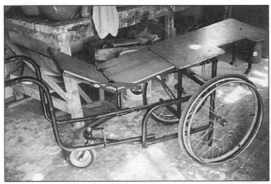

Gurney showing cut out space for the arm, and the cushioned table underneath.

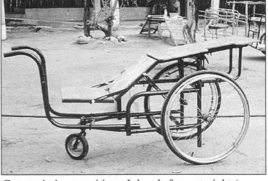

Gurney in bent position. It bends from straight (no angles) to right angles at the hips and knees.

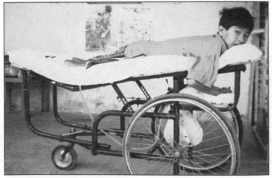

Osvaldo was first placed on the gurney lying in an almost straight position.

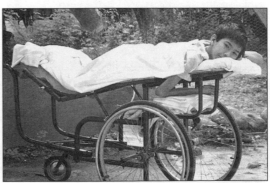

The angles of the gurney were slowly adjusted so that, little by little, his hips and knees would bend.

The steering device for the one-arm-drive gurney

A sliding knob is attached by a pivoting bar to a wire cable. The knob slides up and down to change the angle of the rear wheel. It screws down tightly to hold the rear wheel in the desired position.

The cable, which passes through a series of D-rings, controls the angle of a single, small rear caster wheel.

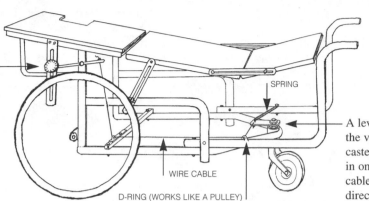

SPRING

A lever arm, attached to the vertical post of the caster wheel, is pulled in one direction by the cable, and in the other direction by a spring.

WIRE CABLE

D-RING (WORKS LIKE A PULLEY)

To move straight ahead, Osvaldo tightens the steering knob to hold the rear wheel straight, and rolls the gurney by pushing the hand rim of the left big wheel. **To make a turn,** he quickly loosens the knob, slides it up or down to angle the caster wheel either to the left or right, and again locks the knob in place. The turn completed, he again moves the knob and locks it in the straight-forward position.

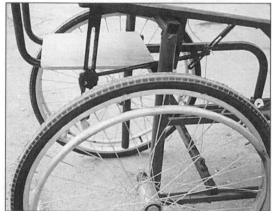

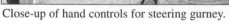

Close-up of hand controls for steering gurney.

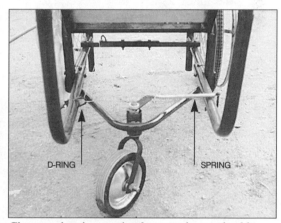

D-RING   SPRING

Close-up showing steering lever, spring, and cable.

Results: Although it had certain problems and limitations, the gurney was a great success for Osvaldo. Through repeated experimentation, and a flood of complaints and suggestions by Osvaldo, the steering mechanism was gradually improved.

At first, too much force was required to make a right turn, and only a very wide turn was possible. But, by placing the D-ring (pulley) nearest the caster further back to provide a pull at closer to 90 degrees, sharper turns could be made, and made more easily. Also, at Osvaldo's insistence, a rack was added on the front of the gurney to hold a large bottle of water (see page 197). This request by Osvaldo reflected his growing interest in making sure he drank enough liquids to avoid further urinary infections.

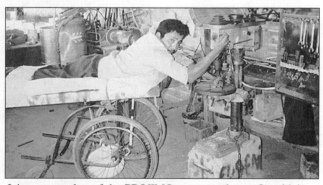

Jaime, a member of the PROJIMO team, works on Osvaldo's wheelchair. As a paraplegic person who works from a gurney, Jaime well understands Osvaldo's needs. He is a marvelous role model for the younger boy.

At first it was very difficult to place Osvaldo on the gurney and to position his hyper-sensitive arm without hurting him. But after a few days, the arm began to get a little more limber and the boy learned to help position both himself and his arm. Once in position, he was soon able to stay comfortably on the gurney for hours.

As the angles of the gurney at Osvaldo's hips and knees were gradually increased, the flexibility of his joints improved rapidly. Osvaldo soon began to spend much of the time on the gurney with his hips fairly straight and his knees bent up. The elevated position of his feet helped to prevent them from swelling. This, in turn, helped his ankle sores to heal.

In summary:

The gurney contributed to Osvaldo's rehabilitation in a wide variety of ways:

- It helped to heal his sores by removing the pressure on them (by his lying face down). Also, his energetic activity on the gurney improved his circulation, which helped the sores to heal faster.

- It protected his hypersensitive right hand by supporting it on a pillow below his body. But at the same time, his activity on the gurney caused some movement of his delicate arm and hand. He tolerated this because his mind was on other things and he was having a good time. Gradually his hand became less sensitive, so that he cautiously began to move it, to wash it himself, and to gently do exercises to get back flexibility. (Although the hand remained paralyzed, some strength returned in his shoulder, and eventually he started using it as a helping hand.)

- The hinged bed of the gurney helped to correct the extension contractures of his hips and knees, by gradually increasing the bend of its jointed sections.

- With its one-arm drive, the gurney allowed him the freedom of self-controlled and self-powered mobility. This greatly improved his outlook on life and on himself.

- Elevating his feet by flexing the hinge at his knees improved the circulation and decreased the swelling of his feet. (This speeded the healing of the deep sores on his ankles.)

- By encouraging physical activity and more drinking of water, the gurney helped to prevent urinary infection and kidney stones.

- Wheeling himself around on the gurney helped to strengthen his more useful arm, providing therapy that was both functional and fun.

- Altogether, the gurney gave him new self-confidence and improved his state of mind. His greater happiness was due partly to being able to go where he liked under his own power, and partly to his participation in designing and improving his own equipment.

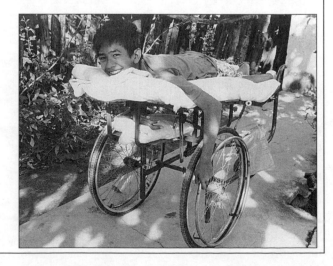

- The role model of other disabled persons who ride and work on gurneys helped a lot.

A One-Arm-Drive Wheelchair

Once Osvaldo's pressure sores had healed and he regained enough flexibility so that he could sit, he needed a one-hand-drive wheelchair.

The problem: Hemiplegic (one-hand drive) wheelchairs are manufactured commercially in the United States and in other rich countries. But they are very expensive and are usually not available in poor countries. Also, the drive mechanism is relatively complex and tends to break down quickly on rough terrain. (The problems with these commercial one-arm-drive wheelchairs are further discussed in Chapter 39.)

Occasionally, PROJIMO has a second-hand hemiplegic wheelchair donated from the cooperating hospitals and programs in the United States. But at the time Osvaldo needed one, none was available.

Solution: Like many rehabilitation programs in the Third World, PROJIMO has a big need for an easy-to-build, low-cost, hemiplegic wheelchair. It occurred to the workers in the shop that the same front-wheel steering mechanism used for Osvaldo's gurney might work for a wheelchair.

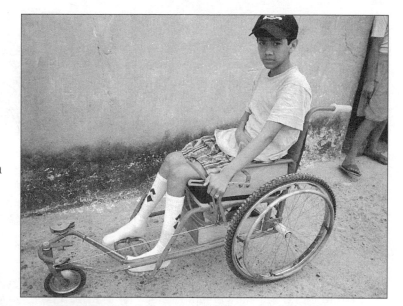

Through a lot of trials and suggestions by Osvaldo, a design was created.

A single front caster was controlled by pulleys and cable to a steering knob mounted on a vertical bracket on the left side of the chair.

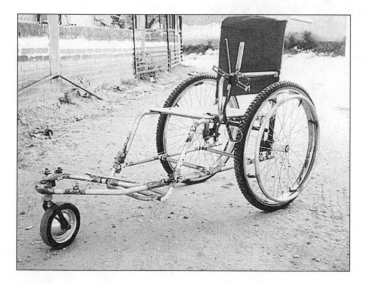

Trial construction, trouble-shooting, and improvements. In the early design, the very small D-rings (improvised front pulleys) gave too much resistance and made steering difficult.

In the modified design, larger, smoother-running pulleys were used. This made steering easier.

Pulling on the lock-knob required too much force for Osvaldo (whose back was still painful). Therefore a longer lever-arm was added.

Design details of Osvaldo's wheelchair:

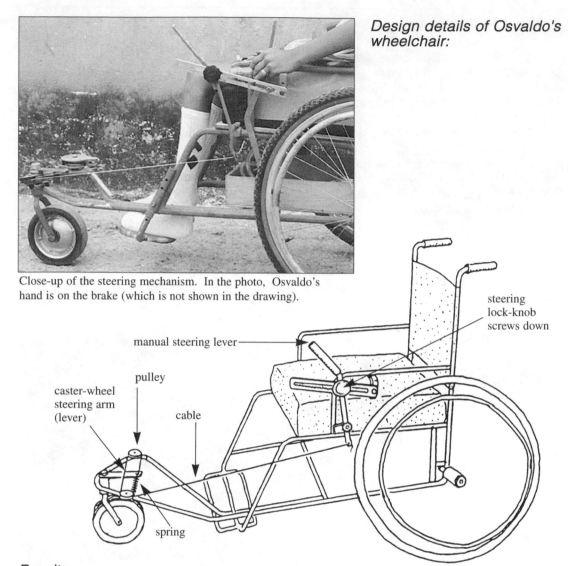

Close-up of the steering mechanism. In the photo, Osvaldo's hand is on the brake (which is not shown in the drawing).

manual steering lever

pulley

caster-wheel steering arm (lever)

cable

spring

steering lock-knob screws down

Results:

After several modifications to make steering easier, Osvaldo found the chair very useful. He learned to steer it with remarkable agility and became relatively independent. The strength in his left arm increased. The removable arm rest on the right side, plus the easy access for his feet, made putting him in and out of the chair relatively simple. He soon learned to help with the transfers, using his left arm.

One disadvantage of this design is its lengthy forward extension to support the steering wheel. This makes moving about in close quarters more difficult (although far less so than the front-wheel-drive tricycles with a bicycle wheel at the front, which are even longer and more cumbersome). On the positive side, the narrowness of the "nose" of Osvaldo's chair, and the small front wheel, make moving about in close quarters somewhat easier.

In conclusion, the Osvaldo one-hand-drive wheelchair provided a relatively low-cost, easily constructed option in situations where standard hemiplegic chairs are seldom available, too costly, and not durable. Although to our knowledge this new wheelchair has not yet been duplicated, we feel it has the potential to help fill the enormous unmet need of hemiplegic wheelchair riders in low-income situations. However, the design still needs to be simplified and improved. One possibility might be to shorten the forward extension to make it easier to move about indoors.

For another, better design of a one-arm wheelchair, see the next chapter (page 253).

Summary of the Combined Methods of Managing Osvaldo's Pressure Sores

Following his accident Osvaldo lay on his back for 5 months without being turned. When he came to PROJIMO he had 11 pressure sores, extending from mid back to his heels. The largest sores were 2 to 3 inches across. Most were fairly shallow (bone not exposed) and his mother had kept them fairly clean. However, there was some dead as well as unhealthy gray tissue on the surface of the sores. The deepest sore, about 2 inches long, was over the heel cord (Achilles tendon) of his left foot; the tendon was exposed.

Complicating treatment of Osvaldo's pressure sores was his hypersensitive paralyzed right arm, which had become rigidly contracted over his chest. This stiff, painful arm prevented him from lying either face down, or on his right side.

SIX STEPS TAKEN TO PROMOTE HEALING OF OSVALDO'S PRESSURE SORES:

1. **Minimize pressure over the sores while lying down.** This was done by:

Putting cushions under his legs to take pressure off his buttocks, lower back, and ankles/heels.

Providing a ring so he could lift himself up.

Using a thick sponge mattress.

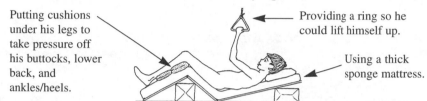

2. **Adequate cleaning of the sores; treatment with sugar and honey.**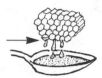

3. **Wheeled mobility while lying face down, with the feet up** (until the sores heal).

4. **Lots of activity to speed up circulation, which causes faster healing.**

5. **Food rich in calories, protein, and iron to strengthen the body and blood, to speed healing.**

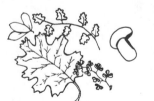

LOTS OF LIQUID—BEST TREATMENT FOR URINARY INFECTION!

6. **Management of the boy's overall health, especially his urinary system.**

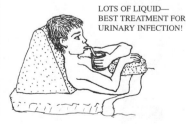

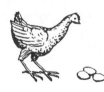

7. **Strengthening the good arm and increasing his ability to change his position.**

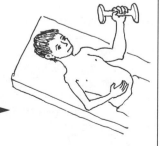

8. **Encourage the boy's understanding and responsibility in healing and preventing pressure sores: above all, changing position and lifting up the body often.**

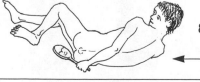

MEDICAL TREATMENT OF OSVALDO'S PRESSURE SORES

Treatment involved **daily washings,** at first brisk enough to remove dead flesh. Once the healthy red flesh was exposed, cleansing became quite gentle so as to avoid damage to the newly forming tissues. After cleaning the sores, a paste of **bees' honey mixed with sugar** was applied to the sores and covered lightly with gauze (see page 156).

Results: With this treatment program, combined with the management techniques reviewed on page 251, the sores healed remarkably fast. Even the deep sore over Osvaldo's heel healed in 3 weeks. The team feels it was the combined actions of treatment and management that led to rapid healing. Surely the change in Osvaldo's attitude made a big difference. He began to oversee and take responsibility for his own care, advising his mother and other attendants about how to place padding to relieve pressure over bony areas, and asking to be turned or moved after a time in one position. His increased physical activity also probably contributed to his quick healing, as did the many hours he spent each day lying face-down on his specially designed gurney.

Comparison of PROJIMO's methods with hospital treatment of Osvaldo's pressure sores. The steel rods surgically placed in Osvaldo's back after his accident came loose, and had begun to poke through the skin. To remove the rods, Osvaldo was taken to an orthopedic hospital in California. During the 2-day drive, a new small pressure sore formed over his sacrum (bottom part of the spine). In the hospital, *Duoderm* (a costly, medicated, absorbent bandage) was put over the sore, and Osvaldo was placed in bed for 24 hours a day. He lay on his back on a special air-flow mattress run by an electric air-pump, so that the pressure over each small area of the body was constantly changing.

In the hospital, with all this costly treatment and equipment, the boy in his space-age bed was deprived of all choice or responsibility for his own care. His pressure sore—smaller and more superficial than ones that had healed in 3 weeks at PROJIMO—took over 2 months to heal.

Ironically, from lying flat on his back for so long in the hospital, Osvaldo's knees and hips were again becoming rigid. A physiotherapist, attempting to restore flexibility, used too much force and broke his right leg. With his leg in a cast for weeks, a new deep pressure sore formed on his right heel. Again, it took over 2 months to heal. During all these months in the hospital, Osvaldo's anger, hostility, and depression—which he had gradually been overcoming—re-emerged. The nurses were at a loss for knowing how to get him to cooperate.

Comparing results of Osvaldo's management at PROJIMO with those at this modern orthopedic hospital, it appears that the comprehensive, action-oriented, *whole-person* approach used at the village center was relatively successful— at least for the healing rate of pressure sores. The rapid healing achieved with Osvaldo's sores has occurred with many (but not all) persons attended at PROJIMO. More comparative study is needed.

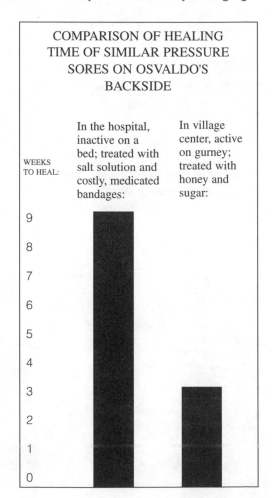

A One-Hand-Drive Wheelchair for Che: A Challenge for Martín

CHAPTER **39**

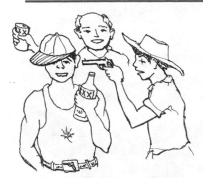

CHE was a policeman until the fateful night he was shot. He and his drinking buddies had decided to play "Russian Roulette," a deadly game where men point a six-shooter pistol with just one bullet in it at each other's head, pull the trigger, and see who gets shot first! Che lost. The bullet left him paralyzed on the left side of his body (hemiplegic).

Luckily, Che's mind and speech were unaffected. He was given a standard wheelchair. But with the use of only one arm, he needed assistance to go anywhere.

Che spent months at PROJIMO for rehabilitation and to learn new skills. A commercial one-arm-drive wheelchair from the United States had been donated to the program. Che loved it, and tried to go everywhere in it. But it kept breaking down.

Commercial one-arm-drive wheelchairs always break. Factory-made hemiplegic (one-arm-drive) wheelchairs are very expensive and seldom seen in poor countries. They have design problems which limit their usefulness. They are built for smooth hospital floors, not village paths. On rough terrain, they repeatedly break—and are hard and costly to fix.

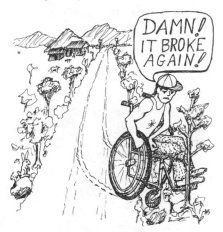

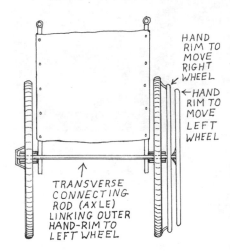

Diagram of wheelchair (seen from behind), showing two hand-rims on the right side, one for each wheel.

This commercial design is nothing like Osvaldo's one-arm-drive chair made at PROJIMO (see page 249). In the commercial chair, the rider delivers power to both rear wheels with one hand. The two hand-rims, one next to and slightly smaller than the other, are mounted on one side of the chair. One rim is fixed to the wheel on that side. The other is connected by a central axle (transverse rod) to the opposite wheel. To move straight ahead, the rider grips both hand-rims at once. To make a turn, he pushes just one hand-rim.

The weakness of the commercial chair is that the axle that transfers power from one side to the other is too thin. It passes (on ball bearings) through the center of the wheel hub on the near side, and is welded to the hub on the far side. Unfortunately, the axle cannot be replaced by a thicker, stronger one because of the small hub-hole it goes through. When modestly stressed, the fragile axle *breaks*.

Need for a Rugged, Low-Cost, One-Hand-Drive Wheelchair. PROJIMO sees a lot of persons who need a one-hand-drive wheelchair. These include folks who have had a stroke or suffered a head injury (like Che), and children with "hemiplegic" cerebral palsy.

Osvaldo's chair with front-wheel steering allowed him to move about town independently and helped him to recover self-direction and the will to live. The design was simple, low cost, and fairly easy to make. But that chair had one big disadvantage. Like hand-driven tricycles, it took up a lot of space. Indoors, it was cumbersome. There was a need for a one-arm chair that was cheap, road-worthy, and compact.

Martín Pérez Designs a Stronger One-Arm-Drive Wheelchair

MARTÍN, the paraplegic wheelchair builder whose gurney is featured in Chapter 37, was aware of the need for a reliable, one-arm-drive wheelchair. Time and again, he had welded and tried to strengthen the weak axle of Che's commercial chair. He also realized that, if the power-transfer mechanism broke while the rider was climbing a steep ramp or trail, it could be dangerous.

During Martín's visit to California, while recovering from surgery, he stayed in the home of wheel-chair designer, Ralf Hotchkiss. When Ralf was away teaching, Martín used Ralf's workshop, which is beautifully adapted for working from a wheelchair (see page 195). One day, Martín began to design and build a one-arm-drive wheelchair that would be compact and low-cost, yet strong.

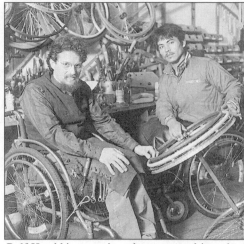

Ralf Hotchkiss examines the one arm drive wheel-chair which Martín is building. The 2 hand-rims are on one side and can be powered together or independently with one hand.

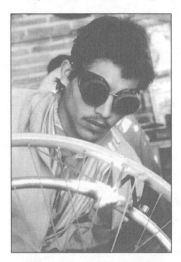

In building the wheelchair frame, Martín followed Ralf's basic Whirlwind design. **For the one-arm-drive mechanism, he used features from the commercial design, but with a much thicker and stronger transverse rod (axle)** to transfer power from a hand-rim on one side of the chair to the wheel on the far side.

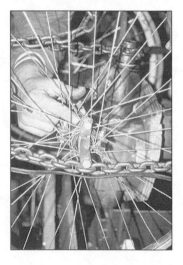

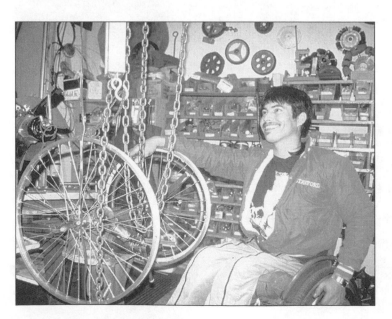

Testing the strength of the new mechanism.
When the chair was done, Martín and Ralf tested the strength of the one-arm-drive mechanism. They hooked a spring scale to the far wheel, and with a block-and-tackle put increasing force on the hand-rim that powered it. To their joy, Martín's heavy-duty axle-rod withstood over 200 pounds of force before it broke. This is much stronger than the commercial hemiplegic system (which breaks at about 30 pounds of force).

Part Five

INNOVATIVE METHODS AND APPROACHES

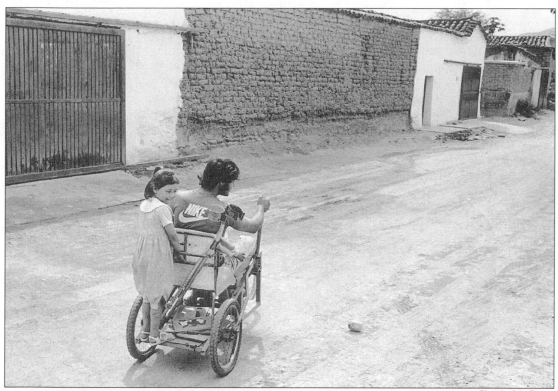

Photo by John Fago

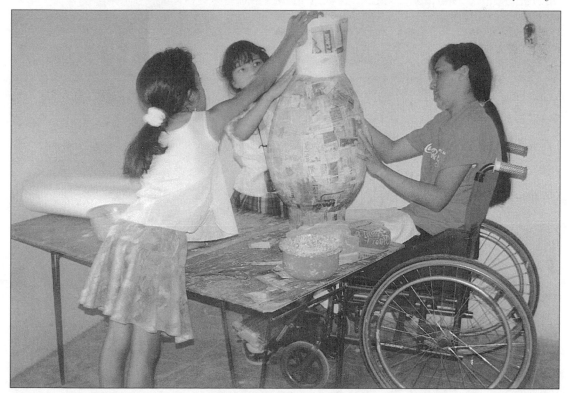

Carmen, who is paraplegic, earns a living making decorative pottery. She covers a big balloon with paper maché (see page 65), then covers that with plaster of Paris designs. Here she teaches two girls at PROJIMO.

INTRODUCTION TO PART FIVE

People Helping and Learning from Each Other as Equals

The importance of physical aids and equipment must not be undervalued. They can be essential for some people to meet their full potential. However, **many disabled persons feel that the most difficult barriers they face are not physical, but social.** Non-disabled people tend to see them as helpless and invalid (not valid). Too often they focus on what disabled persons cannot do rather than on what they can do, on their weaknesses, not their strengths. As a result, many persons with disabilities are denied an equal chance.

To win more equal opportunities will require a community with greater understanding, appreciation, and respect for all people, regardless of differences. This necessitates changes in many people's attitudes and perceptions. In the words of disabled activist Joshua Malinga from Zimbabwe,

"IT IS SOCIETY THAT NEEDS TO BE REHABILITATED."

LOOK FIRST AT MY STRENGTHS, NOT AT MY WEAKNESSES

Soft Technologies. Some important innovations for the enablement of disabled persons are in the realm of "soft" technologies. They include **methods, games,** and activities for **building greater awareness, understanding, and equality** with those who are different. They foster a spirit of caring and sharing, of **looking at other people's strengths, not their weaknesses.**

In this part of the book, we look at examples of soft technologies that help to engender appreciation and equality. But in reality, there is no sharp division between "hard" technologies (which deal with things) and "soft" technologies (methods, approaches, and human processes). The earlier parts of the book stressed the importance of equality and partnership in developing technical aids that meet disabled persons' needs on their terms. By contrast, here we see that some of the best ways for disabled persons to win respect and acceptance in the community are through the **development of practical skills** and by taking action to **assist or defend the rights of others.** Actions speak louder than words.

In the village of Ajoya where PROJIMO is located, the community's growing appreciation of disabled persons has not primarily been due to awareness-raising campaigns.

Rather, attitudes have changed as people have witnessed, in their daily lives, the skills which disabled people have gained and the crucial services they provide.

The fact that both the disability program and the health program are run mainly by disabled persons, and that the whole community benefits, has done much to change people's views about what disabled people can do.

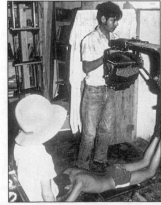

Roberto, who has arthritis, heads the village clinic, delivers babies, and does minor surgery. Here, he operates a donated X-ray machine.

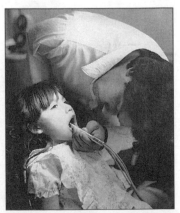

Cleto, a village dental worker who has one arm, drills and fills a child's teeth. Such services help people appreciate disabled persons for their abilities.

A Positive Public Image of Disabled Persons in Society

Appropriate technologies take many forms. One important form of soft technology is **effective communication.** It is important to overcome the image of disabled persons as helpless and tragic persons to be pitied.

Positive images invite positive responses. Where possible, they should show disabled persons who are happy and active, doing worthwhile things with other people, taking initiative, standing up for their rights, and busily getting on with life. **Here are a few examples:**

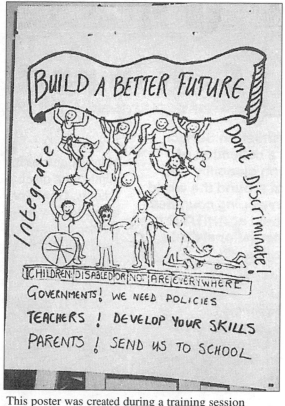

This poster was created during a training session at a *Save the Children Fund* global seminar, 1994.

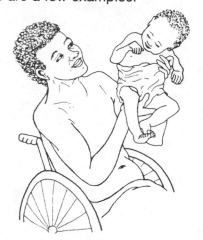

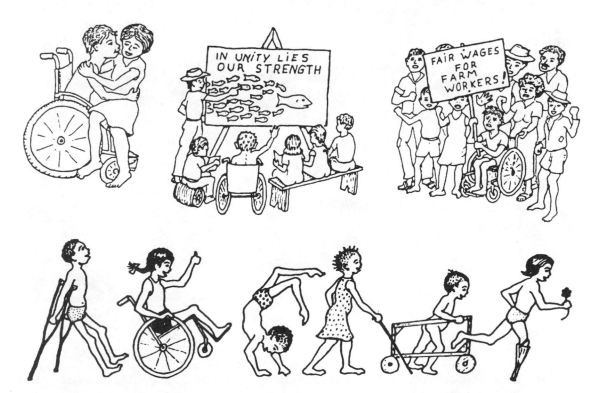

For guidelines on effective communication through printed material, see page 340.

Appropriate Technology for Feeding Babies

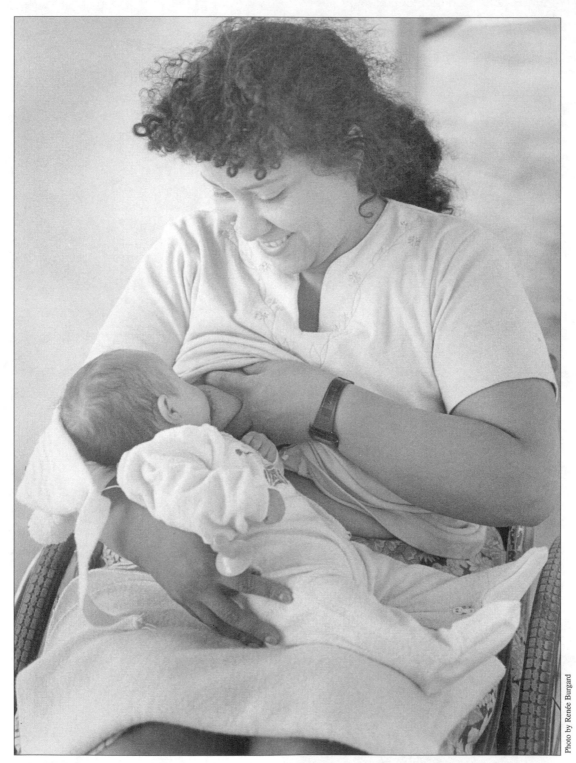

When Mari first came to PROJIMO 2 years after the car accident that made her paraplegic, she was sure that her intimate life as a woman had ended. But that changed when she and Armando grew close and then were married. Mari is wonderful with her daughter Lluvia, and knows that to protect her baby's health *"Breast is Best."* **Mari is a splendid role model for other disabled women.**

Ways Disabled Persons Win Community Respect

Making Unusual Abilities Available. Many persons with disabilities have outstanding abilities. One of the best ways that disabled persons can win the respect and appreciation of those around them is by making their particular abilities visible or publicly available. Here are a few examples.

Welding service and repair shop. Several of the disabled workers at PROJIMO learned welding and metal-working skills in order to build wheelchairs. Because there is no other welding shop in town, farmers began to come to them with broken plows, boys came with broken bicycles, and women arrived with leaking buckets. Completely unplanned, the wheelchair shop has become a village repair shop. People have come to see the disabled workers not in terms of their disabilities, but in terms of their ability to provide services that no able-bodied person there is able to do.

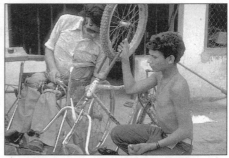

Leopoldo Leyva, a wheelchair rider and builder at PROJIMO, welds a village boy's broken bicycle.

Unusual strength that comes from weakness. One time, when a street light in town burned out, the only person who was daring and able enough to change it was Marcelo.

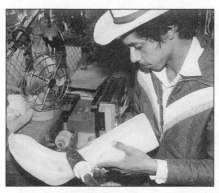

Marcelo's legs are weak from polio. But his arms and hands are very strong because he has used crutches to get about on mountain trails since childhood.

Marcelo is also a master craftsman, brace maker, and limb maker. Here, he makes a plastic leg brace.

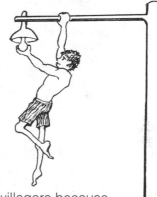

Marcelo has won the respect of the PROJIMO team and of the villagers because he is a peace maker in times of dispute, a loving father to his four sons, and he does not waste his modest income on liquor, as do many of the village men.

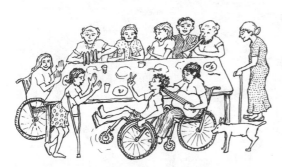

A Christmas dinner for lonely old folks. A few years ago, when disabled youth at PROJIMO were planning a Christmas dinner, someone recalled that of the many elderly folks in town, some were abandoned and alone: "They must feel lonely on Christmas Eve. Why don't we invite them?" Everyone agreed. The occasion was a warm reunion, with music, stories, and lots of conviviality.

The old folks were touched that someone remembered them, as was the rest of the town. The villagers realized that, on this special day, the disabled group showed more social responsibility—more caring and sharing—than did the larger community. The disabled young people provided a good role model for all. Year after year, PROJIMO continues to invite old folks to Christmas dinner.

Courage in the Face of Repression

Abuse of authority in the Sierra Madre. In the mountains of Mexico, almost everyone fears the state police and the soldiers, who are often brutal to those who have committed no crime. One time, I (the author) had to help amputate the hand of a 10-year-old boy who was hit by a high-speed explosive bullet. Soldiers had fired at villagers at an outdoor dance. When someone shouted, "Here come the soldiers!" everyone ran in fear. So the soldiers fired at them. The logic: *If they run, they must be guilty.*

These were anti-narcotics troops, part of the so-called *War on Drugs.* The United States government supplies them with automatic weapons and high-speed bullets. (This violates international law, which prohibits use of such destructive bullets against civilians.)

Such brutality might be more excusable if the War on Drugs were not such a sham. The anti-narcotics troops are notorious for accepting bribes from the large drug growers. They do more to promote than to control the growing and trafficking of illegal drugs. I personally treated a man with broken ribs who was beaten up by the soldiers for *not* growing drugs.

When the US government demands from Mexico a "massive wave of arrests," the Mexican soldiers raid villages and drag men out of their homes at night. They divide their captives into two groups. They torture one group until they sign statements accusing those in the other group of drug growing. One time, those men and boys who refused to "confess" were thrown off the back of a speeding pick-up truck onto a gravel road. A friend of mine was still limping a year after this ordeal. In sum, the illicit drug scene and corrupt narcotics control program is a major cause of violence, death, and disability in the Sierra Madre.

Roberto and other disabled leaders of PROJIMO have publicly protested abuses by the soldiers and police, and have called on the *Commission of Human Rights* and on *Amnesty International* to become involved. Consequently, two of the disabled workers had their lives threatened. However, word of the abuses reached the President of Mexico, who gave orders that the drug-control troops cut back on violence. A period followed in which the worst violence, torture, illegal arrests, and clandestine killings were reduced.

Disabled women protect the village doctor.

The soldiers prohibit health workers from giving medical care to persons wounded by gunfire, and they are sometimes brutal with those who do. One time, four soldiers burst into the village health center and arrested Alvaro, a young doctor who had been a village health worker and who has worked closely with the PROJIMO team. They accused him of having provided emergency care to a man they were hunting and whom they had wounded. The soldiers marched Alvaro out of the clinic and threw him into the back of a pick-up truck.

The villagers, watching from behind closed doors, worried for the well-being and even the life of their doctor, but they were afraid to speak out. However, when word of the doctor's arrest reached PROJIMO, the team took action. In wheelchairs and on crutches, they surrounded the soldiers' truck, which was about to leave. The soldiers ordered them away. But the group refused to move until their doctor was released. The soldiers were taken aback. Reluctant to attack women in wheelchairs, they released the doctor.

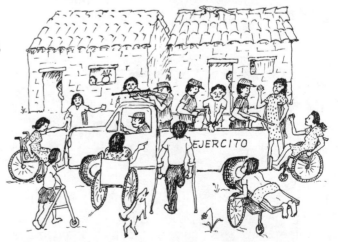

As a result of this action, the disabled people at PROJIMO won even greater respect and appreciation in the village. As one of the village elders commented proudly, "What they lack in muscles, they make up for in guts!"

In Defense of Human Rights

One cannot work for the well-being of poor and disabled persons without becoming involved in human rights and questions of social justice.

As an example, PROJIMO learned of a 12-year-old boy, **ALEJANDRO,** who one day in the slums of a coastal city asked a policeman, "What caliber is your pistol?"

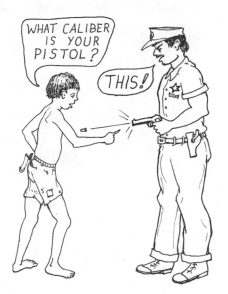

"I'll show you!" said the policeman. Drawing his pistol, he shot the boy through the spine, paralyzing him for life.

PROJIMO has helped young Alejandro with **medical care, schooling, skills training,** and **mobility aids** (see Chapter 31). But the team has also tried to get **legal recourse.** They have not made a great effort to seek punishment for the policeman (which, given the existing power structure, is highly unlikely).

Rather, they have tried to get the city to assume responsibility for the boy's ongoing medical and disability-related costs so that he can stay healthy, attend school, and prepare himself for a reasonable life. It has been an uphill battle, but the city did respond with limited assistance for a while.

More recently, the government's Integrated Family Development Program (DIF) has taken steps to improve the situation of Alejandro and his family, who live in dire poverty. This assistance was spear-headed by an outstanding social worker, **DOLORES** Mesina, who had polio as a child, uses a wheelchair, and is herself a graduate from PROJIMO. Dolores has helped to arrange scholarships for Alejandro to continue schooling, and found funding for a hand-powered tricycle, so that he can get to and from school on the rough roads.

Since Dolores assumed this important post with DIF, there has been much closer cooperation between DIF and PROJIMO.

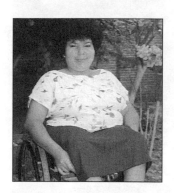

In Defense of Disabled People's Rights. As a wheelchair-riding woman, Dolores Mesina has faced enormous obstacles. In Mexico, it is remarkable that she was able to persevere with her studies and earn a degree as a social worker. That she has obtained a key job in a government program for disabled people is a big breakthrough in the disabled community's struggle to gain strong representation in the decisions and services that affect them. Thanks to Dolores, the motto of the Independent Living Movement, *NOTHING ABOUT US WITHOUT US,* is a little closer to becoming a reality.

Dolores has also started and helped to lead an organization of disabled activists in the coastal city of Mazatlán. This organization has played an active role in the growing **disability rights movement in Mexico,** which has successfully pressured the Mexican government to adopt laws designed to guarantee greater equality, schooling opportunities, and employment of disabled people. Thanks in part to her effort, the barriers to schooling and employment may not be as great for the next generation of disabled youth as they were for Dolores.

In several countries, disabled people have succeeded not only in winning respect for their abilities, but they have won leading and decision-making roles in both government and non-government programs for disabled persons. Examples are Judy Heumann, a polio-disabled woman who now holds a high post in the *Department of Human Services* in the USA, and Beng Linguist, a blind Swedish activist who has a key position in the United Nations.

Disabled Children learn Capoeira in Brazil

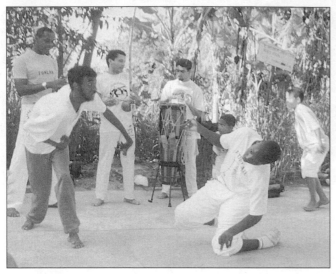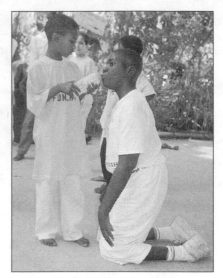

FUNLAR, a community rehabilitation program in the favelas (slums) of Rio de Janeiro, includes disabled children in learning *capoeira,* a ritualistic form of self-defense. Here youths with developmental delay, Down's syndrome and cerebral palsy (boy on knees), perform to music together with non disabled street children.

Jesús Learns Karate at PROJIMO

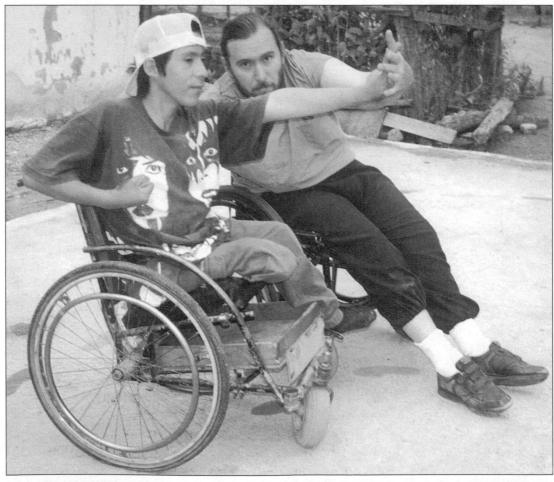

Doug, a visiting North American who has cerebral palsy, teaches karate to Jesús, who has spina bifida and is visually impaired. (See Jesús' story, Chapter 45.)

Karate for Fun (and Therapy) for Children with Cerebral Palsy

CHAPTER **41**

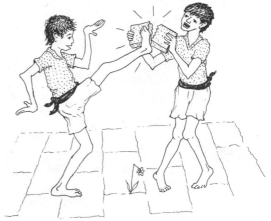

In many countries today, children are fascinated by karate and eager to learn this ancient, artful form of self-defense. Youngsters with cerebral palsy share this fascination with karate—but rarely have a chance to learn it.

In *The Spastics Society of Tamilnadu* (SPASTN), an innovative program in southeast India, children with mild to moderate cerebral palsy are taught karate. They take it very seriously. Likewise their trainers, who are volunteer professional karate instructors, take the children and their learning seriously.

At its best, karate is a physical art which teaches its disciples self-mastery of body and mind, as well as a philosophy of harmony and non-aggressive self-defense. Its guided rhythmic movements conform with many of the therapeutic movements and positioning used for children with cerebral palsy.

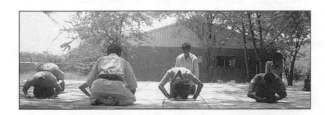

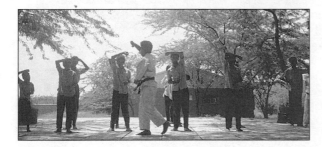

Seeing these children proudly demonstrate their karate skills is a mind-altering revelation, even to those of us who work routinely with disabled kids. It awakens us to the children's hidden potentials. We learn that, when they are challenged with an activity that they passionately want and choose to do, it is astonishing what they can accomplish. Observing their concentration and unexpected grace as they perform this ancient art stretches the boundaries of what therapists, care-takers, and the children themselves dream is possible. For doer and viewer alike, it is a liberating experience.

The karate program at SPASTN was initiated by karate master Shihan Hussaini, who is also trained in social work and guidance counseling. The parents are delighted with the results, and teachers are amazed.

Observable benefits are many: better coordination (both gross and fine), improved behavior and attention span, and a greater sense of personal adequacy, positive self image, feeling of fulfillment, and self-confidence.

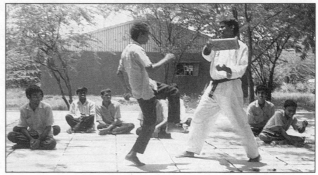

Children with mild to moderate spastic cerebral palsy practice karate with concentration and pride.

Using What Works Best

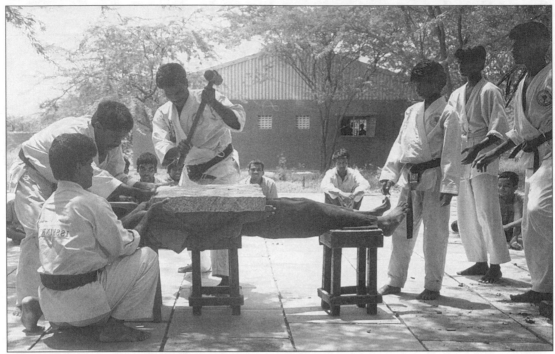

A boy, using his spasticity to good advantage, lies stretched rigidly between stools while a karate master breaks a stone block resting on the fearless boy's body.

In addition to karate, the SPASTN Center assists children with cerebral palsy to expand their capabilities. Rather than trying to "normalize" disabled children to do things the same way non-disabled children do them, they help children learn to do things in whatever way is easiest and works best for them.

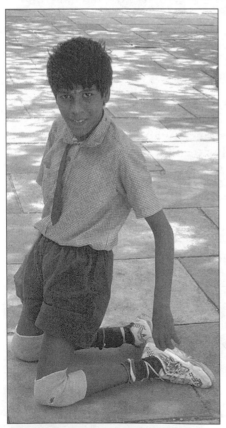

A boy with spastic cerebral palsy walks on knees that are well-protected with padding.

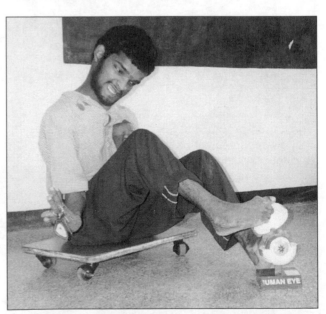

Sitting on his scooter board, this boy skillfully assembles an intricate model of the human eye with his feet.

Need for Independent Living and Women's Liberation: Conchita's Story

The Need for Independence from One's Own Family

In many countries, community based rehabilitation (CBR) has been promoted with its main focus in the homes of disabled individuals. Each home is regularly visited by a "local supervisor," who teaches the family to do rehabilitation activities with the disabled person. In these programs, often there is little encouragement for community centers— even if they are run and controlled by disabled persons themselves. The World Health Organization's guidelines strongly discourage residential centers where disabled children (or adults) are kept away from their homes for rehabilitation and skills training.

Certainly there is a good argument for not taking young disabled children out of their homes and putting them in special boarding schools or in "institutional care." **Usually the best place for a disabled child, like any child, is her or his own home.**

But every rule has its exceptions. **Many disabled children are so over-protected by their parents that they develop little self-confidence or sense of personal worth.** *Especially with teenagers, as long as they stay in their home, they may have a hard time establishing an identity as self-determined adults. As a result, they may become despondent, and appear to lack energy or will power. For some of these youth, a community rehabilitation center—or* **independent living center**—*can help them find their footing and a new sense of self. This was true for Manolo and Luis, whose story is told in Chapter 46, as with many young people who have spent time at PROJIMO. It was especially true for Conchita.*

Conchita's Liberation as a Disabled Person and as a Woman

CONCHITA, who was extremely dependent, depressed, and even suicidal when she first came to PROJIMO, has become one of the program's most capable, caring, and self-reliant leaders. She became paraplegic from a fall as a teenager and spent 8 years at home after her accident. Her family did everything for her, and she had little hope of ever becoming independent, holding a job, or getting married.

When Conchita visited PROJIMO for the first time, she was astounded to see other disabled persons, including spinal-cord injured young women like herself, fully self-reliant and performing a wide range of skills and services. She at once wanted to stay, and had a hard time convincing her protective parents not to stay there with her.

Eventually, Conchita not only became a highly capable leader and technician at PROJIMO, she also married, has two lovely daughters, and manages her own household.

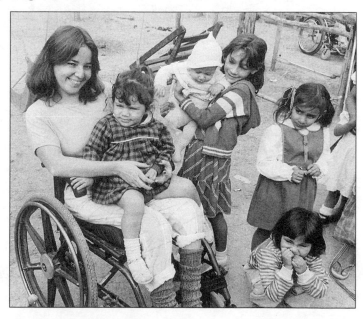

Women's rights. Another one of Conchita's accomplishments is even more impressive: her liberation from male dominance in a Mexican village.

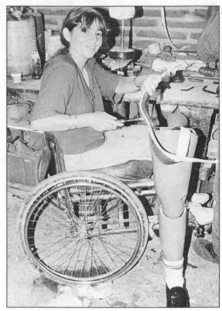

When Conchita was first at PROJIMO, she worked with energy and commitment, giving of herself unselfishly for the well-being of the disabled kids whose needs she helped to meet. She often spoke of her coming to PROJIMO as her "return to life." However, acceptance of her womanhood, with possibilities for love, sex and marriage, took longer. As she saw other disabled persons at PROJIMO having loving relationships and getting married, she began to re-examine her feelings and potentials. A friendship with Miguel, one of the few non-disabled workers at PROJIMO, gradually became more intimate. The mutual attraction began to overcome Conchita's doubts and fears. Eventually she married and moved into a small, lovely home that Miguel built for her. A year later, she had her first baby, Camelia.

Conchita has learned to make artificial legs.

Conchita's husband loves her dearly. But, at first, he treated her like his personal property. He wanted her to do nothing more with her life than to be a good housewife. He insisted that she ask his permission for everything she wanted to do. At the same time, he expected her to suffer in silence his late nights on the town, his drinking habits, and his angry temper.

Influenced by the spirit of equality and self-determination at PROJIMO, in her marriage Conchita was unwilling to settle for the subservient role that most men expect of their wives in Latin American (and in much of the world). She began to demand her rights and insist that her husband treat her as an equal. At first, Conchita's insistence on equality was very hard for her young husband to accept. But she persevered and, in time, Miguel lost a lot of his macho stance and began to treat her with respect. All in all, Miguel has become a more even-tempered, considerate person. He also drinks less than he used to, and is a more responsible and loving father.

Helping other women to stand up for their rights. Conchita and Mari, the two principle leaders of PROJIMO, have both managed to gain equal standing with their husbands in making decisions that affect their lives. In addition, they have helped other girls and young women at PROJIMO to stand up for their personal and sexual rights. The example they have set has had an impact on the whole village, where many women are beginning to speak out, and to refuse to accept double standards from their husbands.

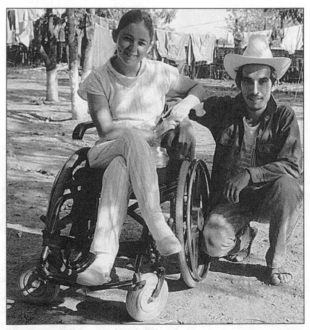

So it is that Conchita has not only emancipated herself by standing up for her rights, but she has also had a liberating and equalizing impact on many of the other women in the village.

Conchita with her husband, Miguel.

Disabled Gangsters Help a Child with Muscular Dystrophy

CHAPTER **43**

Creating an Environment That Brings Unexpected Improvement in Children with Muscular Dystrophy

Muscular dystrophy is a condition in which muscles gradually become weaker and weaker. Most specialists agree that nothing can be done to help the child regain lost strength. This may be true in the long run. But we have seen some children seem to get stronger, at least for a limited time.

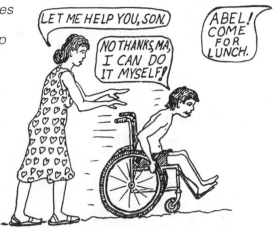

ABEL, for example, is a boy with Duchenne's muscular dystrophy. His arms had grown so weak that he could not push his wheelchair more than a few inches on a flat surface. His parents wheeled him everywhere. While at PROJIMO, Abel gradually regained enough strength to wheel himself around the whole yard. In doing so, he gained a new sense of self-determination.

Over a period of 3 years, as his dystrophy slowly progressed, Abel again lost his capacity to propel his wheelchair. But for years he had achieved greater independence of movement— an ability which he, his parents, and his doctors had assumed was permanently lost.

Although a child with muscular dystrophy has slowly diminishing muscular potential, it appears that, **at any stage of his condition, his strength and physical ability can be increased to more closely approach his potential at that stage.**

Abel's increase in strength and ability at PROJIMO was probably the result of several factors: **increased** *activity,* increased *motivation,* and increased **expectation by others.** At home, his parents had done everything for him. They had kept him away from activities and adventures they feared might tire him. But at PROJIMO, Abel was encouraged to do as much as he could for himself. Also, he had excellent role models, including persons who were quadriplegic (paralyzed from the shoulders down), yet who were largely independent in self-care.

Creating an environment that brings unexpected improvement—in gangsters.

There is an old saying: "Poor Mexico, so far from God and so close to the United States!" Mexico's huge foreign debt, falling wages, growing unemployment, and pressure from the US to weaken Mexican laws protecting small farmers have all increased the hardships for most Mexicans.

Since the start of the North American Free Trade Agreement (NAFTA) in 1994, over 2 million peasants have been forced off their land to join the jobless multitudes in Mexico's swelling city slums. As the gap widens between rich and poor, millions of street children and youth struggle to survive through odd jobs, stealing, prostitution, and drug trafficking. Crime rates, violence, and police brutality have drastically increased. This growing "sub-culture of violence" has brought new difficulties and challenges to PROJIMO. The small village program has had to attend to over 400 spinal-cord injured youths, mostly disabled by bullet wounds, from all over Mexico.

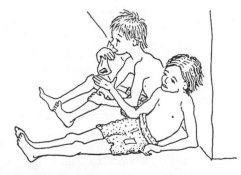

Children as young as 7 years old sniff glue to dull hunger. Many join street gangs.

Dilemma for PROJIMO. When these newly disabled street-youths and gangsters arrive at PROJIMO, most are angry and depressed. Many have been heavy users of alcohol and drugs. Becoming physically disabled does not automatically end their habits of violence, crime, and drugs. PROJIMO has, within the program, had to deal with acts of violence, armed assault, drug trafficking and use, drunkenness, attempted rape, and attempted murder. The team has sought new ways to deal with the complex needs of young men and women (mostly men) who are both physically and psycho-socially disabled.

It has not been easy. PROJIMO has set rules of behavior prohibiting alcohol, drugs, and violence within its grounds. Those who break the rules are threatened with expulsion. But **it is not easy to throw out someone who has dangerous pressure sores or other life-threatening problems.** Many have no home to return to. To send them back to the city streets can be a death sentence. One young quadriplegic man who was expelled from PROJIMO died from pressure sores 3 months later.

One of the worst acts of violence at PROJIMO was when two young men, who had been shot through the spine in gang fights, got high on drugs and booze. They attacked a retired, diabetic school teacher who was being fitted for an artificial leg. They tried to stab him as he lay on his bed. The terrified teacher shielded himself with an electric fan until help arrived.

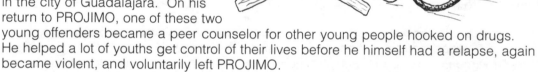

To cope with this problem, PROJIMO sought help from an *Alcoholics-and-Drugs-Anonymous* program run by recovering addicts in the city of Guadalajara. On his return to PROJIMO, one of these two young offenders became a peer counselor for other young people hooked on drugs. He helped a lot of youths get control of their lives before he himself had a relapse, again became violent, and voluntarily left PROJIMO.

What has been wonderful, however, has been the apparent transformation within several of these young gangsters and drug-dealers during their stay at PROJIMO. **Some of the young men, who seemed the most mean-spirited and aggressive when they came, have become among the most helpful and caring members of the PROJIMO team.** In this book's Introduction (on page 3) we mentioned Quique, who was so supportive with José, a mentally handicapped little boy whom no one else was able to reach. Another example is Martín Pérez, who became one of PROJIMO's most gifted wheelchair and gurney designers (see Chapters 37 and 39). Martín showed heart-felt concern for those difficult children whose behavior sometimes led attendants to dislike or neglect them. When Martín, like Quique, was finally thrown out of PROJIMO for repeated drug use, one young girl, Tere, wept. "Martín was always the first to help me if my wheelchair broke, or when I needed somebody to talk to who really listened and cared," she said.

Seeing this kind of change from angry hoodlum to tender care-provider or creative craftsperson has given many of us more insight into human nature. It seems true that *inside every person, however brutish their exterior, there is a hidden seed of goodness,* a seed of compassion waiting for a chance to grow and flower. The longer that core remains dormant and unrealized, the more urgent is its need for fulfillment. Sometimes all it takes to start that seed sprouting is a friendly word, an expectation of good will, a recognition that the person has worth … or a request for help when it is sorely needed. With the right word or touch, the toughest thug may suddenly shed his hard shell and offer heart-warming assistance and concern. And in the process, he discovers joy in doing something loving and lovable.

Angel—a Six-Year-Old Boy with Muscular Dystrophy

ANGEL was brought to PROJIMO by his mother from the village of San Augustine, 40 kilometers away. Mari and Conchita did their best to get the boy to relax and to win his trust. They talked to him in a friendly way and offered him toys to play with. But Angel clung fearfully to his mother and would burst into tears when asked a question or when gently touched.

Angel's mother said the boy had difficulty walking and that his condition was getting worse. She said she had taken him to doctors in the city, who had prescribed everything from painkillers (although he had no pain) to vitamins, calcium, hormones, and injectable antibiotics. But his walking kept getting worse.

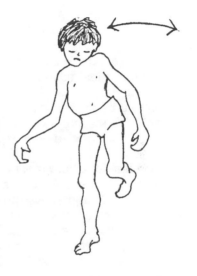

Mari and Conchita asked Angel's mother to walk across the room. She did so, and Angel followed her. He had a waddling gait, throwing his weight from side to side, a sign of weakness at the sides of the hips. His calf muscles were unusually large for his thin body, and he walked slightly on tip-toe. He had trouble lifting his arms over his head. In order to stand up from the floor, he climbed up his body using his arms. Although there was apparently no family history (no relatives with a similar condition), Mari recognized Angel's gradually increasing muscle weakness as typical of Duchenne's muscular dystrophy.

Conchita was also concerned about Angel's emotional and social development. He was very insecure and fearful of strangers. His mother explained that he was not used to strangers. He did not go to school, she said, because other children teased him and said he "walked like a goose." (This made me recall how I was teased as a child, see page 83.)

Possible Actions: The PROJIMO team gently explained to Angel's mother that muscular dystrophy is a condition in which the boy's muscles gradually get weaker. To date, no medical cure has been found. But they helped her to realize that certain things could be done to help her son live a fuller, happier life.

They also discussed with her different forms of "therapy." They stressed that therapy—if used at all—should be approached in ways that help, rather than block, the child's social, emotional, and mental development. They told her about the exciting and rewarding life of the Peraza family, in which 4 children with muscular dystrophy became leaders and teachers in a program for disabled children (see Chapter 48).

Mari also told Angel's mother something about experimental alternatives, including intensive "massage therapy." The PROJIMO team had learned about this from a visiting massage therapist, Marybetts Sinclair. Although they could not promise improvement and the therapy was described as controversial, Angel's mother was eager to try it. Because Marybetts would be visiting again in a few weeks, they invited Angel and his mother to return at that time.

Innovative management of muscular dystrophy: massage therapy combined with physical therapy.

The controversial new treatment for muscular dystrophy mentioned above has been promoted by a self-made therapist named Meir Schneider, who now practices in San Francisco, California. Schneider claims that an intensive program of massage therapy can halt the progression of muscular dystrophy and help to return lost muscle strength. Although many medical professionals are skeptical of Schneider's claims, Marybetts Sinclair, the massage therapist who occasionally volunteers at PROJIMO, has shown the team documents and films supporting his approach. Everyone agreed that perhaps it was worth a try.

Working and playing with Angel. Angel and his mother returned to PROJIMO as agreed. A physical therapist from Australia who was then volunteering at PROJIMO was skeptical about Schneider's methodology. Additionally, he insisted there was "no way" that such an intensive massage program could be applied to a child as fretful and uncooperative as Angel. Everyone agreed that **any attempt at therapy would need to be approached slowly and gently, as much as possible in the form of play, while trying to gradually win Angel's confidence and trust.**

A flexible schedule was developed **combining therapeutic massage and physical therapy.** They began with brief sessions and planned to gradually build up to several hours a day. The challenge was to make the experimental approach interesting, varied, and fun enough for Angel to accept and enjoy it. Sessions of **massage** followed by **exercise games** were followed with **play on the swings, rocking horses, and other equipment** on the outdoor Playground for All Children. To encourage interaction with a variety of people (and to divide up the work), nearly a dozen disabled and non-disabled persons were recruited to help.

The therapeutic massage, in keeping with Schneider's recommendations, consisted of gentle circular motions with the finger-tips over the whole body, concentrating on the most important and affected muscles. At first—as predicted—the boy was fearful of being touched by anyone but his mother. But his helpers were gentle and his mother also took part. The massage was so soothing that the boy gradually relaxed and began to enjoy it. By the third day he was eager for more.

Exercise activities, mostly through play, were combined with and followed the massage. These were designed to encourage a **full range of motion,** as much as possible through **active muscle use, yet without causing fatigue.** Simple games were devised, inviting the boy to touch or hit another person's hand or to kick a ball with his outstretched foot. Each time, he was encouraged to stretch a little farther or reach a little higher. He would proudly count how many times he could repeat each action. (Thus, his counting skills increased along with his physical skills.)

Gangsters as therapists.

Although at first many persons at PROJIMO assisted with Angel's therapy, after a few days fewer people arrived to take part. Among those who showed greatest persistence and concern were some of the "gangsters" and street youth who had been disabled in gun fights. Day after day, three paraplegic young men would circle the couch on which Angel lay, gently providing massage and playful exercise. Angel gradually grew comfortable with them, laughing with delight at the games.

These young men clearly took pride and joy in helping little Angel, and in seeing him respond so enthusiastically to their efforts. It was **good therapy for everyone.**

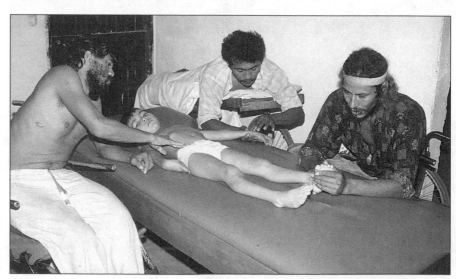

Three spinal-cord injured young men massage Angel. Mario is on the right.

The gentle side of a tough guy.   One of the spinal-cord injured young men who showed the most care and innovativeness in working and playing with Angel was Mario. Perhaps Mario missed his own childhood (which he had never really had). Or perhaps he missed his only child, who had died. In any case, Mario sympathized with Angel's fragile vulnerability.

MARIO had grown up as a street child and, since boyhood, had trafficked in and used drugs. In his 20s he decided to turn over a new leaf. He married and settled down on a ranch. But old gang rivalry caught up with him in the form of a drive-by shooting. The same bullet which left Mario paraplegic passed through his baby daughter in his arms. Weeks later, in revenge, his brothers captured the culprits. From his wheelchair, Mario watched as his bothers tortured them to death.

In retrospect, Mario does not try to justify this action, but sadly explains: "They killed my baby."

For all that, Mario has a gentle side, a depth of caring that is sometimes born of pain. At PROJIMO, where he stayed for a long time while his deep pressure sores gradually healed, Mario learned carpentry skills and began to help in the wood-working shop.

In time, Mario became a skilled craftsperson, making special seating and personalized equipment for children with special needs. He was quite creative. But the main reason that his innovations often turned out well was because **he worked so closely with the child and his parents.** Children liked him because he listened to them and related to them on their terms. He no longer had interest in maintaining the macho (manly) distance and toughness so typical of grown-up males. He'd had enough of all that.

With Angel, Mario was both imaginative and creative—and playful in a non-threatening way. He was constantly coming up with new ideas to turn Angel's therapy into games. Angel loved it, and became very attached to Mario.

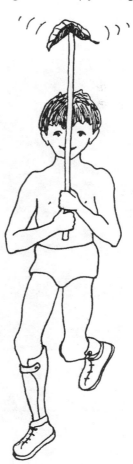

Here are some of the ideas that Mario and his co-workers came up with to motivate Angel and to turn his therapy into play.

The leaf-on-a-stick balancing act, to improve gait.

Although part of Angel's side-to-side pendulum-like gait was due to reduced muscle strength at the sides of his hips, the weakness and outward (varus) collapse of his ankles also was a factor. After Raymundo custom-fitted him with light-weight plastic ankle-braces (AFOs, see page 86), his gait improved. When prompted, Angel could walk without lurching as much from side to side. But, partly due to habit, he would quickly fall back into the old wobbly pattern.

To help him learn to walk without lurching so much from side to side, Mario invented a simple game.

Angel would hold a thin pole upright with a mango leaf bent over its tip. The boy would then try to walk across the room without the leaf falling. To do this, he had to walk smoothly, keep his body steady, and not lurch sideways. When he succeeded (as he did more and more often) everyone clapped. After a few days, Angel's gait showed noticeable improvement, even when he was not playing the game. He also held his head higher.

The truck-under-the-bridge game—to exercise the belly and back.

To help him use his stomach and back muscles, the PROJIMO team asked Angel to lie first on his belly, then on his back, and arch his body upwards. To turn this into a game, Mario asked a group of school children in the toy shop to make a toy truck loaded with brightly colored blocks of different heights.

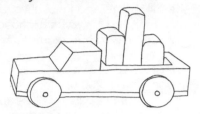

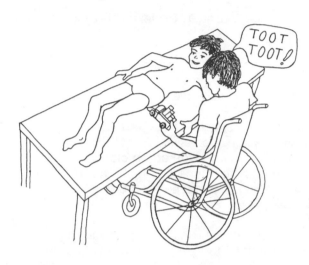

Angel at once fell in love with the truck … and the exercises that came with it. As Angel lay on his back, Mario or another one of the therapy helpers would drive the truck in circles around Angel. They would toot loudly as the truck approached his mid-section. At the toot, Angel would arch his body upwards to let the truck pass under the "bridge" formed by his body. When this game began, Mario started with shorter blocks so that Angel would not have to lift very high. But as his ability to lift his body increased, Angel helped Mario to load the truck with taller blocks. This gave the boy more of a challenge. Angel enjoyed the game and did his best to "lift the bridge" for the tallest truck-load of blocks.

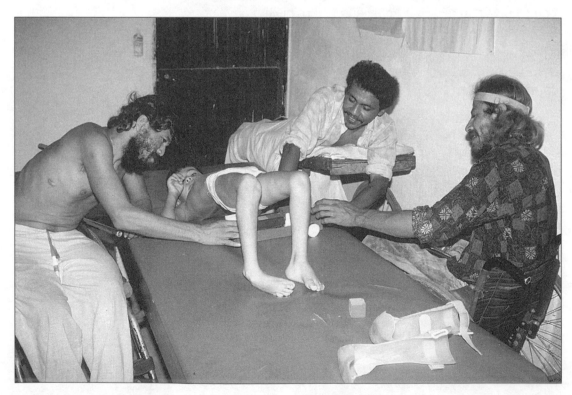

"TOOT - TOOT!"

RESULTS:

On evaluating the therapeutic activities that were used with Angel, it is important to consider their effect on the whole child—physically, emotionally, and socially—not just the specific objectives that the activities were designed to meet.

Physically, the combination of Angel's massage therapy, exercise, and increased activity appeared to have a **limited but positive effect.** During two weeks at PROJIMO, the boy's gait improved visibly. There were also gains in his capacity to do things that involve lifting and moving different parts of his body.

After Angel returned to his home, his mother continued with the massage and exercise games. When Angel came back to PROJIMO 3 months later, many people commented that his walking had improved even more.

We still do not know the long-term outcome. Despite apparent short-term improvements, we can not presume that progressive muscle loss has been reversed or halted. Rather, we suspect that the plentiful stimulation and modest (non-fatiguing) use of under-used muscles helped put his body in more optimal condition, within its given stage of deterioration. It stands to reason that, as the dystrophy advances, reduced activity will add to the degenerative process. By contrast, keeping the body in its best possible physical shape may slow muscle loss and bring at least temporary improvement in body function.

Emotionally and socially, Angel improved enormously. During his stay at PROJIMO, he changed from a whiny, clinging little boy who feared everyone but his mother, into a playful child who enjoyed the closeness and attention of other people.

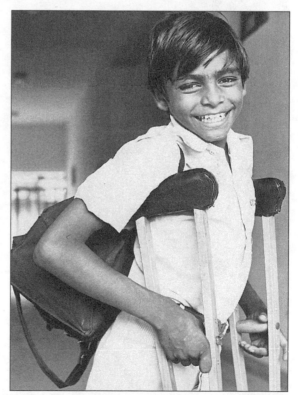

Angel's physical condition will probably continue to deteriorate, possibly more slowly than it might have otherwise. But his mind and spirit will continue to develop—perhaps more openly, fully, and happily than they might have without the warm, friendly touch of folks like Mario at PROJIMO.

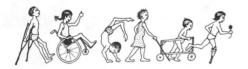

In the last analysis, perhaps the best indicator of an activity's success is the **smile factor.** Certainly, Angel smiles more than he used to!

THE SMILE FACTOR—perhaps the best measurement of a program's success. (Photo: UNICEF/ T.S. Satyan)

WARNING: Though the boy in this photo is smiling now, his poorly adjusted crutches may cause more disability later. With his elbows so bent, he cannot support his weight on his hands, and so he supports himself under his arm-pits. This can damage nerves and gradually paralyze his hands. See the suggestions on pages 12 and 117 . . . *THE SMILE MUST NOT BE THE ONLY MEASURE OF SUCCESS.*

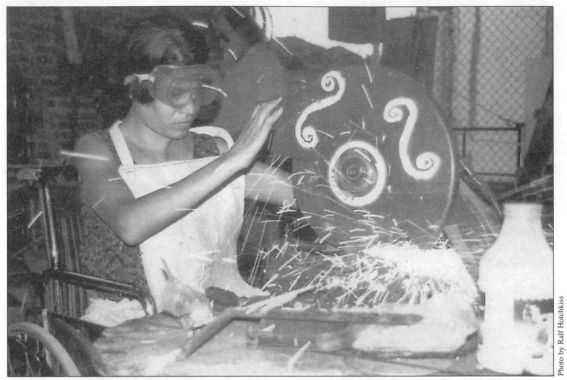

María de Jesús, who is paraplegic, cuts a metal tube for a wheelchair she is making in a training workshop at PROJIMO.

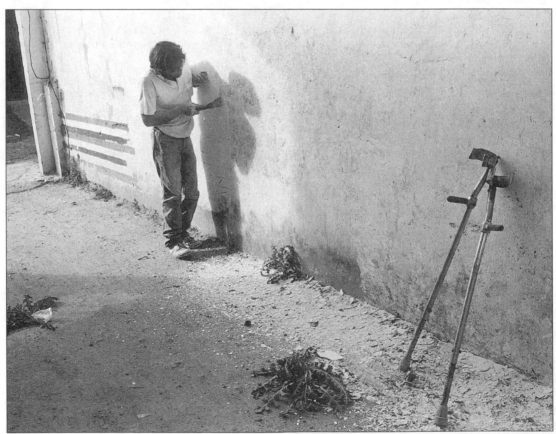

Inez white-washes the mud-brick wall of PROJIMO.

Learning New Ways to Work in the Non-Formal Economy

CHAPTER 44

Work Opportunities for Survival in Hard Times

Every person has a right to contribute to their family, community, and society as best they can. Human dignity and self-determination come, in part, from being able to participate in functions that sustain and enhance life. Life-enabling functions—in addition to acts of love, sharing, art, and nurturing—also include *productive and service-related activities* often referred to as *"work."* As our profit-hungry global economy overshadows sustenance based on caring and sharing, more and more aspects of production and service are performed as *jobs* for pay. Today's money-minded value system—"You get what you pay for"—is systematically marginalizing deeper human values, and the most vulnerable human beings.

Nevertheless, many life-sustaining human activities are still founded on love and sharing. The majority of productive and service-providing work is still done without pay, much of it by women and children in the home. Many disabled people, too, find ways of contributing to the well-being of family and community that are unpaid, yet life-affirming.

Rural areas. In traditional farming societies, survival still largely depends on growing and gathering food, hauling water and firewood, and other physical activities. So physical ability tends to be highly valued (sometimes more than mental ability). In terms of fitting into the life and production of the community **in rural areas, a child with a mental disability may be less socially handicapped than is the child with a physical disability.**

GOYO, a boy with Down's syndrome in Ajoya, the village where PROJIMO is located, regularly went with his father to the fields.

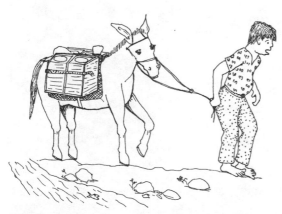

Helping to plant and gather maize (corn) and to cut weeds was repetitive work the boy could learn and do well. He took pride in helping his family. During the long dry season when there was no farm work, Goyo helped to earn a modest income for his family by hauling water from the river for neighbors, in large tins on a donkey. Other boys disliked this hard repetitive work, but Goyo did it with pride. Hauling water was his livelihood until the village modernized and obtained a gasoline pump that piped water into the homes.

In some cases, simple adaptations can help a disabled person, such as this blind child, participate in farm work.
(Photo from Philippines by Robert Jaekle for Helen Keller International)

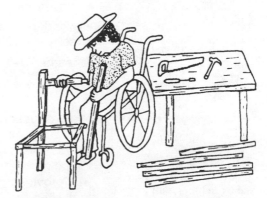

In other cases, it may make sense for the disabled person to learn skills for being productive in other ways, such as furniture making or other work that can be done at home.

Urban areas. In cities, successful integration into society often depends more on mental ability than on physical fitness. Especially for the mentally slow child, schooling may be a major hurdle. A youth who does not graduate finds it hard to find a paying job, even doing physical labor. For these reasons, **although in rural areas more concern is often shown for people with physical disabilities, in urban areas there tend to be more programs for children who are mentally handicapped.**

In the mushrooming cities of the world, **unemployment is a growing problem.** Giant industries, in pursuit of "cost effectiveness" (higher profits), are "down-sizing" (replacing workers with machines). Today, so many persons are job-hunting that it is often hard for disabled persons to compete. Since Mexico's entry into the international free market economy, thousands of small businesses have closed down. Even university graduates and licensed professionals—doctors, lawyers, engineers—beg coins on street corners by selling trinkets or by performing as fire-breathers and clowns.

In today's world of rising joblessness and falling wages, it may be unrealistic to routinely train disabled people for jobs in the *formal economy.* It often makes sense to help them learn skills within the *informal economy:* producing things at home or in neighborhood collectives that they can sell directly on the street or in a stall at a community market.

Several rehabilitation programs that used to train disabled persons for skilled factory jobs, such as operators of lathes and heavy machinery, have changed their approach and now focus on teaching disabled persons skills that enable them to be self-employed or to work in small worker-run cooperatives.

Skills Training at PROJIMO

At PROJIMO, disabled persons are able to learn a variety of skills, mostly in the form of apprenticeships, or **learning by doing.** Some of these skills are related to providing health, medical, and rehabilitation equipment and services to other disabled persons. Other skills are learned as part of income-generating activities. These skills range from the production of various articles for sale, to the management of the village small-goods store, to running a modest welding service or carpentry repair shop.

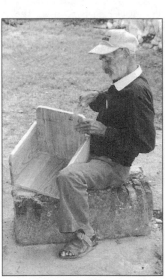

Chon, who is deaf, has become a skilled carpenter. Here, he makes an enclosed seat for a see-saw in the playground.

Income-generating activities at PROJIMO mostly involve the production of low-cost items that can be made with low-cost tools and equipment. Items include such things as:

- **sandals and shoes,**
- **ornaments for festivals,**
- **woven rugs,**
- **wooden toys** and **puzzles** (see pages 290-291 and 322),
- **leather belts** with hand-stitched designs,
- plastic-woven, metal-frame **furniture.**

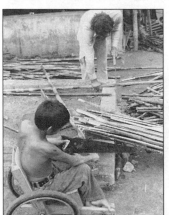

Many skills at PROJIMO are learned by helping with project-related needs. Here, Jorge and Inez build bamboo blinds for the model home (see next page).

The production of these items serves three main purposes. **1)** It provides skills training and productive activities for the disabled people involved. **2)** It produces some income for the program and modest wages for the disabled workers. **3)** It provides disabled persons with work experience, so that when they return to their homes they can set up a small workshop there and help to support themselves and their families.

Home-making skills. PROJIMO provides an environment where young people can perform a variety of home-making skills, ranging from **cooking** to **house-cleaning** to **laundry.** Because the disabled participants run the group kitchen, plan meals, and buy the food, they acquire skills in home economics, learning by doing (and learning from their mistakes).

The Model Home, built by disabled participants with help from the local community, is a disability-adapted, low-cost, mud-brick building. It has many features to help persons with different disabilities be able to keep house more easily. Disabled persons who live temporarily in the model home while visiting PROJIMO can try out its different features, and get ideas for modifying their own houses. Adaptations range from a completely wheelchair-accessible kitchen, to bedrooms with hand-grips hanging from the ceilings for getting in and out of bed. Next to the model home is an outdoor wheelchair-accessible laundry area.

Getting disabled boys and men to help wash dishes and clothes has been a big challenge, but the adapted facilities make it easier.

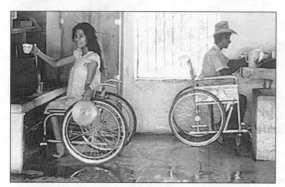

A wheelchair-riding young man washes dishes in the kitchen of PROJIMO's model home.

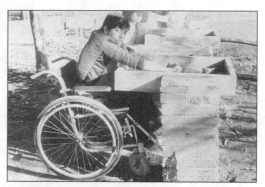

A youth with progressive muscular atrophy, who had been overprotected at home, washes his own clothes.

Skills learned in making assistive equipment can be applied to many kinds of community work. On page 259, we gave the example of how the wheelchair-making shop turned into a village repair service where farmers came to repair their broken plows, and children their busted bicycles. As another income-producing venture, the workers in the welding shop began to make metal chair frames from metal building rods (re-bar). Other disabled persons learned to weave the chairs with plastic ribbon.

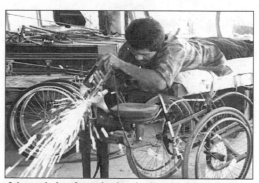

Jaime grinds a farmer's plow in the wheelchair shop.

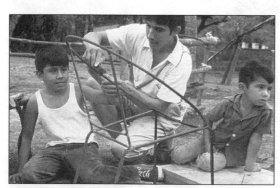

Big Miguel helps Miguelito (a boy with cerebral palsy) paint a chair frame, welded in the wheelchair shop.

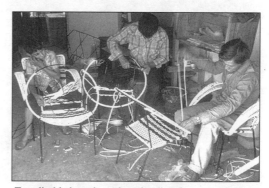

Two disabled youths and a schoolboy learn to weave plastic-ribbon upholstered chairs at PROJIMO.

These woven chairs sold well in local villages. One boy, Rubén, later set up his own chair-weaving business at his home, and soon earned twice as much as his brother in a factory.

Disabled people helping one another provide a lot of the skills-learning at PROJIMO. Some young persons who first came for their own rehabilitation have stayed on at PROJIMO to learn the craft, organizational and rehabilitation skills that most interest them. Several have become very capable therapy-workers and craftspersons. One example is INEZ, who first came as an abandoned street child, with one leg paralyzed by polio. Inez has become a skilled therapy worker, having been taught by visiting physical therapists.

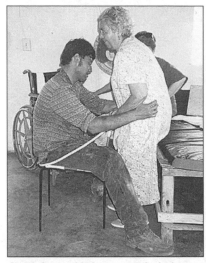

Inez helps an elderly woman who had a stroke, and then broke a hip, begin to stand up and regain her balance.

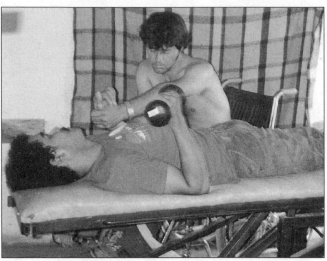

Inez helps Che—the left half of whose body was paralyzed by a bullet wound in the head—maintain range-of-motion in his weak left arm and increase the strength of his right arm. (See story, page 253.)

Inez became such a capable therapist and rehabilitation worker that, after a few years at PROJIMO, he set up his own successful physiotherapy practice in the city of Mazatlán. In time, however, he gave up the private practice and returned to PROJIMO. He preferred working as part of a community-based team to help those with limited resources. Inez married another PROJIMO worker, Cecilia, and has two energetic daughters.

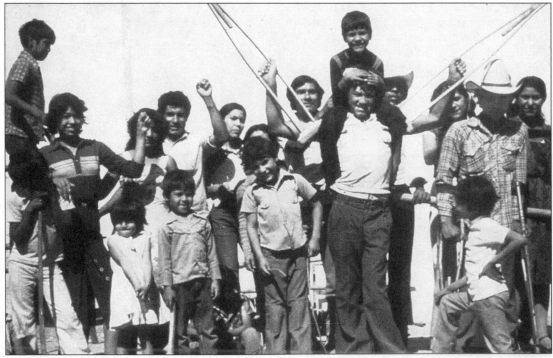

With a disabled child on his shoulders, Inez raises his crutches in a sign of victory. This scene is from a village theater skit to raise public awareness about the potential of disabled persons. It portrays Inez's own story: how he first came to PROJIMO as a boy for rehabilitation, and later became a skilled therapist helping others.

Carpentry skills. The PROJIMO wood-working shop is where many disabled youth apprentice in making all kinds of equipment for disabled children, ranging from special seating and standing frames to educational toys. With the skills learned in this shop, some of the disabled young people have gone on to set up their own carpentry shops. Others have joined rehabilitation programs where they can put both their carpentry and rehabilitation skills to good use.

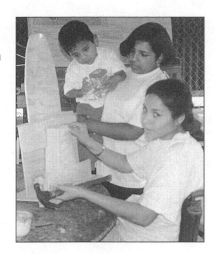

Marielos, who is paraplegic, makes a special standing frame for a child, who watches with interest from his mothers arms. Marielos also makes doll-house furniture, for which she has more requests for sales than she can meet.

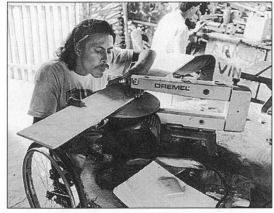

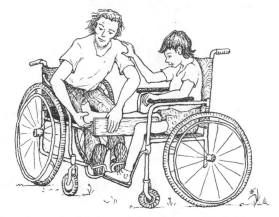

Mario, a street youth who became paraplegic from a bullet wound in the spine, learned carpentry skills while helping to make special seating and other equipment at PROJIMO.

But what makes Mario an outstanding worker is his heartfelt understanding and concern for the children he works with (see page 270-271). Here, he adapts a support for a girl whose leg is casted.

Even some of the young people who are quadriplegic (with paralysis of their arms and hands as well as legs) have become skillful carpenters and toy makers. The first obstacle for them to overcome is their feeling (and fear) of incapacity. The beauty of PROJIMO is that new-comers have excellent role models to follow. They dare to try new things and to test—and stretch—their limits.

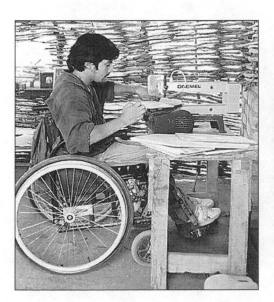

When Rafa, who is quadriplegic, came to PROJIMO, he was convinced that his hands were useless. But, in the wood shop, he learned he could do far more than he dreamed. In time, he became an excellent toy and puzzle maker.

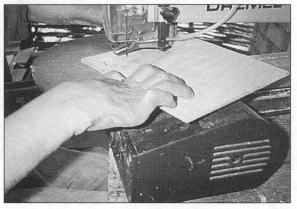

Business skills. Several disabled persons at PROJIMO who collectively run the program have also learned some **organizational skills,** and also **book-keeping.**

Conchita studied accounting before she became paraplegic. Now she is a coordinator of the program and manages the financial records. She has taught other workers to help with accounting and program records. These skills can be useful for those who later set up their own small workshops or cooperatives.

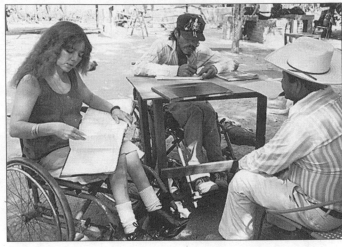

Conchita Lara, with Mario's help, works on the monthly financial report of PROJIMO. For more about Conchita, see Chapter 42.

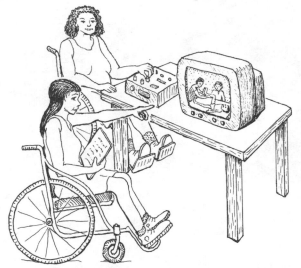

Conchita and Mari edit a video film they have made of range-of-motion exercises for disabled children.

Video skills. Some work opportunities are unplanned. The PROJIMO team decided they should make educational video-tapes of aspects of rehabilitation and therapy where movement is important, and where words and drawings are not sufficient. So they raised money to buy a video camera and recruited a skilled filmmaker to come teach them how to use the equipment, and put together and edit a film. Mari and Conchita, the two main coordinators of PROJIMO, mastered these skills.

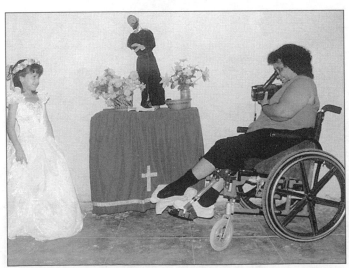

As an income generating community service, Mari makes a video of Flora's first communion.

Video cameras and film making was a new and exciting event for the local villagers. There are 3 or 4 video cassette players in town. Local people begged to have pictures taken of themselves and their families. Having acquired the needed skills, Conchita and Mari soon found themselves invited to take videos of events such as baptisms, weddings, and the coming-of-age parties of 15-year-old girls. **Making and editing of videos has become one of the more successful income-generating activities of PROJIMO.**

Maintaining PROJIMO's grounds and buildings.

The maintenance of PROJIMO provides skills training and practice at a range of tasks useful for maintaining a home or business.

Cecilia, who is now married and runs her own household, helps to clean up PROJIMO's consultation room.

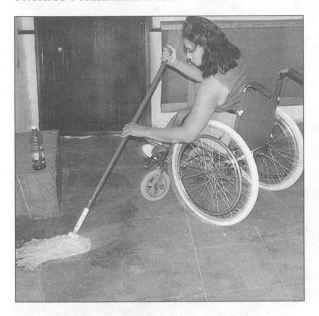

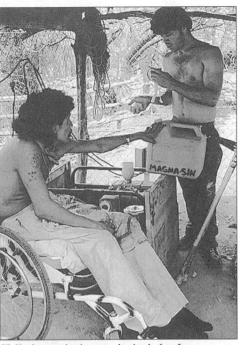

Heliodoro, who is paraplegic, helps Inez repair the project water pump, and in the process he learns a useful skill.

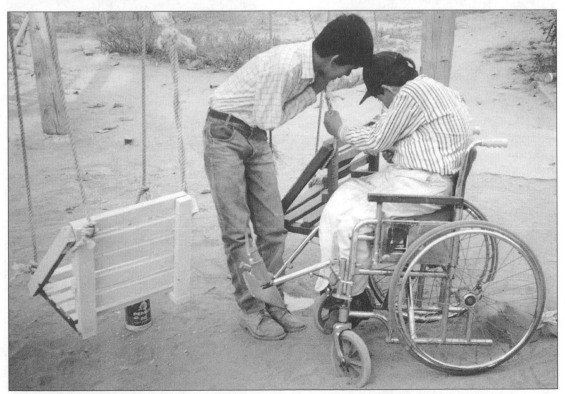

A schoolboy helps Jesús, who is almost blind, to paint the swings in PROJIMO's Playground for All Children. (See more on Jesús in Chapters 16 and 45.)

The Spanish Language Training Program run by disabled villagers. For persons whose disabilities extensively limit the use of their bodies and hands, finding work opportunities can be quite a challenge. This is especially true for those who have little or no formal education—which is often the case.

One skill such persons do have in Mexico is speaking Spanish. So the PROJIMO team decided to start an intensive Spanish language training program. For the first classes they invited foreign students who, in exchange for being taught conversational Spanish, would help teach their teachers how to teach. PROJIMO especially welcomes language students who are disabled activists, rehabilitation workers, or progressive health workers. (If you are interested, send for a brochure. Fees are modest and help support the program.)

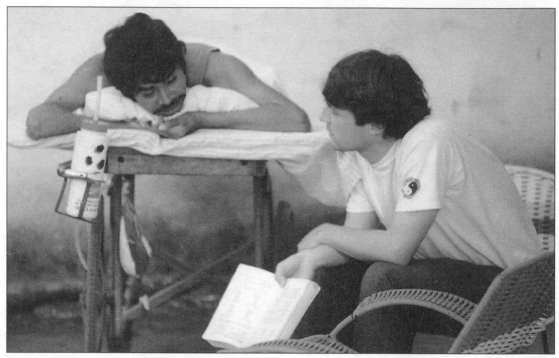

Quique, who was quadriplegic, had almost no control of his hands. He was one of the teachers in the Intensive Spanish Language Training Program. Here, he is teaching an idealistic young North American physiotherapist. He is lying on a wheeled cot, or gurney, to allow the pressure sores on his backside to heal.

VICTOR, a young doctor, gave PROJIMO one of its biggest rehabilitation challenges. Soon after graduating from medical school, Victor broke his neck in a car accident. He spent months in a hospital, where he developed pressure sores and urinary infections. He had become suicidal. He was sure he could never work as a doctor.

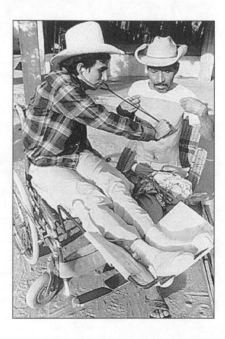

At PROJIMO, Victor gave the village team a hard time. He did not believe that a group of uneducated villagers—disabled ones at that—could do anything for him. But, little by little, his sores healed and his health improved. He learned to use his hands to grip things by bending his wrists backwards. In time, he started to provide medical services to sick villagers. Victor became one of the exceptional doctors in Mexico who choose to work in a poor and rural community. (In Mexico City there are over 5000 unemployed doctors who refuse to go to the poor rural areas where they are needed.)

ALL WORK AND NO PLAY MAKES JUÁN A DULL BOY

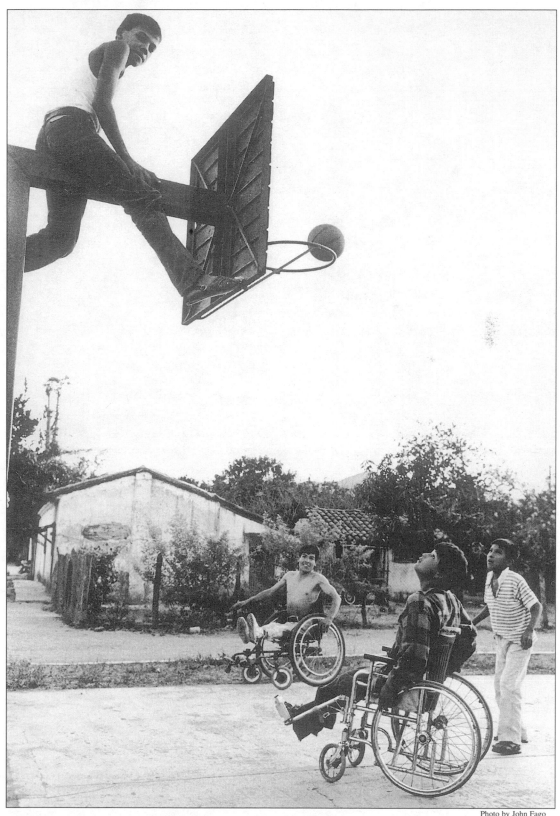

Photo by John Fago

Note: The different work activities shown in this chapter represent only a few of many possibilities. We have focused on some of the more innovative examples, mostly from PROJIMO. Clearly, the examples shown here only touch the surface of what is possible.

A Time for Play and a Time for Work

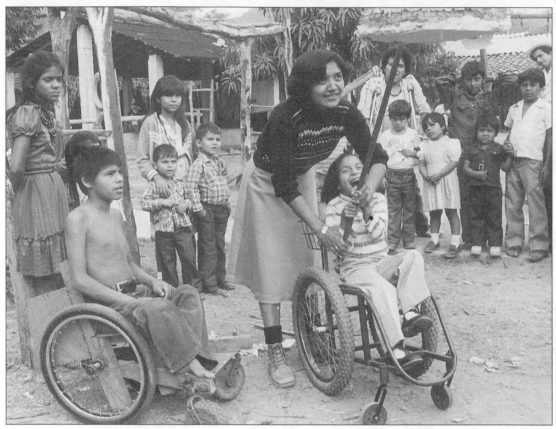

Lina tries to break a *piñata* full of candies, while Jorge and other children wait their turn.

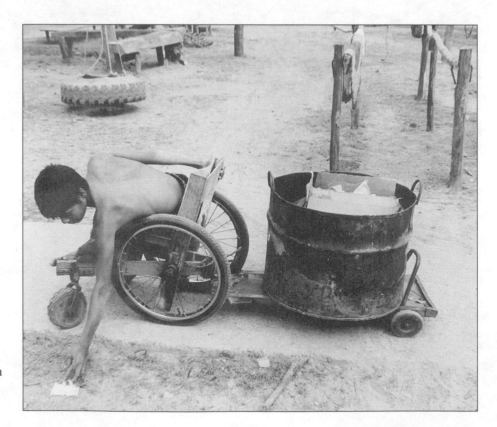

After the fun comes the clean up.

Part Six

CHILD-TO-CHILD:
INCLUDING DISABLED CHILDREN

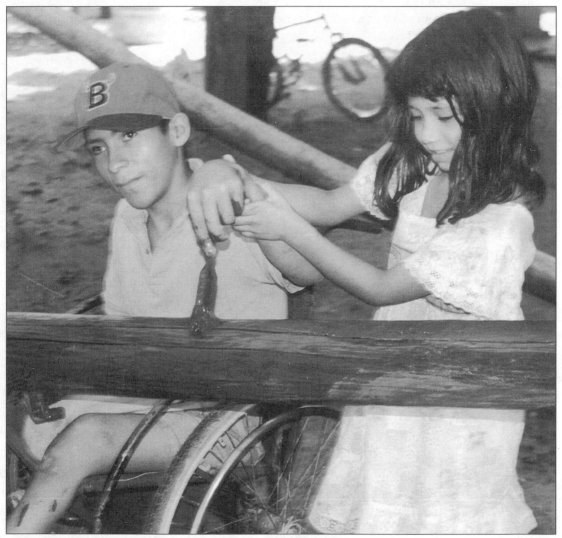

Inez's daughter, Bianca, helps Jesús, who is blind, to paint a see-saw in PROJIMO's Playground for All Children.

INTRODUCTION TO PART SIX

Helping Children Respond Creatively to the Needs and Rights of the Disabled Child

Part Six of this book focuses on Child-to-Child activities, where disabled and non-disabled children interrelate and learn from each other through play, work, joint adventures, and creative problem-solving.

About CHILD-TO-CHILD and Discovery-Based Learning

Child-to-Child is an innovative educational methodology in which school-age children learn ways to protect the health and well-being of other children, especially those who are younger or have special needs.

Child-to-Child was launched during the International Year of the Child, 1979. It is now used in more than 60 developing countries, as well as in Europe, the USA, and Canada. Many early Child-to-Child activities were developed in Project Piaxtla in Mexico, the villager-run health care program that gave birth to PROJIMO. Key to this adventurous approach was Martín Reyes Mercado, a village health promoter who worked with Piaxtla, and then with PROJIMO, for 2 decades. Martín now works with CISAS in Nicaragua, facilitating Child-to-Child throughout Latin America.

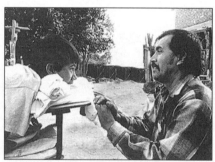

Martín Reyes befriends Osvaldo, who was unhappy and withdrawn after his accident.

CHILD-TO-CHILD FOR DISABLED CHILDREN

Children can be either cruel or kind to the child who is different. Sometimes it takes only a little awareness-raising for a group to shift from cruelty to kindness. One of Child-to-Child's goals is to help non-disabled children understand disabled children, be their friends, include them in their games, and help them to overcome difficulties and become more self-reliant.

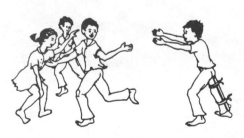

To give school-aged children an experience of what it is like to have a disability, a few of them can be given **a temporary handicap.** To simulate a lame leg, a stick is tied to the leg of the fastest runner in the class, to give him a stiff knee. Then the children run a race and the "lame" child comes in last. The facilitator asks this temporarily handicapped child what it feels like to be left behind.

Finally, all the children try to think of games they can play where a child with a lame leg can take part without experiencing any handicap: for example *marbles* or *checkers*.

A variety of activities can also be designed to **help children appreciate the strengths and abilities of the disabled child,** rather than to just notice their weaknesses. For this, **skits or role-plays** can be helpful. Here is an example. ➔

Various role plays, games, and activities to sensitize children to the feelings and abilities of children with different disabilities can be found in the Child-to-Child chapter in the book, *Disabled Village Children* (see page 343).

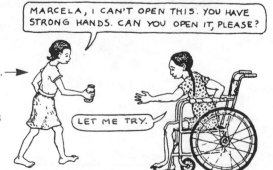

MARCELA, I CAN'T OPEN THIS. YOU HAVE STRONG HANDS. CAN YOU OPEN IT, PLEASE?

LET ME TRY.

The need to include disabled children in activities concerning disability

Many examples of Child-to-Child activities have been discussed in two of the author's earlier books: *Helping Health Workers Learn* and *Disabled Village Children.* (See more complete references to these books on pages 339 and 343.)

Some of the activities focus on **what children can do to prevent accidents.** →

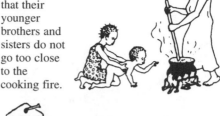

• Make sure that their younger brothers and sisters do not go too close to the cooking fire.

• Keep matches out of the reach of small children. (Older children can make a small basket or shelf for matches to be stored high on the wall.)

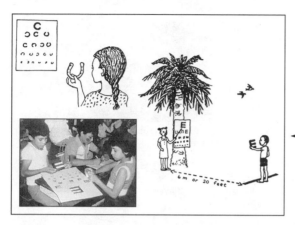

← The books also suggest enjoyable ways in which school children can **test the vision and hearing** of those who are beginning school, as well as things they can do so that the handicapped child can participate and learn more effectively.

Unfortunately, in many countries, disability-related Child-to-Child activities are frequently conducted in ways that do not include disabled children in central or leading roles. Too often activities are *about* disabled children, not *with* them.

In Child-to-Child events led by PROJIMO, disabled children often play a central role. They make it a point to involve school-aged children—disabled and non-disabled together—as helpers and volunteers, and as "agents of change" among their peers.

Child-to-Child, at its best, introduces **teaching methods that are learner-centered and "discovery-based,"** not authoritarian. It encourages children to make their own observations, draw their own conclusions, and take appropriate, self-directed action. This problem-solving approach emphasizes **cooperation rather than competition.**

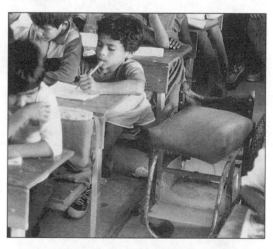

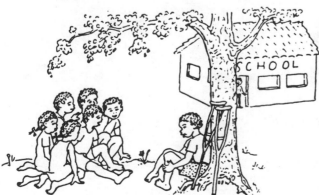

PROJIMO makes an effort to get disabled children into normal schools. It uses Child-to-Child activities to help both school children and teachers appreciate and build on the strengths of disabled children. It designs activities to address the needs, barriers, and possibilities of individual disabled children in the school and community setting.

Disabled activists—some of whom are disabled school children—often take the lead in this process.

Encouraging Disabled and Non-Disabled Children to Play and Learn Together

Two of the ways that PROJIMO encourages interaction between non-disabled and disabled children are the *Playground for All Children* and the *Children's Toy-Making Workshop*.

PLAYGROUNDS

A great playground—but NO CHILDREN!

The idea for making a low-cost rehabilitation playground came from a refugee camp in Thailand. That playground had a wide range of fine equipment, made with bamboo ... But when the author visited the playground, there was one big problem: NO CHILDREN! The playground was surrounded by a high fence with a locked gate. The reason, the manager explained, was that the local, non-disabled children used to play there, and constantly broke the equipment. So the local kids were locked out. Too often, however, so were the disabled children!

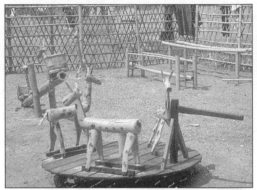

The rehabilitation playground in Thailand: beautiful, but without children.

A Playground for ALL Children.

To avoid such a problem, PROJIMO, in Mexico, invited local school children to help build and maintain a playground, with the agreement that they could play there too. The children eagerly volunteered, and the playground has led to an active integration of disabled and non-disabled kids.

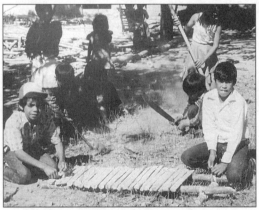

Out of poles they collected from the local forest, school children make a ramp as part of the equipment for the playground.

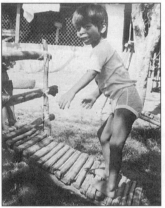

A boy with cerebral palsy plays on the ramp, encouraged by other children. The ramp stretches his tight heel cords. This "therapy" will help him walk better—not on tip-toes like this.

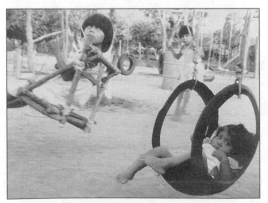

Disabled children play in enclosed swings made by village schoolchildren (See pages 32 and 57.)

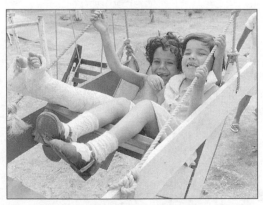

This extra-wide swing allows two children to swing together, one assisting the other.

Making therapy functional and fun. When a piece of equipment in the playground seems to provide a child with helpful exercises, he or she is encouraged to play on it. And because it is easy to build with cheap local materials, the family can make one at home.

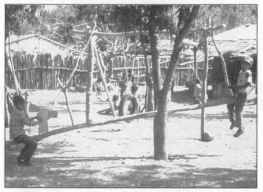 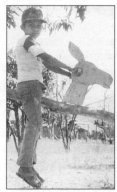 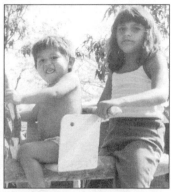

A teeter-totter (see-saw) in the crotch of a mango tree has a donkey on one end. The other end has an enclosed seat, with space behind it where a non-disabled child can sit and help support the disabled child.

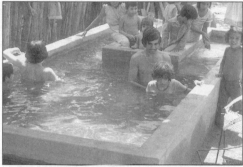 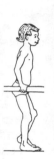 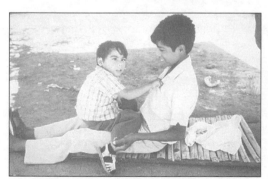

This water-therapy tank is also a small swimming pool. Young village children can learn to swim, play in the water, and help with the therapy of disabled playmates.

The parallel bars help disabled children learn to walk, and also function as gymnastic bars for non-disabled and disabled children alike.

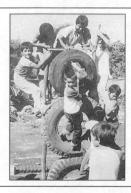 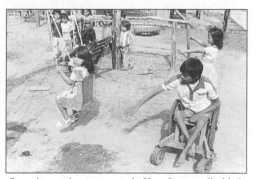

An older brother helps a child with developmental delay improve his balance while sitting.

Sometimes roles are reversed. Here Jorge, a disabled (but very capable) child, swings a non-disabled child.

Good Ideas Spread.
The idea of a *Playground for All Children* has spread to other villages. Here disabled and non-disabled children from Ajoya, where PROJIMO is located, help children in another town make their own playground.

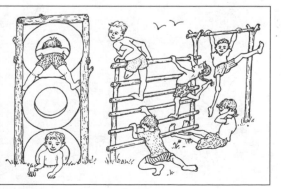

THE CHILDREN'S TOY-MAKING WORKSHOP

The children's toy-making workshop at PROJIMO serves a number of purposes. It helps disabled young people to develop manual dexterity and useful skills. It attracts local school children to come make fascinating playthings together with disabled children. And it provides a supply of simple, attractive, early-stimulation toys and wooden puzzles. These are useful for children who are developmentally delayed or who need to develop hand-eye coordination. The sale of some of the playthings also brings in a modest income.

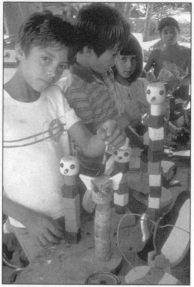

The toy shop is coordinated by teen-age village girls and disabled young women, who produce high-quality toys themselves and who guide the work of the younger children. They have an agreement with the local children: the first toy a child makes goes to a disabled child who needs it. The second toy she makes can be taken home for a younger brother or sister. (After all, early stimulation toys and activities enhance the development of any young child. This way, the process of children helping children—Child-to-Child—extends into the wider community.)

In the Children's Toy-Making Workshop, disabled and non-disabled youngsters make early stimulation toys for babies and young children who need them.

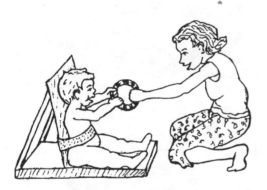

A school girl uses a rattle made in the toy-shop to help a multiply-disabled child respond to different stimuli and to use his eyes, ears, and hands.

A wide range of toys and playthings are made. Some of the simplest toys are rattles and brightly colored objects that can be shaken or hung in front of a baby or a child whose development is slow.

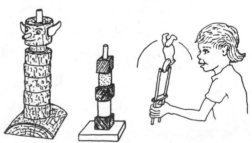

Other play-things include toys and games for the development of manual coordination, for learning relative sizes, shapes, and colors, and for learning numbers and letters.

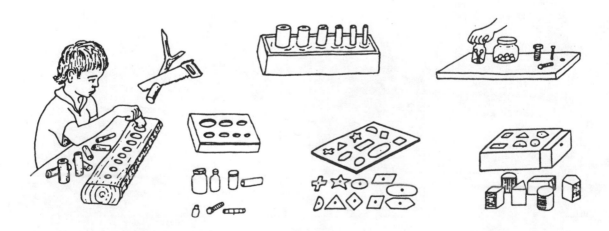

The toy-makers also produce a wide variety of wooden puzzles, from simple to complex, to match the abilities and needs of different children.

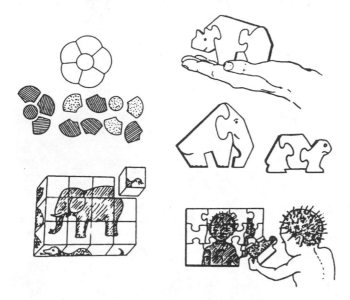

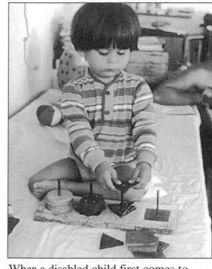

When a disabled child first comes to PROJIMO, she is invited to play with puzzles or toys to help her to relax and know that people care. It also helps the worker evaluate the child's mental, physical, and social abilities.

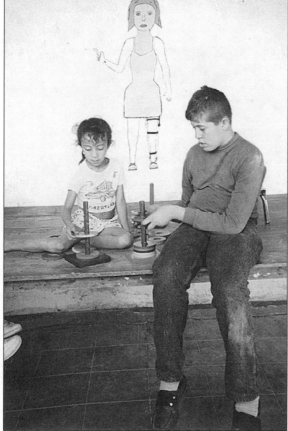

Lluvia—daughter of PROJIMO's disabled leader, Mari—teaches an older boy to use a toy, for better hand control. Brain-damaged from meningitis, the boy is mentally slow (but very friendly). He makes little use of his spastic left hand. To remove the colorful rings from the toy, he needs to rotate them past small pegs on the upright post. ➞ This helps him gain more skill with his hands. Lluvia makes it fun. Like her mother, she is a good teacher.

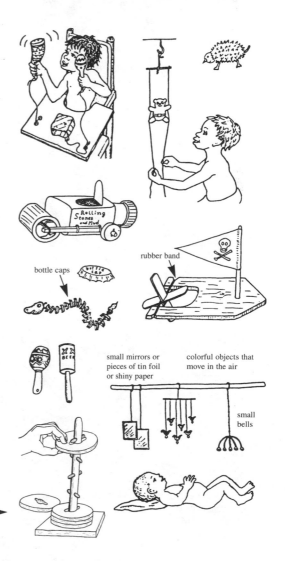

bottle caps

rubber band

small mirrors or pieces of tin foil or shiny paper

colorful objects that move in the air

small bells

CHILDREN HELP WITH THERAPY AND EQUIPMENT

After school and on weekends, some of the school children not only work in the toy-shop, but they also help disabled children with exercises, play, and other activities. Sometimes a school child will help make a wooden walker or special seat for a disabled child, and then become involved in helping that child learn to use the equipment.

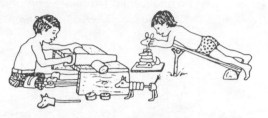

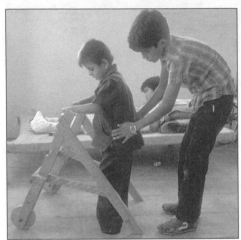

A school boy, Efraín, made this wooden walker for a disabled child visiting PROJIMO, then proudly helped him learn to use it.

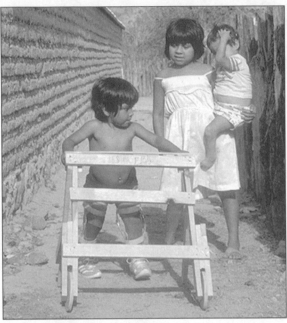

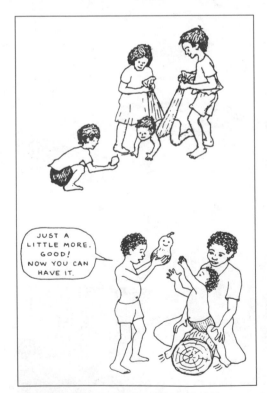

Children are encouraged to play with their disabled brothers and sisters, and to teach them how to help with exercises, stimulation, and skills-learning activities.

Standing behind Jésica (with the walker), a school-girl called Gordi holds little Toni. Born with club feet, Toni spent several months at PROJIMO. (His mother had troubles and could not care for her child.) Gordi became very attached to Toni, and Toni to Gordi. Gordi bathed Toni, dressed him, and in a playful way helped with stretching exercises for his hands and feet.

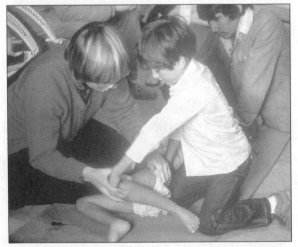

A therapist visiting PROJIMO, Ann Hallum, teaches the older brother of a girl who is disabled by polio how to do stretching exercises to correct a hip contracture. Many children are taught in this way to be "therapy assistants."

CHILDREN ADAPT A SPECIAL SEAT FOR A CHILD WITH A VERY LARGE HEAD

JACINTO was born with spina bifida (see page 131) and hydrocephalus, a condition where liquid in the brain makes the head very large. Jacinto's mother, Cata, brought him to PROJIMO for rehabilitation, then decided to stay and work there for several months. Having a disabled child of her own, she was very able and loving with other disabled children.

Juán, a disabled craftsman, made Jacinto a special seat with wheels so that Jacinto's mother, Cata, could push it. (She lived at the far end of town.) It had a removable table to hold toys and food. Above the table, Juán mounted a bar from which rattles and colorful toys could be hung, to encourage Jacinto to use his eyes and hands and lift his head.

But the design had a problem. The seat-back and head-rest were both on the same plane, tilting back a little. For many children this would be OK.

But Jacinto's head was so big that the head-rest bent his head forward. This made it hard for him to keep his head upright. Because the hydrocephalus caused his eyes to angle downward, it was impossible for him to look up at the toys that were hanging in front of his face.

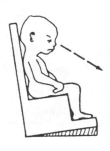

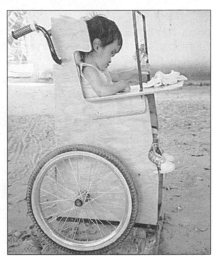

Head-rest straight. Head tilted down.

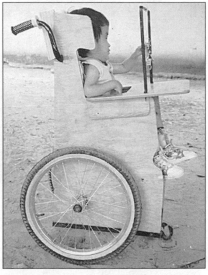

Solution. To allow Jacinto to lift his head more, the head-rest needed to be positioned farther back (behind the plane of the back-rest). Juán was busy on another project. So a couple of school boys who often came to PROJIMO to fix their bikes and help with odd jobs, offered to make the adjustments. They cut a rectangle out of the part of the seat back that supported Jacinto's head and mounted it further back by adding bits of wood on either side.

Then they put Jacinto in the seat. What a difference! Now he could lift his head and see the world around him. He could look at the toys hanging in front of him. The boy reached out to play with them.

The two "junior rehab technicians" felt proud that they had been able to help. They were eager to help more.

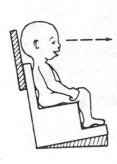

Head-rest tilted back. Head well positioned.

Disabled Child to Disabled Child

PROJIMO is based on a give-and-take approach, where disabled persons help and learn from each other. **Peer assistance can—and often does—start quite young.** A child with a disability not only tends to better understand the needs, feelings, hopes and fears of another disabled child, but can also be an **excellent role model.**

Several examples of ways that disabled children assist, teach, and care for each other have been seen in previous chapters. Chapter 32, for example, shows how **CARLOS,** a boy who has a combined physical, visual and mental handicap, helped another boy, **Alonzo,** learn to walk.

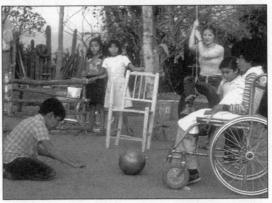

MIGUELITO, who has cerebral palsy, helps TERESA, a girl with arthritis, to strengthen her legs by kicking a ball he rolls to her. This makes therapy fun, and both children benefit.

Part 6 of *Nothing About Us Without Us* tells a number of stories about ways that disabled children assist one another. In such relationships, often both the receiver and the giver of assistance benefit greatly.

Chapter 45 describes **JESÚS,** a boy with spina bifida who is also nearly blind. Jesús was first helped by his classmates, through Child-to-Child activities, to be accepted and treated more fairly by his teacher. Later, Jesús himself becomes a facilitator of Child-to-Child, helping two children with muscular dystrophy in another village to be appreciated and assisted by their classmates.

Chapter 46 tells how **JORGE,** a boy in a wheelchair, helps **MANOLO,** a mentally slow but physically strong teenager, to speak and act for himself. After his integration into PROJIMO, Manolo takes pride in assisting physically impaired children. Then a friendship develops between Manolo and **LUIS,** who has cerebral palsy but is mentally bright. By bringing together the brawn of Manolo and the brains of Luis, the two indulge in adventures which neither could have accomplished on his own.

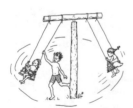

Chapter 47 tells of how **VANIA,** a spirited 9-year-old girl with a spinal-cord injury, provides nursing care and friendly companionship to 6-year-old **JÉSICA,** who is similarly paralyzed.

Chapter 48 shows how the remarkable Peraza family—with 4 children who have muscular dystrophy, including **SÓSIMO**—plays a leading role in a program run for and by disabled young people.

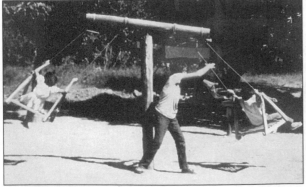

This circular swing helps 2 developmentally delayed children to gain better balance and body control. TACHO, the boy pushing the swing, has cerebral palsy. The twisting motion helps to reduce his spasticity. Good therapy for all. And good fun!

Another of these 4 children, **DINORA,** studies English with a disabled young teacher, so that she, in turn, can teach her disabled friends.

Chapter 49 explains how **FERNANDO,** a boy with cerebral palsy, is helped by **MANUEL** and other playmates to learn a variety of skills and to gain greater self-confidence.

Chapter 50 describes how **MARIA,** a mentally handicapped girl in Brazil, learns to provide care and therapy for **EMA,** a multiply disabled child.

From Beneficiaries to Facilitators: Ramona, Jesús, and Child-to-Child

CHAPTER **45**

Looking at Strengths, Not Weaknesses

One of the shortcomings of games that give non-disabled children a temporary, imaginary disability (such as tying a stick to one leg) is that it only allows them to experience the difficulties and frustrations of being disabled, rather than to appreciate the ways that disabled persons develop new strengths and abilities to cope with their difficulties. Thus, the game can result in pity rather than appreciation.

To encourage a group of youngsters to focus on strengths rather than weaknesses, **it helps to include disabled children in the games.** The importance of this became clear during a Child-to-Child training program held in Nicaragua in 1990.

RAMONA, a timid teenaged girl, was one of the disabled participants. One of her legs was paralyzed and contracted from polio, and she walked on the other leg using crutches. When the time came to play a "simulation game" to help non-disabled youngsters to experience disability, several children were asked to tie one foot to their backside and to stand on one leg. Other children were asked to find a pole or improvise crutches, so that their "disabled" playmates could walk. Then they held a race. To everyone's surprise, Ramona shyly asked if she could join the race.

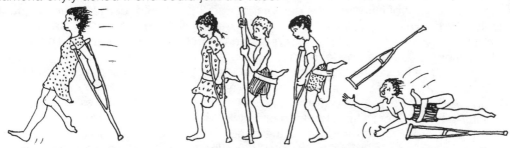

Ramona, of course, won with flying colors. The other children, rather than feeling sorry for her, marveled at her speed and agility.

This game was not only an eye-opener for the children, it was a liberating experience and a turning point for Ramona. In the various activities that followed, others treated her with new respect. And Ramona, losing much of her shyness, participated enthusiastically.

Ramona has come a long way since then. As a health promoter with CISAS,* she has become a leader in her community and a strong defender of women's and children's rights. She traveled from Nicaragua to Mexico to take part in a PROJIMO workshop on disability rights. (While there, the PROJIMO team straightened her knee contracture with a series of plaster casts, then made her a light-weight plastic brace.) Back in Nicaragua, Ramona has formed and leads an organization of disabled persons. She has also become an outstanding facilitator of Child-to-Child activities, in which she helps young people in her town look at the strengths of disabled children, not their weaknesses.

Fingers that see. At the same Child-to-Child workshop in Nicaragua where Ramona won the race, other disabled children participated. A blind girl showed other children how she could read Braille (tiny raised dots on a page) with her fingertips (see page 5). The other children were amazed at her ability, especially when she explained how she did it and then had them try it. Far from feeling pity, they marveled at and admired the blind girl's ability.

* CISAS is a Nicaraguan health education program that has done a lot to promote Child-to-Child and human rights. See p. 341.

Classmates Help a Disabled Child to Stay in School

In January, 1995, PROJIMO hosted a four-day workshop on the management of small community based programs. (Lack of management skills is a common problem.) Participants came from 13 programs in Mexico and Central America. Ramona, described above, came from Nicaragua. The PROJIMO team was delighted to have her back.

JESÚS, one of the disabled children staying at PROJIMO, rolled up to the study group in his wheelchair, interrupting a lively workshop that was being held under a giant laurel tree. He asked for Conchita, one of PROJIMO's coordinators who was participating in the workshop. The 13-year-old was obviously distraught. "This is the last day I'm going to school!" he declared.

"Why?" asked Conchita, rolling over to him in her own wheelchair.

"Because the teacher is mean to me," said Jesús. "When I ask her what is written on the blackboard, she scolds me for disturbing the class!"

"Doesn't your teacher know you can't see?" asked one workshop participant, herself blind.

"I've told her, but it's like she doesn't hear me. Or doesn't believe me." said Jesús. "She treats me as if it were my fault I can't see!"

Jesús, who is multiply disabled, has had a hard life. He was born with spina bifida, a defect of the spinal cord that causes reduced strength and feeling in his lower body (see page 131). With a lot of help from his parents, at age 3 Jesús did learn to walk, although awkwardly. Then, when he was six, he fell ill with meningitis. This left him nearly blind and with muscle stiffness (spasticity) that reduced control of his movements. The stiffness gradually lessened, and the boy learned to walk again, with crutches and dragging his feet. But due to the lack of feeling in his feet, he developed a deep sore on his right foot. This led to a chronic bone infection and, at age 7, his right leg was amputated. Jesús went back to crawling, and gradually developed flexion contractures of his hips and remaining knee. From sitting too long on his buttocks (which also lacked feeling), he developed large pressure sores, down to the bone. His lack of urine and bowel control (due to spina bifida) made the sores hard to keep clean, and they had worsened, year after year. (A device to help heal the sores on Jesús' foot is described in Chapter 16.)

When Jesús was 13 years old, his mother brought him from their home in the distant city of Mazatlán to PROJIMO, in the village of Ajoya. On examining Jesús, the team told him that with an artificial leg—which they could make—he could probably walk again. But first his hip and knee contractures must be corrected. This, they explained, would require weeks or even months of gradual stretching while lying on a wheeled cot, or gurney. In any case, lying face-down would be necessary to allow his large pressure sores to heal. Jesús was so eager to walk that he agreed. His mother did, too. So plans were made for him to stay at PROJIMO for an extended time.

While in Ajoya, Jesús had his first opportunity to attend school. His excitement about school overcame his fear of being away from home. His mother and older sister had already taught him the alphabet. He could read the letters and numbers if they were drawn very large and if he held them two or three inches from his face. So Jesús was enthusiastic about learning more. At first he went to school on his wheeled gurney.

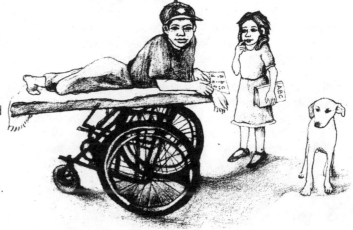

Jesús is obviously bright and has an inquisitive mind. In spite of his poor vision, he learned so fast that, within a few weeks, he was advanced to the 2nd grade. Unfortunately, his new teacher had little understanding of his special needs. She regarded the disabled child more as a nuisance than as a challenge. Because Jesús was unable to read either the blackboard or his books, and because his teacher scolded him when he asked for help, the boy had grown discouraged. "It's no use," he complained. "I'm going to quit school. I want to go home."

When Jesús announced that he was quitting school, the workshop participants tried to think of ways to help the boy find the courage and will to continue. Three participants were from a program for visually impaired persons, and one was blind herself. They suggested ideas for helping Jesús learn more easily, and offered to talk with his teacher.

Then Ramona from Nicaragua exclaimed, "Why don't we try a Child-to-Child approach? It could help both the kids and teacher understand his problem better and look for ways to assist him with his studies?" The workshop participants knew little about Child-to-Child, but wanted to learn more. Those working with blind persons were eager to take part in Jesús' class. Arrangements were made with the school Director and the second grade teacher to do the activity the next afternoon.

A Child-to-Child activity.

Ramona led the Child-to-Child activity. Her spritely manner at once captured the children's attention. First she explained a bit about Child-to-Child and introduced the visitors. Then she told the children that she wanted to explore with them what it was like to be blind, or partially blind, like Jesús. When she said this, all the children looked at Jesús, who sat in his wheelchair at the side of the classroom. Sensing their attention, he sat up importantly and smiled back at them.

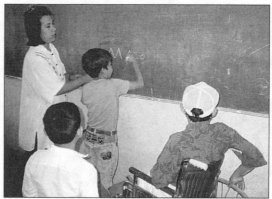
A child "teacher" writes big letters on the blackboard.

Ramona called for volunteers to take part in a role play. Two children played the role of blind pupils. Two others took turns playing the role of a visually impaired pupil like Jesús. And two others played the role of school teacher. The two "blind" children had bandanas tied tightly over their eyes, and could see nothing. They tried to find their way around the class-room and to follow the instructions of the "teacher." These children bumped into things and got confused. They said it was like trying to find their way in a dark room at night.

The other children helped by giving them clues or guiding them. They also played a trick on one of the "blind" boys. The "teacher" asked the boy to find a girl named Eliza and bring her to the front of the class. Feeling his way, the boy made his way to Eliza's seat. But as he approached, Eliza quickly swapped seats with the girl next to her. The boy took the other girl by the hand, led her forward, and presented her to the teacher. "Here she is," he said proudly. "Are you sure this is Eliza?" asked the child playing the teacher. "Yes!" said the boy. "Take off your blindfold and have a look," said the "teacher."

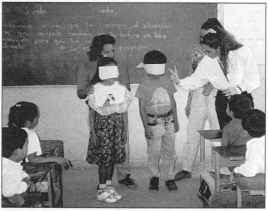
Blindfolded children learn what it is like to be blind.

The boy took off the blindfold off and stared dumbfounded at the girl he had thought was Eliza. "They tricked me!" he shouted. The class burst into laughter.

In the next role play, a pupil experienced **partial blindness:** a cotton shirt was draped over her head. (Ramona had tried different cloths until she found one that limited vision similar to Jesús' visual loss.) The "teacher" then asked the pupil to read from her book. Only by holding it close to her face could she read the largest letters. Then the "teacher" wrote a word on the blackboard, and said, "Read it." To read, the pupil had to go very close to the blackboard. By making the letters bigger and bolder, the weak-sighted child could read the word from farther away. But she still had to go close to the blackboard.

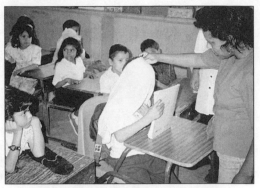

A cotton shirt over this girl's head gives her the experience of visual impairment.

After this role play with simulated visual impairment, another "pretend teacher" asked Jesús to read a word on the blackboard. Jesús rolled forward. To read the words he had to grip the armrests of his wheelchair and lift himself upright so that his face was almost touching the word, which he read proudly.

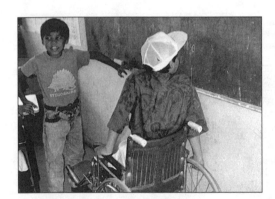

After the school children saw the difficulty Jesús had reading, both from the blackboard and from his school books, Ramona asked them, "Can you think of ways that you, Jesús' classmates, can help him understand his lessons and get the most out of school, in spite of his disability?"

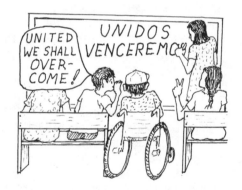

The children came up with a wide variety of creative suggestions:

• Be sure that Jesús sits at the front of the class, near the blackboard.

• Write and draw very large on the blackboard.

• Have Jesús sit next to a pupil who whispers in his ear what is written on the blackboard.

• Our teacher, or one of us, should always read out loud what is written on the blackboard.

• One of us could copy into Jesús' notebook what is written on the blackboard.

• And we should write in his notebook in big, dark, clear letters.

• Maybe Jesús could use an extra-big notebook and a black marking pen, so he can read for himself what he writes.

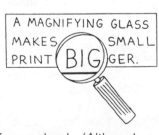

A MAGNIFYING GLASS MAKES SMALL PRINT **BIG**GER.

• Would it help if Jesús had a **magnifying glass?**

• We children could take turns after school, helping Jesús with his homework and reading to him from his books.

• Some of us can also take turns helping to bring him to and from school. (Although Jesús has learned to find his way without trouble, there is a steep slope on the way to school, and Jesús appreciates the assistance and the camaraderie.)

With a little prompting, the children came up with yet more ideas:

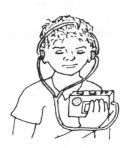

- What about a **tape recorder?** We could record the lessons from his books, and that way he could study them whenever he wants.

- When we are given tests and exams, couldn't Jesús whisper the answers in the teacher's ear? (In other words, **take exams orally.**)

After this discussion, Ramona asked the visually impaired visitor if she had any further ideas. She suggested a way to make writing easier for Jesús (and the results more legible for the teacher). They could give Jesús **writing paper with extra dark lines.** A visually impaired person simply cannot see the very thin pale lines on ordinary lined paper. If paper with dark, thick, widely separated lines could not be obtained, she suggested, the children could create such paper for Jesús with a ruler and a marking pen.

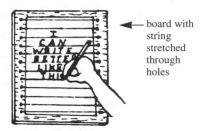

board with string stretched through holes

Another good idea. This way Jesús can feel the lines on the page

Then the blind visitor made a suggestion that fascinated the class. She told them that, with a little help, **Jesús could learn to read with his fingers.** From her bag she pulled a large sheet of **Braille script,** and showed the children how she could read it with her finger tips (see p. 5). She let every child feel the tiny bumps on the paper. Then she let Jesús try it, guiding his finger over the paper. She gave Jesús a sheet with the Braille alphabet. Next to each Braille letter she printed a large dark letter, so that Jesús could begin to learn Braille. The children were fascinated, and Jesús was so excited he trembled. The visitor explained that the Braille system had been invented many years ago by a blind schoolboy in France.

Judging from the children's response, this Child-to-Child activity was a big success. Jesús decided to stay in school. The teacher asked Jesús to sit next to a mischievous boy who had made many suggestions of ways to help Jesús with his learning. A few of his classmates began accompanying Jesús to and from school. Some even helped him with his homework. And now Jesús has both a magnifying glass and a small tape recorder. A girl at PROJIMO, who also has spina bifida and an amputated leg, offered to help tape his lessons.

Clearly, not all the problems are solved. Rather than helping Jesús to do his homework himself, his helpers at first tended to do it for him. But the whole Child-to-Child process has been a rewarding experience for all. **Both Jesús and his classmates are learning more than just their lessons. They are learning the joy that comes from bridging barriers to understanding, from creative problem-solving, and from helping one another.**

Jesús finished the school year in Ajoya, where he became more self-confident and independent. His mother, who had previously been reluctant to send him to school, was convinced he should continue.

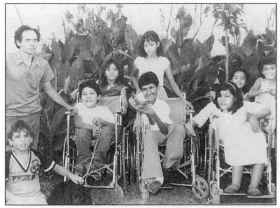

Sósimo (in center wheelchair) with a group from Los Pargos.

Jesús, who had begun to learn Braille, was eager to learn more. During the summer vacation, the PROJIMO team arranged for Jesús to study Braille in Mazatlán with the help of a young man with muscular dystrophy, named *SÓSIMO*. Since he was a young child, Sósimo had been active in Los Pargos, a program run by families of disabled children (see Chapter 48). Although his health was very delicate, Sósimo was still an active leader of the program. He had studied Braille in order to teach blind children. Jesús could not have had a better teacher—nor a better role model.

Jesús Becomes a Child-to-Child Facilitator

In spite of his early difficulties, after the Child-to-Child experience, Jesús liked school so much that he chose to return to attend school in Ajoya the following school year.

Jesús now helps to facilitate Child-to-Child activities in other villages. His first involvement concerned a family from a village called Limón, 50 kilometers away. The family had come to PROJIMO with two children, CHIRO and RICARDO, who had muscular dystrophy (see page 317). The brothers, ages 9 and 11, walked awkwardly and were very shy. Two years before, their parents had tried sending them to school. But the boys no longer attended because they had been teased by the other children.

The PROJIMO team thought that introducing Child-to-Child to the school children in Limón might help. They invited Jesús to go with them. He eagerly accepted.

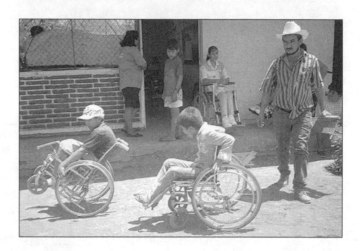

Arriving at Limon, Jesús and the PROJIMO team first visited the family of the two brothers, who rather reluctantly accompanied them to the school. It was a tiny primary school with 3 rooms. The teachers were intrigued by the arrival of the disabled troupe, and gladly interrupted their classes.

Ricardo and Chiro watched from a safe distance. They were astonished when Jesús ran in a wheelchair race with the most athletic children in the class. Skilled in wheelchair use, the disabled youngster left his competitors far behind. Excited, the brothers moved closer.

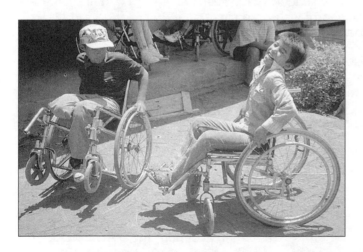

Having won the respect of the children by winning the race, Jesús did "wheelies" (balancing on the chair's back wheels) and whirled in circles on two wheels, gracefully dancing. The able-bodied riders tried to imitate Jesús, with upsetting results. Everyone applauded Jesús, who thrived on the attention.

Overcoming their fear, the two brothers, Ricardo and Chiro, came closer to get a good look.

After the activities, the PROJIMO team discussed with the class and teacher the importance of treating disabled children as equals, and of helping them to build on their strengths rather than pitying or teasing them for their weaknesses. The school children appeared eager to befriend and assist the two newcomers. And the brothers, after watching the children's admiration for the blind boy in a wheelchair, lost some of their fear of school. Arrangements were made for the boys to attend school next term.

All benefitted from this experience—not least, Jesús. **Not only did he win admiration from his peers, but he discovered the joy of helping other children with special needs to gain new self-confidence and hope.**

CHAPTER 46

An Unusual Friendship: Manolo and Luis

Some of the best things that take place in a community based program, as in life, are completely unplanned. They take place because the program and its facilitators are flexible and relaxed enough to let spontaneity flourish and heart-felt adventures happen.

In this chapter we reprint an article from Newsletter from the Sierra Madre #20.* *It is the true story about a unique friendship between two disabled young people at PROJIMO, as told by Oliver Bock, a California orthotist (brace maker) who has made several trips to the program to share his skills with village rehabilitation workers. The innovation described here is* **the way that persons with very different disabilities can complement and assist one another.** *It also raises the question of recruiting able-bodied but mentally handicapped young persons to be helpers or "attendants" of those who are able-minded but physically handicapped.*

Following the story, we give a bit of background about how Manolo joined PROJIMO and how another disabled child managed to reach him, when others could not.

Manolo and Luis

by Oliver Bock

Manolo feels caught. Once again, he doesn't know what to do. He is sure that a joke is being played on him, and he is confused. Lacking the tools for understanding, Manolo resorts to his tried and true response. "Don't look at me!" he demands. And, with a jerk of his head away from the insult, he trundles off, looking for more hospitable company.

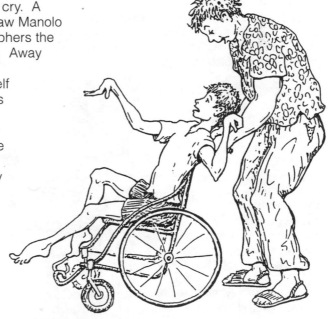

Seeing Manolo retreat from the brace shop, sad-eyed Luis lets out his unmistakable cry. A throaty bellow and waving limbs draw Manolo to his side. Intuitively, Manolo deciphers the message that Luis needs company. Away from his family for the first time and having a hard time at making himself understood, after three days, Luis is somewhat desperate.

Manolo is gentle with Luis, but there are others who love to tease him. One of the favorite games they play with Luis is asking him if he misses his mother. Then his beautiful brown eyes look at you with wrenching sadness as his head drops into a crook of his elbow. With tears running down his face and arm, Luis sobs quietly until he is comforted.

---

* The *Newsletter from the Sierra Madre* is published 2 to 3 times a year by HealthWrights and covers innovations and ideas from community based health and rehabilitation programs in Mexico and elsewhere. It also looks at issues concerning the politics of health and the basic rights of disadvantaged and oppressed peoples, from both local and global perspectives.

Manolo doesn't know how to play that kind of game, but he does know how to push a wheelchair. He is strong and enjoys pleasing his passenger. Luis loves going for rides, so the two of them head up the narrow path leading to the main street of Ajoya. It is a hot day. The mangos are almost ripe. The dust lifts easily, and quietly coats everything. The younger kids, almost impervious to heat, are playing, while the men tilt back against shaded adobe walls, waiting patiently.

The squeaking of dry bearings and a cloud of dust temporarily interrupt the magic stillness. Nearly indifferent eyes follow the pair as Manolo pushes Luis' wheelchair through the hot sun. Wheelchairs inhabited by all varieties of disabled bodies have become so commonplace in Ajoya that they no longer generate curiosity or fear in the villagers.

The overwhelming heat finally forces the two companions to seek relief. Manolo's round, soft body is shining with perspiration while Luis' angular, contracted body sticks uncomfortably to the vinyl seat and back of his chair. "Shall we go to the river?" Manolo asks hopefully. Luis eagerly agrees to the promise of adventure and escape from the oppressive heat.

With sweat streaming, the two companions make their way to the end of town and down the treacherous path toward the river. Boulders, erosion ruts, and deep sand turn the half mile into a monumental expedition. At times, Luis has to slide his spastic body out of his chair and drag himself over impassable obstacles while Manolo handles the progress of the chair. In one spot, Manolo has to carry Luis across a deep ravine, set him down on the far side, and then return for the wheelchair.

The patient determination of the two companions builds a feeling of friendship that is both wonderful and foreign to them. Twice Manolo asks Luis if he wants to abandon the mission. Both times, Luis answers Manolo with his deep expressive eyes, as if to say, "Let's go on. I know it's a lot of work for you and you must be tired, but I'm so excited. I love you for being able to take me with you like this." Manolo interprets the response correctly, and the two slowly labor on toward the river.

When they finally arrive, Manolo, hot and dusty, splashes into the slow-moving, tired river.

The small stream of water looks insignificant as it cuts its narrow path through the huge riverbed. Soon, when the rain comes, this calm trickle will become a raging torrent, at times filling the entire riverbed with a powerful flow of boulders, branches, and silt-filled water carried down from the high valleys of the Sierra Madre.

Manolo splashes his face with the tepid, green river water and looks upstream at the town he now thinks of as home. He can't remember how he got to Ajoya, but he knows it is where he is happy—happier than he has ever imagined possible. He thinks about the important jobs he has. He washes people who can't wash themselves and dresses them in clean clothes so that they can look nice. He fetches sodas for clever men who make amazing things in the workshops. Sometimes they even give him jobs in the shop, and that makes him feel very proud.

People like him here. Sure, they tease him, but he's used to that—and besides, here they tease with a smile. And those around him have problems, too. Many of them have bodies that don't work right. Some have shriveled legs and walk with crutches, and some sit in wheelchairs all the time and can't feel in their legs. There are others, like Luis, who can't control their bodies and have to live with twitches and jerks that keep them from talking or moving the way they want to … For his part, Manolo has a good, strong body. He can help in a lot of ways, but his thinking doesn't work right. He doesn't understand many things, and he has a hard time remembering. But when something is clear, Manolo is happy to do it. He loves to write. He fills pages of notebooks with sentences that have been written for him to copy. He can't read and he doesn't know what he writes, but it doesn't matter. He is doing useful work!

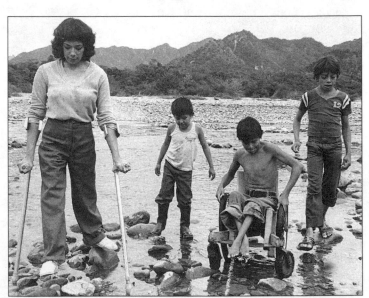

The river provides play and adventure for disabled and non-disabled children alike. The boy in the wooden wheelchair is Jorge, Manolo's first friend in Ajoya.

A loud splash brings Manolo out of his thoughts. Luis has slid out of his chair and dragged himself into the river. Happily splashing away the heat and dust, he gives Manolo a huge grin. Manolo is a bit worried because Luis is wearing all his clothes and they are getting soaked. Luis smiles as if to say, "Its fine, my clothes are hot too." Manolo laughs and plops down in the river next to Luis. Luis splashes uncontrollably and Manolo imitates. The two friends are soaking wet and thoroughly enjoying the fruits of their difficult trek.

Across the river, on the bank overlooking the bathers, a wealthy landowner watches the scene. Sitting astride his horse, he contemplates the wheelchair. Watching the two friends, he realizes what a good thing it is that these children have a place to be where they can enjoy life and be valued for their ability to smile, laugh, play, and be helpful in whatever way they can.

Moved by a sudden impulse, the horseman spurs his beast down toward the two boys just as Manolo is lifting the joyous Luis back into his chair. Surprised and scared by the approaching rider, Manolo almost drops Luis and becomes confused about whether to run, fight, or remain still. Fear fills Luis' eyes as he senses Manolo's anxiety. With fewer options available, Luis sits and waits to see what will happen.

"Don't be afraid, my friends. I will not harm you." Manolo and Luis slowly look up at the horseman. He smiles at them and swings down off his horse. He is a small man, much smaller than Manolo, but he has the strength of someone accustomed to having power. "My name is Chuy. I was watching you two play in the water, and I thought you might like some help getting back to Ajoya." Manolo is uncertain. The friendly offer confuses him; he is torn between temptation and fear. Luis, on the other hand, is thrilled. His quick mind has already determined that he is about to get a ride back home. Manolo still can't make up his mind. Decisions are a threat to him, especially when they involve responsibility. Fortunately, Chuy resolves Manolo's confusion by helping Luis lift himself onto the horse.

Loading a spastic child onto a horse is no easy task, especially when the child is nervous and excited. Manolo quickly sees that his assistance is needed. Chuy is barely able to lift Luis, much less lift him onto the horse and try to pry his legs apart enough to straddle the horse's back. After several exhausting attempts, Luis proudly sits on the horse, with his hands tied together around Chuy's waist to keep him from falling off. When drool starts running down the man's back, he momentarily questions his generosity. But as they head back to Ajoya, with Luis groaning happily and Manolo gleefully pushing the empty wheelchair, Chuy feels glad that he decided to help.

Long shadows and cooling temperatures greet the trio as they enter the village. Thirsty, they buy and drink three sodas. At least half of Luis' soda makes a sticky mess down his front, and onto the saddle and horse. This time, Chuy doesn't even flinch. He knows it can be cleaned up, and he doesn't want to disrupt the mood.

A group of small children trail along after the trio as they enter the PROJIMO yard. The workers in the metal shop stop work to watch and yell out greetings. Other children playing in PROJIMO run over to the horse and riders. Manolo proudly helps Luis down off the horse and returns the joyous child to his chair. Luis is overwhelmed with excitement as tears of happiness run down his cheeks. Chuy wheels his horse around, waves goodbye, and rides away content and a little embarrassed by Luis' tears. It's a moment he will never forget.

Manolo, on the other hand, has already forgotten where they have been and why they returned the way they did. He does know that he feels happy and proud when Luis smiles at him.

Later that night, when Manolo lifts Luis out of his chair onto his sleeping mat, Luis manages to get his arms wrapped around Manolo's back. When the time comes to let go, neither one of them does so. For a moment, the two friends hold each other quietly. When they do release their embrace, their eyes meet. Something they can't explain has happened, and they know it is important.

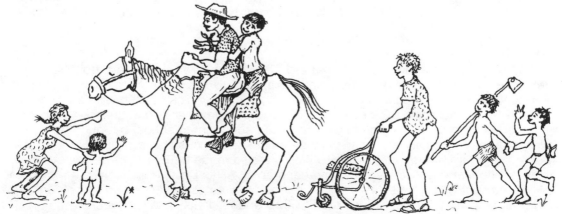

Manolo's Transition at PROJIMO

PROJIMO began as a program run by physically disabled villagers for physically disabled children and youth. But after a time, disabled persons of every age and with every kind of disability began to arrive. So the PROJIMO team tried to expand their knowledge and abilities to help persons of all ages and disabilities to meet their needs. With the help of visiting special educators and counselors they have learned something about mental handicap and developmental delay. But the team feels they still have a great deal to learn.

When Manolo was brought to PROJIMO by his mother, Mari and Conchita took charge of the consultation. Manolo was 14 years old but full grown and heavy set. His mother led him into the room and told him to sit down. Manolo silently obeyed, but he looked unhappy and angry. He did not answer when Mari greeted him; he just stared at his feet. His mother told Mari that Manolo gave her nothing but problems. "Yes, he can speak a few words," she said. "But usually he doesn't say anything ... especially around strangers."

Mari turned toward Manolo "What things do you like to do, Manolo?" Mari asked him in her friendliest voice.

"Nothing!" replied his mother. "He does nothing."

"Manolo, do you like to play games?" asked Mari, putting her hand on his broad shoulder.

"No!" said his mother. "He doesn't like to do anything. When he was little, I tried sending him to school, but he learned nothing. After 3 weeks the teacher sent him home. She said the other children were afraid of him."

"Do you like to watch T.V.?" Mari asked Manolo.

"No!" said his mother. "He doesn't like to do anything ... except to eat."

"What foods do you like, Manolo?" asked Mari.

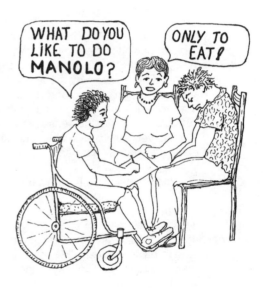

"He eats everything!" said his mother.

Mari turned to her. "Give him a chance to answer for himself," she suggested gently.

"He won't say anything." answered his mother. "He doesn't talk to strangers."

It seemed she was right. His mother now kept silent and Mari tried to interest Manolo in a variety of things and to get him to say something. He didn't respond. Mari was unsure what to do next. Then, suddenly, Jorge rolled into the room with a loud whoop. Jorge was 14 years old but small for his age. He had two flail legs from polio and used a wooden wheelchair. On seeing that a consultation was in process he at once turned to leave.

"Jorge!" Mari called after him. "Please come here."

JORGE paused in the doorway. "What did I do wrong now?" he asked, frowning defensively. Jorge was a great mischief maker and always getting into trouble. He had first come to PROJIMO for leg braces and a wheelchair (which he much preferred). Two years later he had come back because his aging grandmother with whom he lives in the city said she couldn't manage him. She would send him to school but often he would spend the day—and sometimes the nights—in the streets or saloons. At times the police would bring him home drunk. In PROJIMO he also made trouble. But he went to the village school and was learning income-generating skills. Despite his pranks, he was a lot of fun and got along well with other children. He was especially good at befriending children who had recently arrived at PROJIMO and felt lonely and homesick.

"I need your help," said Mari. Jorge grinned. "I've been trying to learn what Manolo here likes or wants to do," Mari explained. "But he's shy and won't answer. Can you take him outside and show him the playground and shops. Maybe something will catch his fancy."

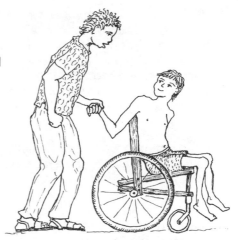

Jorge boldly rolled up to Manolo and took his big hand. "Come with me, compadre," he said. "I'll show you around." Manolo, looking gloomy, slowly rose and followed Jorge out the door. Although they were the same age, they looked like David and Goliath.

Mari stayed behind talking with Manolo's mother, who explained that she was worried because Manolo was so big and so bad tempered.

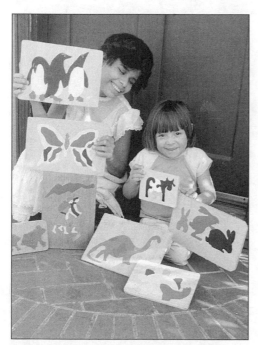

In the children's toy-making workshop, Jorge made wooden puzzles like these.

"Sometimes I'm afraid of him," she said. "He's so strong he could really hurt someone. And he's too big for me to control."

After a quarter of an hour the door burst open and Manolo came dashing in, followed by Jorge. "Mama! Mama!" He shouted. "Look at this!" He held up a colorfully painted wooden jigsaw puzzle. "Jorge make this!" he exclaimed. "I want make this! Jorge teach me!"

Manolo turned to Mari. He seemed a totally different person than the one she had been trying to get to speak a few minutes before. "Can I stay and make?" he asked Mari loudly.

"I hope so," said Mari. "We'll see what we can arrange."

Later that day, Mari asked Jorge what he had done to get Jorge to speak. "You won't be angry if I tell you?" asked Jorge. Mari shook her head. "I asked him if he wanted a cigarette" said Jorge, grinning devilishly. "That hooked him!"

Manolo stayed at PROJIMO for almost 6 months. As it turned out, he never did learn to make jigsaw puzzles. Although Jorge and others tried to take him through the process step by step, it proved too difficult for him. But he did learn to do many things, to live with a group outside his own family, and to gain a bit of self-respect.

One of the first jobs done by Manolo won him strong appreciation by the team. The tar-paper roof of the wheelchair shop had begun to leak and needed replacing. The tar-paper is held onto the wood struts with small nails. To prevent the tar-paper from tearing loose in the wind, bottle caps from soda bottles are used to give the nail heads a broader base. For this, each bottle cap has to first have a hole punched in it with a nail and hammer. One day, José was in the shop with a sack-full of hundreds of bottle caps, starting to punch the holes. Manolo was fascinated. "What you do?" he asked. José explained the chore. "I help!" said Manolo. José taught Manolo how to center a bottle cap over an iron sheet with a small hole in it, hold the nail in the middle of the cap, and hit it with the hammer. He guided Manolo through the first dozen or so caps. Then Manolo took over the job.

Manolo would punch holes for a while and then get distracted. But soon shouts would come from those on the roof asking for more bottle caps. With this feedback and encouragement for his work, Manolo persevered. When the new roof was completed, everyone celebrated. Manolo was praised along with the rest for getting the job done so quickly and well.

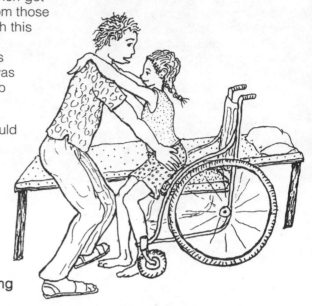

Manolo began looking for other things he could do to help. Because he is able-bodied and strong, and most of the PROJIMO staff are physically disabled, they would often call on him to help lift Quique (who was quadriplegic) out of bed and onto his wheeled cot. He also helped others who cannot move themselves. **It was not long before Manolo became a real attendant, pushing the wheelchairs of those who needed help, and even assisting them with changing clothes and bathing.**

For Manolo, this was a complete reversal of roles. From someone who was dependent and considered useless, he had suddenly become someone who had physical strength and ability others lacked. He was genuinely needed for this unusual ability!

When his mother came to visit she could not believe how her son had changed. When she took him home, she at first had a hard time readjusting to the new Manolo. For a while, both mother and son slipped back into the old pattern of accusation and apathy. But after a longer second visit by Manolo to PROJIMO, and some long discussions with his mother, things began to go better at home too. Manolo began to help with jobs around the house and even to help neighbors with simple tasks. But his real love was to be an attendant to physically disabled persons.

Manolo, by now, has probably forgotten Luis. And Luis may have forgotten Manolo. But Manolo gave Luis a degree of freedom, adventure, and joy of life he had not known before.

Jorge's fate. As for young Jorge, he went through some difficult times. In time, he was thrown out of PROJIMO for drunkenness, and ended up as a vagrant street youth. Fortunately, years later, Jorge was "rescued" by Leopoldo, another disabled youth who was expelled from PROJIMO (for shooting at a rival who was courting his girlfriend). Eventually Leopoldo became a leader in a self-help program of disabled youth in the city of Hermosillo, where he opened a wheelchair repair shop. On one of his travels, he happened upon Jorge in the northern border town of Tijuana. Jorge was sick from hunger and drugs and in despair. Leopoldo took Jorge back home with him to Hermosillo and arranged work for him in the workshop of the disability program.

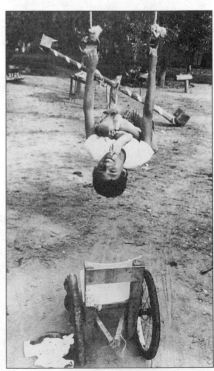

The last we heard, Jorge was off drugs, healthy, self-reliant, and about to get married. Like many of us, he has had his ups and downs.

Jorge playing on the rings during one of his first visits to PROJIMO.

CHAPTER 47

Vania and Jésica:
A Ten-Year-Old Doctors a Younger Child

JÉSICA is a lively, high-spirited little girl from a poor barrio in the city of Mazatlán. But at age 5, when her mother first brought her to PROJIMO, her condition was critical.

*Three days after Jésica was born, a doctor had injected her in the backside (her mother does not know why). An **abscess** formed at the injection site. The infection spread to her spinal cord, leaving her **paralyzed from the hips down (paraplegia).***

Jésica spent most days alone in the family hut. Her father was a fisherman, but when there was no work, he spent most of his time drinking. Her mother was often gone all day trying to earn money to feed the children.

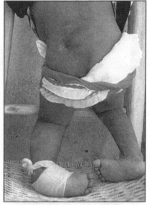

Note the scar on Jésica's buttock where the abscess was drained. The infection caused paralysis of her legs and also clubbing of her feet. Trying to stand, she developed a pressure sore on top of her foot.

Because of her spinal-cord injury, Jésica had **reduced feeling in her lower body** and she **lacked urine and bowel control,** which had resulted in **chronic sores on her genitals and near her anus.** Poor hygiene had made the sores worse. She would sit all day in her urine and poop, which aggravated her sores. Yet she did not complain, because she felt no pain.

Jésica also had **a large, infected sore on top of her left foot.** This had formed from trying to stand. She would hold onto a chair and pull herself up. But her ankles flopped over so far that she stood on the tops of her feet.

A decision was made for Jésica to stay at PROJIMO long enough to heal her sores, straighten her clubbed feet with a series of casts, and to equip her with leg braces so that she could walk. A family in the village agreed to take care of Jésica, because her mother needed to return to Mazatlán to care for the other children. But fortunately Jésica's mother was able to stay in the village for a few days, until Jésica felt comfortable with her new care provider, who was a very motherly woman known as Doña Toña.

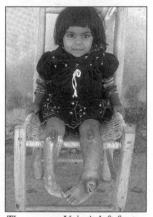

The sore on Jésica's left foot was infected and her whole leg was swollen.

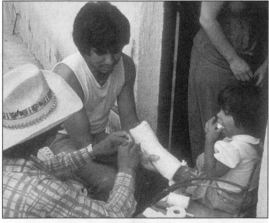

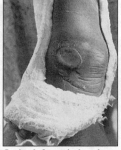

Javier left a window in the cast so that the sore on Jésica's foot could be cleaned and treated.

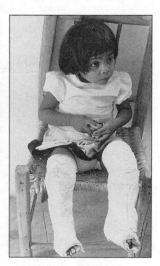

Javier (who also had a chronic pressure sore on a foot when he first came to PROJIMO) made a series of plaster casts for Jésica's legs, to gradually straighten her bent over ankles.

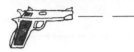

VANIA is another little girl who had a hard childhood. She was born in a squatter settlement in Culiacan (the state capital). When she was 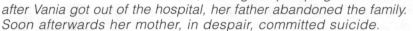 *one year old, there was a gun-fight in a neighboring shack. A bullet passed through the card-board walls of the shacks and hit her in the back, leaving her paraplegic. Two weeks after Vania got out of the hospital, her father abandoned the family. Soon afterwards her mother, in despair, committed suicide.*

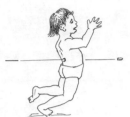

Vania was taken in by a great-aunt who was so old and frail that she had trouble caring for the disabled child. The little girl almost never left her aunt's home, never had a wheelchair, never went to school. She was nine years old when her aunt learned about PROJIMO and sent her there with neighbors. At that time, Vania was little more than skin and bones. Her head was crawling with lice, and she had severe pressure sores on her backside. Yet her warm smile and courage quickly won everyone's heart. At PROJIMO she saw people with spinal-cord injuries similar to hers, who were riding about independently in wheelchairs, working, and enjoying life. She decided she wanted to stay. Her great aunt gave permission.

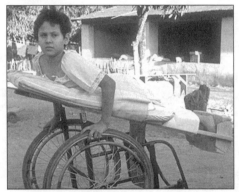

Vania on her wheelchair gurney.

Mari took charge of caring for Vania. She got rid of her head lice and began treating her pressure sores. The sores were large and deep. Mari cleaned them daily and packed them with a paste made of honey and sugar. They began to heal fairly quickly (see page 156).

The wheelchair shop workers made a small gurney, or wheeled lying-board for Vania. The board was mounted on a specially built wheelchair, for her to use after her sores healed.

At PROJIMO Vania discovered new life and hope. The whole village loved her. Mari and Conchita were like mothers to her. Because both women were paraplegic, vibrantly alive, and self-determined, they were excellent role models.

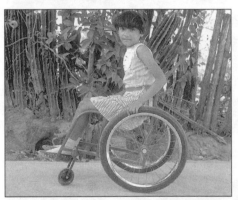

Vania in her wheelchair with the gurney removed.

Vania soon began going to the village school, first on her gurney, and after her sores healed, in her wheelchair. She learned quickly.

After school, Vania enjoyed learning and working in the children's toy-making workshop with both disabled and non-disabled children.

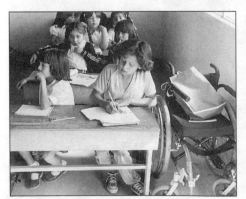

Vania at the village school after her sores healed.

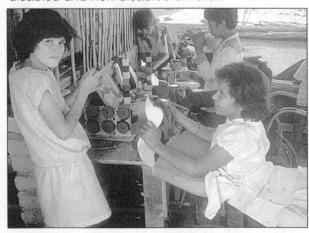

Vania with other children in the toy-making shop.

Vania provides nursing care to a donkey. One afternoon, Mari was working in the treatment room cleaning Jésica's pressure sores. Suddenly, little Vania rolled in on her gurney and said importantly, "Do you have any more supplies for treating sores?"

"Over there on the table" said Mari. "Why?"

"I need to use them," said Vania mysteriously. Mari watched as the girl rolled over to the table and carefully transferred soap, a bottle of boiled water, gauzes, a small jar of honey-and-sugar, and a pair of surgical forceps (still in their sterile paper wrapper) to the edge of her gurney and wheeled out of the room. Curious, Mari wheeled to the doorway and looked out at her.

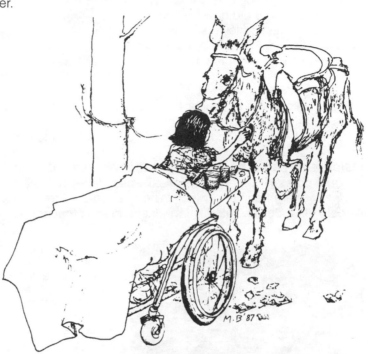

To Mari's amazement, Vania rolled up to a tree where a visitor had tied his donkey. The donkey had a big open sore on its neck, probably the result of a fight with a rival donkey. Fearlessly, Vania parked in front of the donkey, patted his nose, and talked to him tenderly. Then she began to gently wash the sore. The donkey flinched when she touched the sore, but let her continue. Dumbfounded, Mari watched as the girl carefully packed the sore with honey-and-sugar paste and covered it with gauze.

"We have a natural-born nurse here!" Mari exclaimed to members of the PROJIMO team, after Vania had carefully washed and returned the instruments. "We are so overworked, and we especially need additional nursing help." She turned to the little girl on the gurney. "Would you be willing to help us, Vania?" Vania's face lit up with delight.

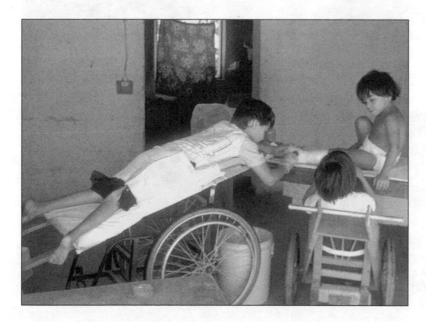

Vania as Jésica's nurse. After a few days of instruction and guidance by Mari, Vania took over the nursing care of Jésica. Every day, she carefully washed and packed the sore that could be seen through the hole in the cast on the younger child's foot. Little Jésica enjoyed being treated by another girl with similar needs. Under Vania's care, the sores healed rapidly, without complications.

Jésica's bowel program. Vania helped the younger girl with another essential service. Jésica had no control of her bowels. At unpredictable times of the day and night, she would dirty her clothing or her bed clothes and foul her sores. To reduce the likelihood of accidents, Mari taught Vania how to do a "bowel program" with Jésica. Shortly after breakfast each morning, before Vania went to school, she would have Jésica lie on some old newspapers. Putting on a plastic glove, she would stimulate Jésica's rectum with a finger. This caused a reflex which made her bowels move.

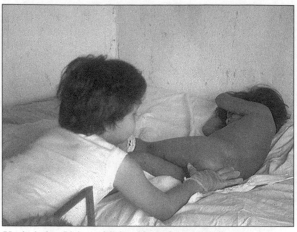

Vania helps Jésica with her "bowel program."

With this help in emptying her bowels at the same time each day, Jésica was able to be active all day without much risk of "accidents." Her regular bowel program became even more important when, some time later, Jésica began to go to kindergarten.

Jésica and Vania both show great improvement. With Vania's help, Jésica's pressure sores healed rapidly. Meanwhile, Javier adjusted the casts on Jésica's feet to gradually straighten her ankles. When her sores were healed and her feet were straight, Marcelo fitted Jésica with full-leg plastic braces (calipers).

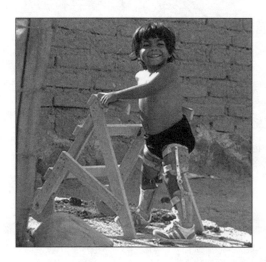

School children helped build a **wooden walker** for her, and she proudly began attending kindergarten.

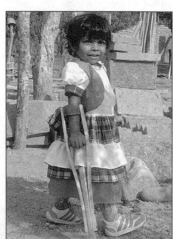

In time Jésica learned to walk with **crutches**. In the process she became more self-confident.

For Vania, being able to help Jésica gave her a new sense of personal worth and confidence. **At an age when most little girls are playing "nursy-nurse" with dolls, Vania was providing real nursing services to a real child.**

Equally important was the role model that Vania provided for Jésica. The girls became close friends, and helped each other in many ways.

Vania's story illustrates **PROJIMO's** goal: *to help children go beyond what they are usually expected or allowed to do, and come closer to realizing their full potential.*

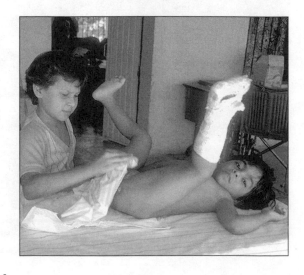

CHAPTER 48

Four Siblings with Muscular Dystrophy Lead a Program for Disabled Children

Progressive weakness. Many health and rehabilitation workers look at muscular dystrophy as one of the more difficult and discouraging disabilities. It tends to be familial, often affecting brothers. It is progressive and, within current medical knowledge, incurable. Duchenne's muscular dystrophy (the commonest type) begins in early childhood and causes increasing muscle weakness. The child—usually a boy—develops trouble walking, and eventually needs a wheelchair. As the weakness progresses, his arms get too weak to push his wheelchair or lift his hands to feed himself. Eventually, the weakness affects his breathing and, usually in his late teens or early 20s, he dies, often from pneumonia.

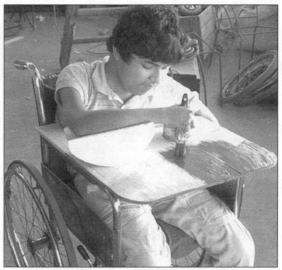

With the help of an arm rocker made of foam plastic, a boy with muscular dystrophy paints the table on his wheelchair.

*The good news. Despite all this, when given encouragement and a supportive environment, **many children with muscular dystrophy live full and adventurous lives,** even though they may die young. In this chapter, we tell the story of a remarkable family, the Perazas. Of their 7 children, 3 boys and one girl—CACHITO, SÓSIMO, JUANILLO, and DINORA—had muscular dystrophy. All were in wheelchairs by age 10. Today, only Dinora is still alive. The boys all died in their teens or early 20s. But, in their short lives, they did some amazing and fulfilling things.*

THE PERAZA FAMILY lives in a poor *barrio* of Mazatlán city. When the parents realized that several of their children had muscular dystrophy , they wanted to do all they could for them. In those days it was impossible to get such children into the public schools. Yet the Perazas felt that their children had the same right as other children to attend school.

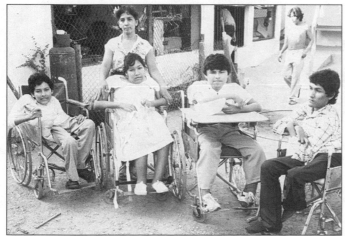

Three of the Peraza children, with a friend who also has muscular dystrophy, on a visit to PROJIMO.

So the family created their own school. Helped by an exceptional social worker, Teresa Paez, the Perazas met with families of other disabled children in the community and collectively started their own education and rehabilitation program for their children. The children themselves decided what to name their group. They called themselves *Los Pargos*, the name of a local fish which the elite consider inferior, although it provides a good source of food and a livelihood for local fisher folk.

Los Pargos

The Los Pargos school was organized as a cooperative, in which the disabled children and parents were participating members. Most families were quite poor. To raise money for school supplies and transport, the families made colorful crafts to sell. Outstanding were designs with artificial flowers, mostly made out of fish scales.

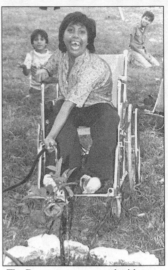

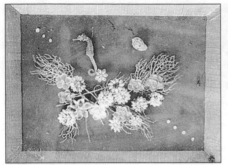

A framed design with flowers made with fish scales and sea shells, made by the Pargos and their parents.

Parents and children went on **work picnics** to the sea-shore where fishermen cleaned fish. They collected sackfuls of fish scales. These they washed and sun-dried. Then they stained them various colors and glued them together to make delicate bouquets of flowers.

The Pargos are concerned with ecology and wildlife. Here, they take part in a tree planting project.

With the help of Teresa Paez, Los Pargos convinced the city government to let them use a local school building after the official school day was over. Eventually the Education Department agreed to pay for a teacher. But the Pargos had trouble finding a teacher who respected and knew how to work with disabled children—until they found Victor.

VICTOR, **the teacher,** was born with athetoid cerebral palsy and began to walk when he was 8 years old. He stands and walks with great difficulty and falls often. When excited (which he usually is) his arms and legs jerk this way and that. He has a slight speech problem. But Victor is avidly independent. From primary school through college, he had to struggle to be accepted. Yet he was a gifted student. He won a scholarship to medical school, but had to drop out because the campus was far from home and his family could not afford bus fare. Since then, he strove to improve his mobility. He and a friendly mechanic invented strange and wonderful wheeled devices: walkers, motorcycles, and even a hand-controlled auto.

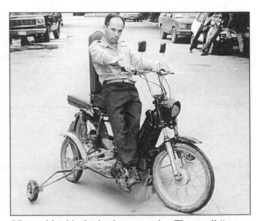

Victor rides his 6-wheel motorcycle. The small "outrigger" wheels keep his jerking body from upsetting it. He removes them to pass through narrow doors.

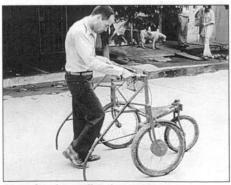

Victor found no walker that could keep him from falling—until he created this five point system. The rear pipes add stability and act as extra brakes, along with the hand brakes.

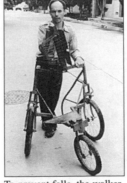

To prevent falls, the walker must be very wide. Victor shows how it folds for narrow doorways.

Victor majored in biology and math, and has a teaching degree. For several years he taught at the Pargos school, where he was a wonderful example. He had loving concern for his students, yet did not pamper or spoil them. He challenged each child to do his or her very best.

With a role model like Victor, many of the disabled students became junior teachers and creative facilitators for younger children and those who needed more assistance.

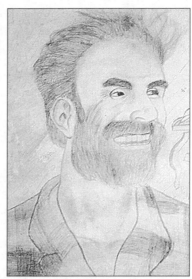

In this peer teaching process, **the Peraza children took the lead.** By the time they reached their teens, their dystrophy was advanced. Yet *CACHITO* and *SÓSIMO,* the older two brothers, had become very capable organizers and teachers of the Pargos. Sósimo even learned how to read and write Braille, so that he could teach blind children. The Peraza siblings also loved to draw and paint. With practice, they became gifted artists. One day when I (the author) was meeting with the Pargos, Sósimo drew the pencil sketch of me shown here. ➡

With care and patience, the Peraza children taught other children to draw and paint creatively. When the Pargos had enough pictures painted and fish-scale flowers made, they periodically held a public sale.

Pencil drawing of David Werner by Sósimo

The Peraza children led Los Pargos in the defense of endangered wildlife, with which they somehow identified. One summer, they led a city-wide **Campaign to *Protect the Sea Turtles,*** whose numbers were rapidly diminishing due to relentless hunting of both turtles and eggs. The Perazas asked each *Pargito* (disabled child) to do a painting of sea turtles as best as he or she could. The resulting collection of paintings was astounding: adult turtles, turtle eggs, and baby turtles of every size and color, swimming, dancing, playing, laying eggs—and being hunted and butchered—in the sea and on the beach of Mazatlán.

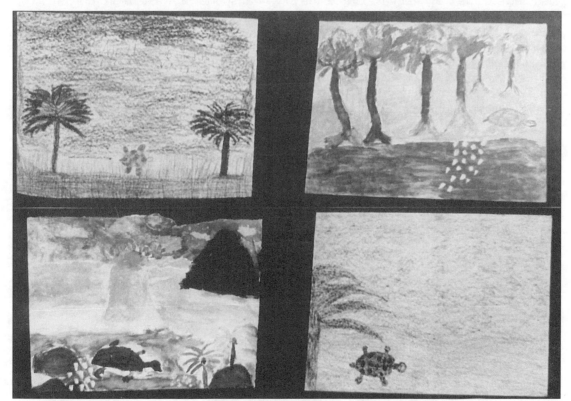

Paintings by the Perazas and other disabled children, as part of their campaign to protect endangered sea turtles.

With the cooperation of the city authorities and local artists, a public event was held to display the sea-turtle paintings (which sold like hot-cakes) and to raise the awareness of the larger community. In their defense of the sea turtles, Los Pargos won people's respect and appreciation for the abilities of disabled children.

All four of the Peraza siblings became gifted artists and craftspersons. But Sósimo was the most outstanding. Like the other *Pargitos,* he had a fascination with the ocean and its creatures. One of his most haunting paintings is the portrait of a woman in the bottom of the ocean. After Sósimo had died, his sister Dinora told me he had painted it "because when people die they go to the bottom of the ocean, and that is what makes the waves."

Evolution of Los Pargos. Eventually, Los Pargos gained enough public attention to pressure the local public schools into accepting some less severely disabled children. Even so, many of the Pargitos who began to attend public schools continued to come to Los Pargos' group in the afternoons. Several of the older Pargos took over the management, activism, and teaching responsibilities of the program. Among these were the Peraza siblings, whose leadership skills and ability to motivate others grew with time, even as their physical ability and health declined.

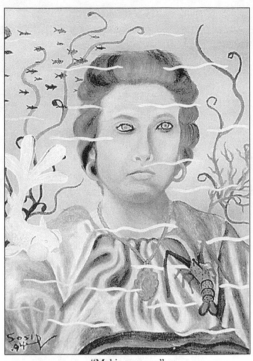
"Making waves."

As the years went by, Los Pargos grew and expanded. Children with all kinds of disabilities—physically disabled, mentally handicapped, epileptic, deaf, blind, and multiply disabled—came daily from all parts of the city. Transportation was a big problem. At last, with money they earned plus donations by well-to-do patrons in the city, the Pargos were able to buy a second-hand bus—which they named the *Pargobus.* Periodically the Pargobus would make trips to PROJIMO, in the village of Ajoya, about 100 miles from Mazatlán. The outings served as visits to the countryside and a chance for the children to enjoy the games and equipment in the Playground for All Children. The visits also provided an opportunity for children to be fitted with wheelchairs, orthopedic appliances, special seating, and other assistive devices. Again, the young Perazas often played a leading role in helping to organize these trips.

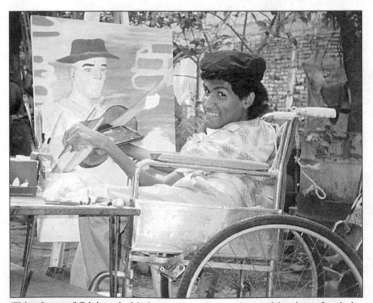
This photo of Sósimo in his late teens reflects his combination of artistic ability, self-determination, and his radiant joy in the creative process. I wish all children with muscular dystrophy, and their parents, could have had a chance to know and learn from Sósimo and his family.

It was amazing what these four youths with muscular dystrophy managed to do, and the pride and joy they took in doing it, even as their physical condition gradually deteriorated.

But for all their creativity and problem-solving skills, they could not halt the progress of the disease. Over a period of several years, one after the other of the 3 Peraza brothers died from pulmonary problems. Today only their sister, Dinora, is still alive. **But the dignity, caring, and leadership skills they developed and shared with their peers live on.**

At present, Los Pargos is managed and run by disabled graduates of the program, some of whom are continuing with their formal schooling and some of whom have jobs. (One of the first members of the Pargos, Miguelito, who has physical and speech difficulties, works in an automobile repair shop, skillfully taking dents out of damaged cars.) Occasionally, the disabled youths who run the program call on the assistance of special educators, teachers, doctors, and therapists when they think their help is needed. But overall, the group takes pride in its autonomy and independence.

DINORA BECOMES AN ENGLISH TEACHER—WITH HELP FROM JOSÉ ANGEL

Recently I (the author) visited the Peraza home and had a long talk with *DINORA*. She is now almost 20 years old. Her muscle weakness has progressed so that she can not lift her arms. However, she creates lovely hand-sewn crafts by balancing her forearms on the armrests of her wheelchair. She still is active with Los Pargos. Although travel by bus to the Pargos center is now too difficult for her, she teaches English to several of the *Pargitos* who come to her house.

I asked Dinora how she had learned to teach English. She said she had studied at the *ACADEMIA DE INGLES THE GOLDEN GATE*, a few blocks from her home. Her father took her there daily in her wheelchair.

"David, I wish you could meet my teacher, who runs the Academia," said Dinora. "He's a wonderful person. He's disabled."

"Is his name José Angel?" I guessed.

"Yes!" said Dinora. "Do you know him?"

"Years ago, when he was a boy, we took him to Shriners Hospital in California for surgery," I replied. "I haven't seen him for years, but I heard he was teaching English in Mazatlán."

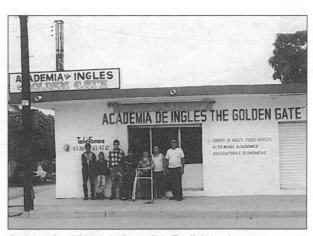
José Angel and friends in front of his English Academy.

That afternoon, Dinora's father took me to visit *JOSÉ ANGEL* Tirado. The Academy, next to his father's house, is a great success, with 3 classrooms and 3 teachers. José Angel, who has a rare degenerative bone disease, made many trips to Shriners Hospital in California for surgery when he was a child and an adolescent. Now he has artificial hips and knees. On his many visits to the USA he learned a lot of English.

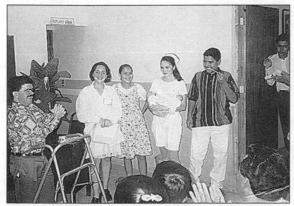
José Angel's creative teaching methods make learning English fun. Students perform role plays in English of many basic events, such as a mother who delivers a baby in a hospital.

Once back in Mexico, José Angel began tutoring classmates in English, and he eventually started teaching small groups. He was a good teacher who knew how to make learning fun. More and more students wanted him to teach them. So, his father rented a room next door, and that was the start of the Academy. Today, there are 80 students and a long waiting list. Financially, the Academy has been so successful that José Angel paid for a full renovation of his father's house. He charges enough to make a good living. **But for disabled people who want to study at the Academy, he gives full scholarships.**

A close community. The Peraza family and the Pargos, together with disabled role models and teachers and like Victor and José Angel, form a close community of peers and friends who help, challenge and provide inspiration to one another. Despite their difficulties, there is an aura of warmth and even joy about the Peraza home. Every time I visit the Peraza's, I come away with new energy and hope—not so much hope for a wonder drug to cure muscular dystrophy (although that would be marvelous), but rather, hope for humanity.

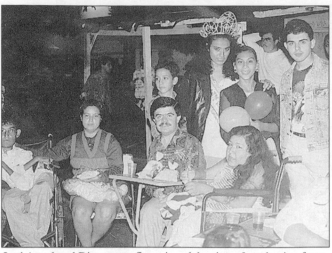

José Angel and Dinora at a fiesta in celebration of graduation from the English course at the Academy.

The Peraza family and their children with muscular dystrophy somehow found unusual strength and vitality. The children made the most of their lives, however short, finding pleasure in helping others in need. We can learn a lot from them.

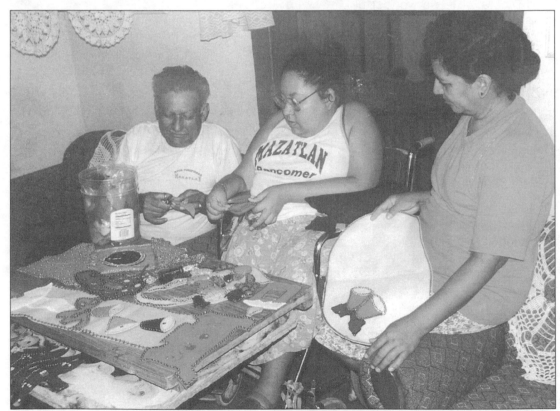

Although Dinora can no longer lift her arms from the armrests of her wheelchair, she helps support the family by sewing colorful ornaments and designs. Here her mother and father admire her work and give suggestions.

Their spirit lives on. Three of the four Peraza children are no longer physically present. But each of them, until very shortly before his death, found great pleasure and dignity in helping other children in need. The remarkable abilities they developed were not limited to their artistic creativity. They inspired disabled and non-disabled people to do their best, and to bring out the best in one another. Their short lives, far from being tragic, were full and rewarding—with joys, sorrows, challenges, and adventures—as life should be.

Innovative Therapy Aids for Other Children with Muscular Dystrophy

CHIRO and RICARDO are two brothers with muscular dystrophy, from a village called Limón. (Child-to-Child activities to help school children be more accepting of these boys are described in Chapter 45, on page 300.) When their parents brought the brothers to PROJIMO, they were at a loss as how to help their sons. They had taken the boys to a rehabilitation center in the city where they had been given a number of exercises to stretch their tight heel cords and to try to maintain their muscle tone. But the boys whined and complained when their parents tried to apply the exercises, which were anything but fun.

At PROJIMO, Mari encouraged Jesús and some of the other disabled children to introduce Chiro and Ricardo to different activities in the Playground for All Children. Playing on the ramps and swings, the boys engaged in exercises that stretched their tight heel-cords and helped them use many muscles of their bodies. And the boys enjoyed it.

Inspired by the PROJIMO playground, the boys' father decided to build at home some of the playground equipment that his sons most enjoyed, and which provided necessary exercise. The following photos show some of the equipment he built, with the help of his sons, behind the family hut in their village.

Exercises to stretch the heel cords help to prevent or delay the awkward tip-toe gait (way of walking) which many children with muscular dystrophy develop.

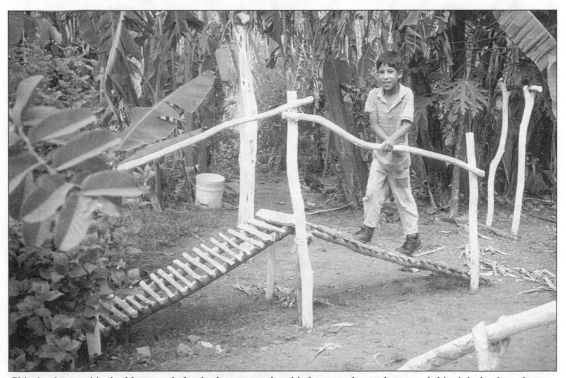

Chiro's play on this double ramp helps both to strengthen his leg muscles and to stretch his tight heel cords.

Heel-cord stretcher. This apparatus, invented by their father, also helps Ricardo and Chiro stretch their tight heel cords. This is done by stepping on the pole on the ground with the front part of the foot, and then rocking back and forth.

The device also helps exercise the child's shoulders, arms and hands.

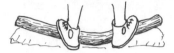

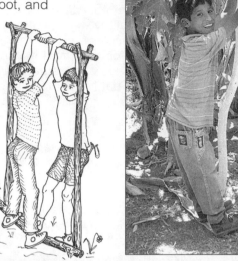

Standing with the fore-foot on the pole on the ground helps to stretch tight heel-cords. The bend in the pole—so that it slants down to the center from either side—helps combat inward (varus) deformities of the feet.

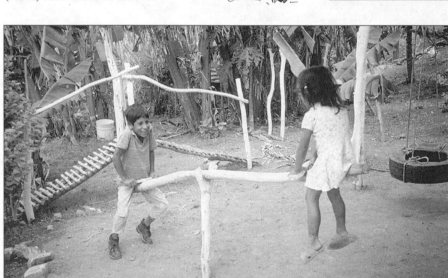

Chiro plays with his sister on a see-saw. The play helps to exercise his arms and his legs.

The tire-swing and the other exercise equipment are so much fun that not only the boys with muscular dystrophy, but also their sister (and other children) like to play on them.

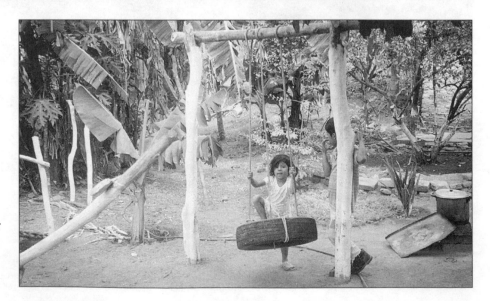

CHAPTER 49

Playmates as Therapists:
Helping Fernando Learn New Skills

CHILD-to-child

In Chapter 45, we saw how Child-to-Child activities helped Jesús' classmates and teacher to better understand his needs and possibilities. Here, we see how the playmates of another disabled child succeed in helping him to learn useful skills and activities that adults had been unable to teach him.

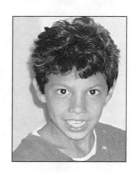

FERNANDO is slow to trust adults. He has good reasons. Since he was a baby, he has been hurt in different ways by grown-ups who wanted, in their own way, to help him.

Fernando's mother grew up in a small village, but in her early teens she went to the city to study. There she was courted by a young man, whom she soon married. Months later, a baby was born and they named him Fernando. He was a lovely child with golden curls. At first, the signs of his cerebral palsy were not very obvious.

After three difficult years, the marriage broke up. Both parents fought to keep the child. One night, Fernando's father came home to the village, very drunk. He kidnapped the little boy from the mother's family at gunpoint. But as the child grew, spasticity and other signs of cerebral palsy became clearer. He began walking at the age of 4, with a spastic, knock-kneed gait. He has never been able to talk. Unwilling to accept that his son was disabled, his father took him to one doctor after another, seeking a cure. Some doctors said the boy's condition was hopeless: nothing could be done. Others performed costly tests and prescribed costly medicines. Unwilling to raise a son whom he considered "minusvalido" (less valid), his father took Fernando back to his mother.

But by this time, the boy's mother had another lover who, like his father, did not want an "invalid." In the end—as often happens—Fernando's grandmother took the child in. She loved him and wanted the best for him. But her own husband had died (of tuberculosis and alcoholism), and she had trouble maintaining her small store to make ends meet.

Fernando's grandmother lives in Ajoya, where PROJIMO is located. The PROJIMO team offered her advice and, when Fernando was 5, encouraged her to put him in kindergarten. Year after year, he attended school, but he never got beyond the first grade. The boy was alert and in some ways seemed intelligent. But he had a learning-disability with talking and reading. After repeating first grade for 5 years he still could not write his name.

Rather than focusing on the "3 Rs," the PROJIMO team thought it might be more enjoyable and useful for Fernando to learn some practical skills. They made repeated efforts to include the boy in activities at PROJIMO: in the *Playground for All Children,* and the *Children's Toy-Making Workshop.* But even at age 11, the boy was still very timid, especially around adults.

One day when a physical therapist was visiting PROJIMO, Fernando's grandmother took him there for another evaluation. Terrified, the boy clung to Grandma's dress, his head down. Trying to win his confidence, Mari asked him if he would like to play on the swings or the merry-go-round. Fernando shook his head "NO!" and burst into tears at the thought of it. He was still very fearful of adults.

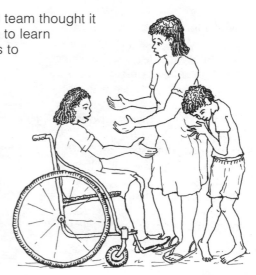

Playmates as Therapy Helpers

The PROJIMO team thought that Fernando's manner of walking might be improved with gait and balance activities. But despite their best efforts, Fernando refused to cooperate.

One day, Mari, who has helped to facilitate Child-to-Child activities with school-aged children, had an idea. "Fernando is so fearful with us adults," she observed, "even when we try our hardest to befriend him. Yet, outside his house, I often see him playing with other little boys with whom he is wild and fearless. Why don't we invite his young friends to come to PROJIMO, and bring Fernando with them? We can explain some play activities to his friends that could help Fernando improve his walking and balance. Maybe they can also get him involved in the toy-making shop, where they can all learn to make and paint toys together. That way Fernando could start learning useful skills."

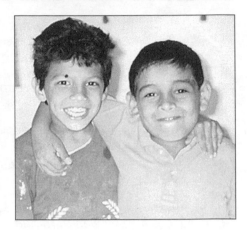

Everyone thought this was a splendid idea. Conchita talked to Fernando's young friends, and to their mothers. Fernando's playmates were excited with the idea and wanted to help.

The Board-Walk Balance Game

The next day the two young boys, Manuel y Chito, arrived at PROJIMO, followed—somewhat nervously—by Fernando, who lurched awkwardly from side to side as he tried to keep up. Mari suggested a game to help Fernando improve his foot-control and balance. Directing from her wheelchair, she asked the children to bring several boards down from the loft, and to place them over bricks to form narrow walkways.

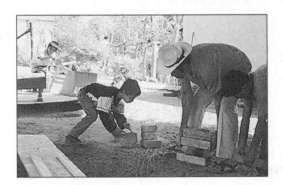

Fernando, following the example of his friends, helped to carry the bricks and place them on the ground to support the boards. This was not easy for him. But somehow he managed to bend down, pick up the bricks with his spastic hands, carry them with his scissored gait, and place them under the giant fig tree. **This way, not only the play-therapy activities, but also his involvement with his playmates in preparing the equipment, helped Fernando to develop body control.**

When the "boardwalk" was in place, Mari asked the children to **"follow the leader,"** walking back and forth on the boards. The 10-inch-wide boards were about 6 inches above the ground. The two able-bodied boys bravely "walked the plank," and Fernando fearlessly followed. He tipped precariously this way and that, looking as if he would surely fall off. But, to everyone's amazement, he kept his balance, grinning happily as he followed his friends back and forth. Everyone applauded.

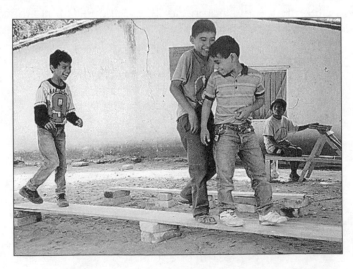

Mari knew it was a good idea to have started Fernando with an activity he could succeed at easily. It gave him confidence. But this was too easy. He needed more of a challenge. So Mari had the boys arrange 3 long boards, each only 2 inches wide, in a triangular path.

Mari challenged the boys to walk as many rounds on the boards as they could without falling off. Fernando, despite his wobbling back and forth, waving his arms wildly to keep his balance, did amazingly well. At first, he—and occasionally also one of the other boys—sometimes lost their balance. But he rapidly improved until he rarely lost his footing on the narrow board.

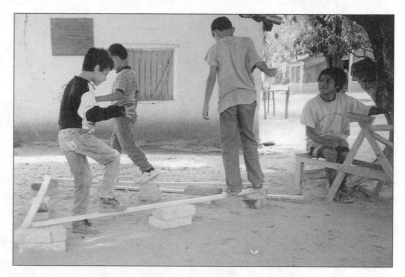

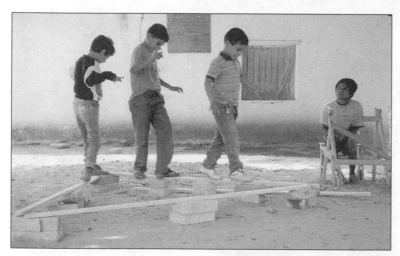

Mari laughed at herself. "I thought Fernando needed to improve his balance!" she declared. "But he has incredibly good balance—better than I had before my accident!" She realized that he needed—and had developed— exceptionally good balance to be able to walk and run with legs that only imperfectly followed his wishes.

Important as these activities were for Fernando's balance and positioning of his feet, they were equally important for his growing sense of confidence among a mixed group of children and adults.

He very quickly appeared to be a very different child than the one who had arrived a few days before and had hung miserably to his grandmother's dress.

Spontaneous play and inter- action with other children had as much therapeutic value, both physical and social, as did the specially designed activities.

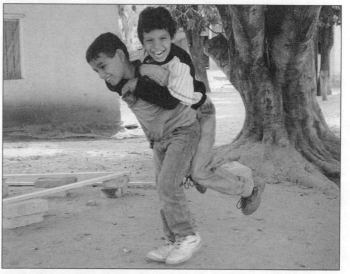

One of his friends gives Fernando a piggy-back ride after playing "walk the plank" together.

Introduction to the Toy-Making Workshop

After their play on the "board-walk," the three boys were eager to do something different. Mari led the way to the toy-making workshop. This small shop was set up to involve disabled and non-disabled children together in making early-stimulation toys and puzzles, especially for children with developmental delay. (See pages 290-291.)

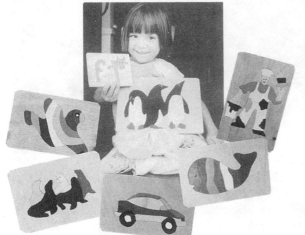

WOODEN PUZZLES MADE AT PROJIMO

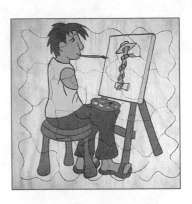

To interest the 3 boys in making toys, Mari asked the help of Manuella, a village girl who works in the toy shop. Manuella agreed to cut out wooden figures of animals or persons for each of the 3 boys, which they could sand and paint. The boys asked her to cut out figures of themselves. David (the author of this book) drew the boys, each posed in the position he wanted to appear in.

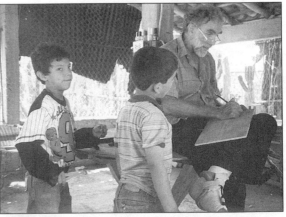

Then the boys watched, fascinated, as Manuella cut out the figures on the electric jig saw. The figures emerged: Chito in a Karate pose, Manuel as a muscle man, and Fernando dancing.

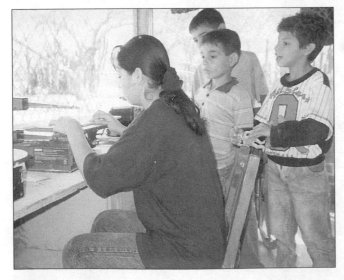

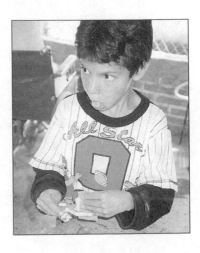

The boys carefully sanded the wood figures. With his spastic hands, Fernando had difficulty holding the figure and trying to sand it. But the other boys showed him how. Fernando did his very best.

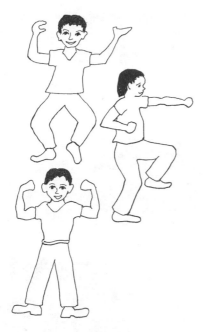

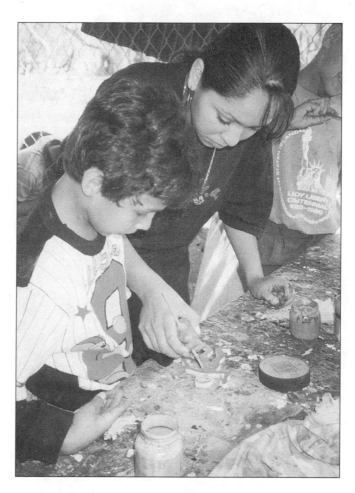

Next the boys painted the wooden figures of themselves. At first, Fernando had trouble holding and controlling the brush, and Manuella helped him by guiding his hand.

At last the boys finished painting the figures of themselves, and held them up with delight.

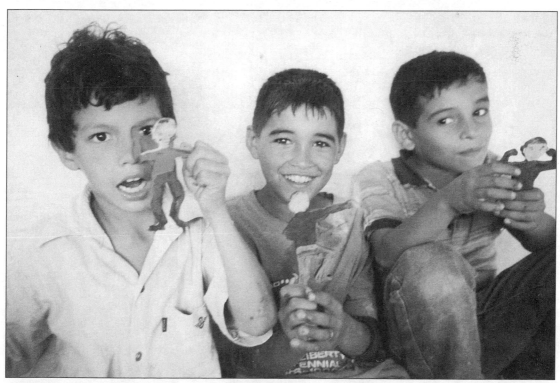

Although Manuel and Chito greatly enjoyed the activities themselves, they also took their job of helping Fernando to learn new skills quite seriously, and they felt proud when they saw him manage to do new things.

Making other toys. The children wanted to make other toys in the workshop. They asked Fernando if he wanted to make an animal, and began to name different kinds: A chicken? A dog? A cow? A cat? A raccoon? Fernando shook his head "No!" at each suggestion. Then the boys said "A Horse?" Fernando grinned and nodded. Chito and Manuel said that they, too, wanted to make horses. Excited, Fernando had yet another idea, but unable to speak, he had trouble communicating it. Everyone asked him questions about other animals or figures he might want to make. He kept shaking his head.

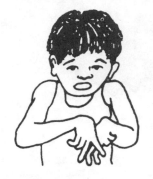

At last, Fernando made a gesture, as best he could with his spastic hands. It was something like ← this.

"He wants a rider on his horse!" cried Manuel.

"Then a horse and rider you will have!" said Manuella. She created a simple design. The rider was made of 3 pieces of wood: the body and two legs. The movable legs were attached to the hips with a small nail, so that the rider could be seated firmly on the horse.

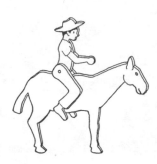

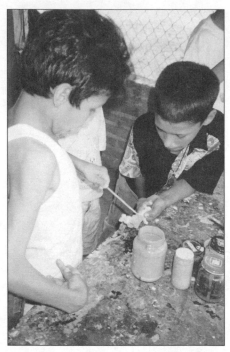

Of, course, all of the boys wanted a horse and rider. Again, they sanded and painted them lovingly. This time, one of the boys held the pieces while Fernando carefully painted them. He now seemed to have more hand control, which perhaps came partly from greater confidence.

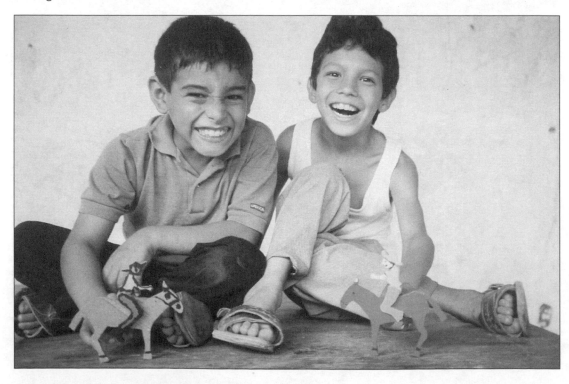

Helping Fernando Walk with His Feet Pointing Forward

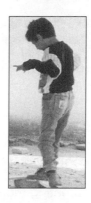

The following morning all 3 boys were back at PROJIMO at the crack of dawn, eager for more. Now no one needed to coax Fernando to take part. The big challenge to Mari and others was to find new playful ways for Fernando's playmates to help their friend master new skills.

Fernando's manner of walking was awkward. His arms flailed with every step, and his body pitched from side to side. His toes pointed inward more than a pigeon's. As his knees jerked past one another it looked as if he would surely trip himself up and fall. But he seldom did.

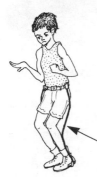

Despite his spasticity and strange movements, the PROJIMO team felt that Fernando had adapted to his physical disability amazingly well. The goal of rehabilitation should not be to make him *walk normally* but to help him to *function at the best of his potential.*

Nevertheless, Fernando's turned-in feet did occasionally get in the way and sometimes he came down with a crash. Years before, his father had taken him to specialists. He had been given braces with *torsion cables* to try to position his feet so they would point forward (see page 110). But he hated them, and he fell more often.

Now that Fernando had therapy-helpers (his young playmates) whom he enjoyed, he was more open to learning new skills. The team thought it might be useful to experiment with activities to teach Fernando to point his feet forward rather than inward as he walked.

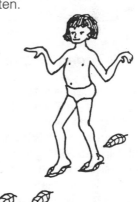

Mari had seen pictures from the *Sarvodaya Community Rehabilitation Program* in Sri Lanka, where a village worker used mango leaves to help a child learn to take more even steps. The worker placed a row of leaves on the ground at even intervals, and asked the child to step on these as she walked. (The method worked well when there was no wind.)

Based on this technique, the PROJIMO team devised two different methods that might help Fernando learn to take more regular steps with his feet pointing forward.

1. *Painted footprints.* Instead of using leaves (which can blow away or move out of place when stepped on) the team decided to paint footsteps on the ground. The new outdoor court for wheelchair basketball was a perfect place to paint them.

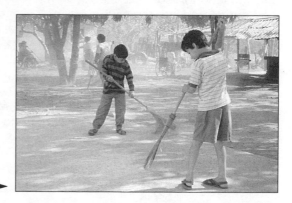

Fernando and his playmates were eager to paint the footprints, so Manuella and Mari invited them to do so. By now a dozen children also wanted to help paint. But first the basketball court needed to be swept. →

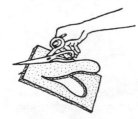

To make the footprints the right size and shape, Manuella made stencils (shapes to trace around) from thick cardboard and from thin scraps of wood. On these she traced a child's sandal and cut out a foot-shaped hole. The children placed the stencils on the cement basketball court and painted different bright colors in the open foot-shaped spaces.

Some older boys from the village (who had come to play basketball) helped guide the younger children in correctly spacing and positioning the footprints. At first one boy held the wooden stencil for Fernando and helped guide him in painting the footprints. But soon Fernando did it all by himself. Creating the stepping aids was as much a learning experience for the boy as was using it.

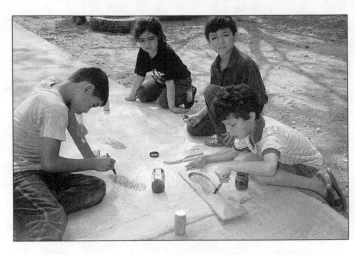

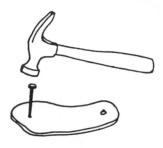

When the paint had dried, all the children wanted to walk on the footsteps along the winding course on the basketball court. They played **follow-the-leader,** each imitating the child heading the line. Sometimes they walked fast, but more often they walked slowly, taking care to step precisely on the footprints. They encouraged Fernando to do the same. Fernando tried hard to place his feet correctly, and succeeded in taking more evenly positioned, forward-pointing steps.

2. *Wooden footprints.*

An alternative method was developed to help train Fernando and children with similar gait problems. One of the girls cut more than 20 footprints from scraps of thin boards. The children, including Fernando, painted them in bright colors. A hole was drilled in both ends of every footprint. The footprints were positioned on the ground in a pattern similar to the foot paintings on the basketball court. To hold the footprints firmly, 3-inch nails were placed through the holes in them and hammered into the earth. Again, the children—a dozen or so including Fernando—played follow the leader.

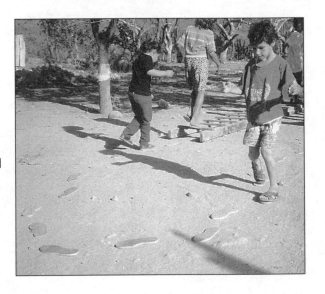

The wooden footprints have several advantages over the footprints painted on cement. First, because the thickness of the wood raises them above the ground slightly, children make a greater effort to step on them precisely. Second, they can be easily transported. And third, they can be adjusted according to the needs of the individual child.

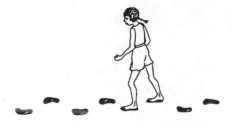

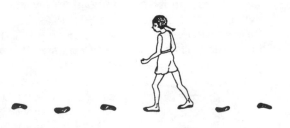

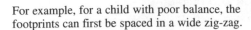

For example, for a child with poor balance, the footprints can first be spaced in a wide zig-zag.

As the child's balance and control improves, the prints can be repositioned into a straighter line.

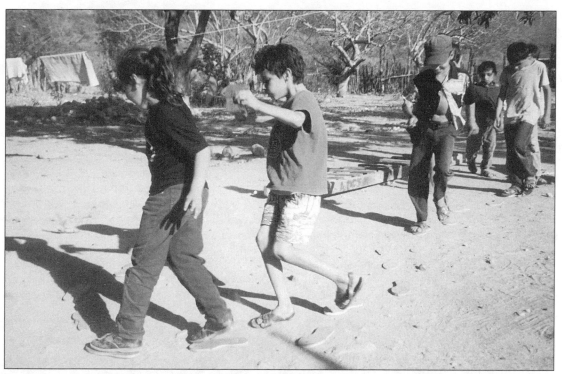

At first, Fernando stepped on the footprints with his toes turned in. But, with the children's encouragement, he found he could position his feet more exactly over the footprints, thus pointing his toes in a straighter (less pigeon-toed) position.

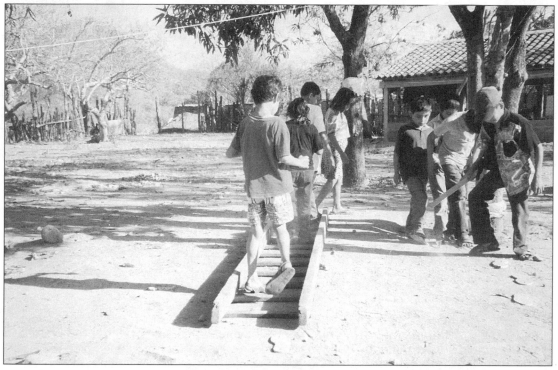

Stepping between the rungs of a ladder. Another simple method to help Fernando improve his foot control also comes from a CBR program in Sri Lanka. As a part of the marching-on footprints game, the team placed a long wooden ladder on the ground. The children were asked to step in the spaces between the rungs. To do this, Fernando had to lift his feet high and place them carefully. Again, the children played follow-the-leader. At first Fernando followed, but by the end began to proudly lead the other children.

Playing Ball to Improve Coordination

To help Fernando improve hand and arm control and reduce his spasticity, the PROJIMO team encouraged his playmates to play ball with Fernando. They made up a game similar to volleyball, throwing a large lightweight ball over a fishing net between two trees.

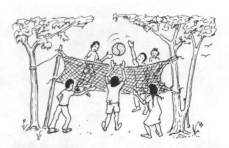

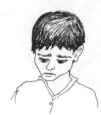

But to everyone's surprise, Fernando's closest friend, 8-year-old Manuel, refused to play. Following his friend's example, Fernando also refused. Mari and I begged Manuel to join the game. We explained to him how beneficial it would be for Fernando to throw and catch the ball. But Manuel still stubbornly refused to play. The PROJIMO workers wondered why young Manuel, who up to now had been so eager to involve Fernando in learning games and activities, had suddenly become so uncooperative.

Finally, we gave up on volleyball and decided to try a simpler game. We asked the children to stand in a circle and toss the ball to the person next to them. This time, Manuel stood up to join in. He glanced at his friend Fernando. Then, all smiles, the two boys entered the circle.

Although much easier than volleyball, this new game was a big challenge to Fernando. Even when the ball was thrown to him gently from a close distance, he had a hard time catching it. At first he usually missed the ball, his arms and hands flailing. The boy's frustration was obvious. But soon he learned to catch the ball by pressing it against his chest with both arms. Each time he caught the ball he grinned happily. Then he would twist around to throw it to the child on his other side. (Twisting the body like this often helps to reduce spasticity.) Fernando's ability to throw the ball increased rapidly. He was delighted.

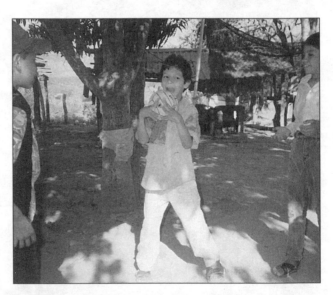

The Wisdom of a Child

Watching Fernando, the PROJIMO team gained insight into why his young friend Manuel had so stubbornly refused to play volleyball. Manuel was protecting his friend from failure and possible ridicule. He was aware of his friend's lack of ability for a fast, competitive game like volleyball. Rather than see Fernando humiliated, Manuel simply refused to play. He guessed that his friend would take the clue and do likewise. However, the new ball game was easier and less competitive. Manuel seemed to sense that Fernando could successfully take part without losing face.

Young as he was, Manuel intuited one of the basic lessons for helping teach a disabled child (or any child) new skills: **Introduce new activities in small steps that the child can master quickly, to experience success.** Somehow the boy sensed that to plunge Fernando into a volleyball game with able-bodied peers would be too difficult for him, the pressure too great. It would draw attention to Fernando's weaknesses, not his budding abilities. Manuel did not want us well-intending adults to subject his disabled friend to another disheartening experience.

We learned a lot from Fernando's playmates. Children often have a secret wisdom. If we humble ourselves and take the trouble to listen to them with an open mind, we can learn a lot.

Ball Games Where the Ball Can't Fall

For children like Fernando who have trouble catching a ball, there are various ways to keep the ball from falling. Here are 2 possibilities.

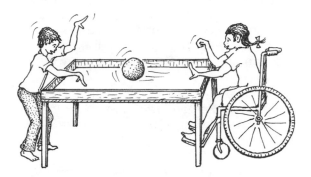
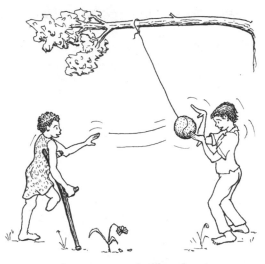

Karate and Horse-Play

In Chapter 41 we saw the example of how, in India, Karate is used with children who have cerebral palsy—both as excellent physical therapy and as an exciting adventure for them.

Fernando and his playmates were fascinated by Karate, and loved taking poses, kicking high, and challenging one another in play. It was quite remarkable how Fernando could take and hold hard positions. Self-chosen therapy—and lots of fun!

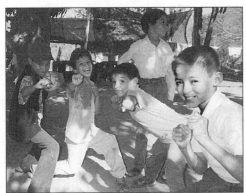
Fernando and friends pose as "Karate kids" for the camera.

Wrestling

One of the best activities for increasing Fernando's strength and control was developed by the children themselves in, of all places, PROJIMO's therapy room. On seeing the large platform with padded mats, Fernando and two of his playmates were inspired to wrestle. As the boys tumbled and twisted this way and that, Fernando used almost every muscle in his body, in a bizarre but surprisingly coordinated way.

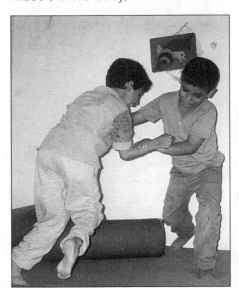

It would have been hard for us adults to have designed any therapy program that would have been as effective, or half as much fun.

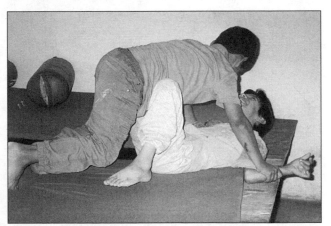

Learning to Use Pictures to Communicate

The idea to use pictures to help Fernando communicate arose out of the activities in the toy-making workshop. Manuella had asked the boys to name an animal they wanted to make out of wood. Fernando, who cannot speak, had difficulty communicating what he wanted. At last, making improvised signs with his hands, he was able to tell her that he wanted a horse and rider. But to communicate other things, at times Fernando had more difficulty. Mari loaned Manuella a picture book of animals, from which Fernando could pick by pointing. Creating a game, the children began to say the names of different animals, and asked Fernando to point to them on the page. He did this remarkably well.

Although Fernando could not read, write, or speak, he obviously had good perception of spoken words and pictures. The team saw that, at times, Fernando was anxious to try to communicate things that were important to him. But he had difficulty. He could use a few simple hand signs, but the spasticity in his fingers limited him.

Then his playmates had an idea. Why not use a series of pictures of common things and events to help Fernando to communicate his needs? The children had seen Andrés using a "picture board" with José, a man who had lost his speech as result of a stroke (see Chapter 23). Carefully designed picture boards might work with Fernando, too. With Fernando's help, his young friends and Mari selected lists of foods, common objects, and various things and actions that Fernando most wanted to "say." They organized these into groups and drew pictures of them, as best they could.

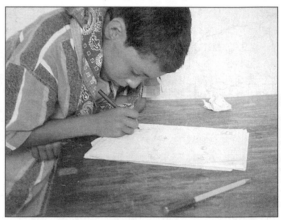
Dionicio makes a "picture board" for Fernando.

Mari suggested they write the name of each thing below its picture. Fernando had been unable to learn to read in school. But if, in the form of play, he were to repeatedly see the written word associated with each picture and its spoken name, perhaps something would stay in his mind.

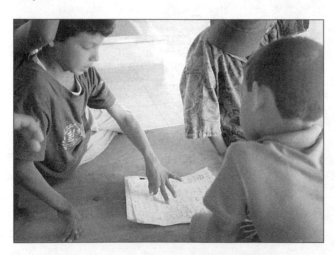

When the picture board was finished, Fernando's playmates began naming the different foods and objects drawn on the board. They asked Fernando to point to them. He recognized and pointed at once to many of the objects, such as FISH, CHICKEN, SPOON, TORTILLA, and ICE CREAM. He had more trouble recognizing other objects, such as SUGAR, POTATO, and BREAD. But after being told what they were, he did not forget. Soon he could identify every figure on the picture-board.

Fernando enjoyed the learning game as much as his young friends enjoyed teaching him. Thanks to the help of his playmates, the use of picture-boards opened up a new realm of communication for Fernando.

The next step was to introduce the method to his grandmother and school teacher.

How a Caterpillar Taught Fernando to Count (with Manuel's Help)

In many areas, Fernando's mind seemed to be quick and intelligent. In others, he had trouble learning. In school he had repeated first grade for 5 years. He still could not read or write. Learning to read numbers was especially hard. On his fingers, he could count up to 10 (although holding his fingers in the position he wanted was a big effort).

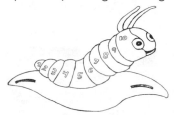

But Fernando had a good sense of space and proportion. He surprised his friends with his ability to assemble some of the wooden jigsaw puzzles made at PROJIMO. One day, Manuel challenged him to put together a puzzle of a caterpillar, the segments of whose body were numbered from 1 to 10.

At first it was hard for Fernando to position the pieces because they were similarly shaped. Then Manuel pointed out that they were numbered in order. Fernando looked at Manuel in surprise, as if discovering for the first time that printed numbers had some real use. First Manuel guided him, and little by little, Fernando seemed to recall the numbers that had repeatedly been taught to him in school. Fernando practiced and practiced. Soon he was able to assemble the puzzle quickly, and to hold up the number of fingers written on each segment of the caterpillar.

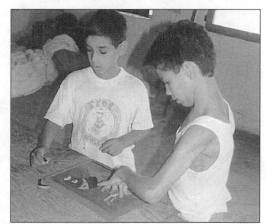

Alternating Work with Play

Although Fernando enjoyed learning to read numbers and use picture boards with his friends, he could not stay quiet for long. Neither could his friends. They would teach Fernando for a few minutes and then suddenly begin to frolic or rough-house. The *Playground for All Children* at PROJIMO remained a constant inspiration for new games.

Rocking Horse

Not long ago, Miguel (Conchita's husband) made a new kind of rocking horse out of an old tire and a huge spiral spring from a dead truck. He designed the horse to resist the wildest play of unrestrained children.

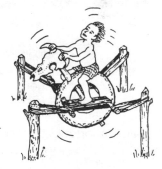

The former rocking horse →
in the Playground—made by
hanging an old tire with inner-
tubes between 4 upright
poles—was always breaking.

The old design, with the tire suspended by inner-tubes, kept breaking.

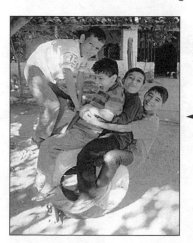

← The new rocking horse had strong bars welded to the base of the spring, and cast into a broad cement base that was buried in the ground. The spring, which passed through one side of the tire, → was firmly attached to the tire with heavy iron bands.

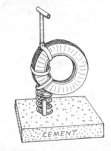

Children, disabled and not, loved the new horse that rocked wildly up and down and in all directions. But none gave it a more energetic work-out than Fernando and his playmates.

The new design, with a steel truck-spring instead of rubber tubes, withstood even Fernando and his friends.

Improvements

With Manuel and his other playmates as his therapy assistants, Fernando blossomed. It is hard to measure how much Fernando has gained physically in terms of improved gait, posture, or hand control. But in terms of his self-image and confidence, he has come a long way. Many people in the village comment on the differences. "He used to be so withdrawn and fearful, especially around grown-ups. Now he seems ready to take on the world!" "He looks so much happier and full of life!"

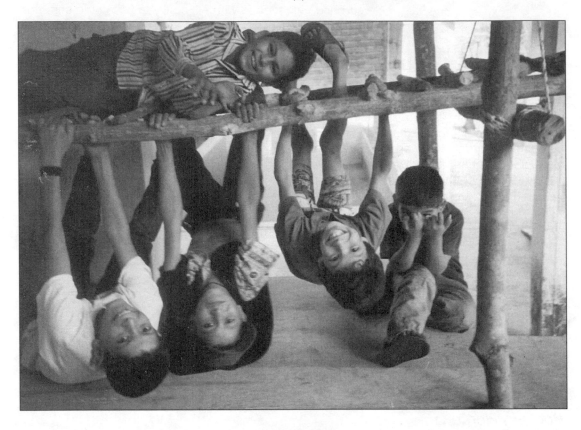

Not only is Fernando learning new skills, but he is learning to relate well with other people: mostly children, but increasingly even adults. Equally important, the many children who have worked and played with Fernando have come to accept and enjoy him as just another kid, playful and adventurous like themselves. When they grow up, they will understand disabled persons better than most adults. Maybe they will become agents of change for a fairer and more understanding world.

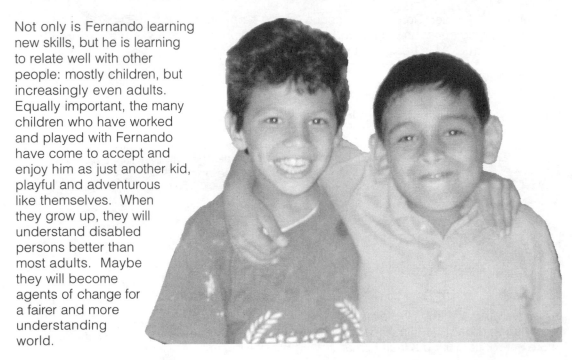

Mentally Handicapped Girls Assist Multiply-Disabled Children:
Outcome of a CBR Training Course in Brazil

Helping Rehabilitation Professionals Listen to and Work as Partners with Disabled Persons

Brazil is a vast country of diverse cultures and striking contrasts. A small percentage of people are enormously wealthy. Millions live in poverty. Big cities have a few modern, highly sophisticated rehabilitation centers. But most disabled persons—especially those living in shanty towns and rural areas—receive little or no assistance beyond what their families can provide. Big barriers, both physical and social, lie in the way of full community integration.

An effort to improve this situation is being made by CORDE, a branch of the Ministry of Justice concerned with the integration and needs of disabled persons. CORDE is now committed to introducing Community Based Rehabilitation (CBR) throughout Brazil.

In November, 1996, CORDE invited me (David Werner) to the coastal city of Recife to facilitate a one week course for future "multipliers" of CBR. According to an early plan, most course participants were to be rehabilitation professionals from government institutions. However, experience in many countries has shown that **many of the most successful CBR programs are started from below by those who are most concerned: by groups of disabled persons and families of disabled children.**

Therefore, to facilitate a partnership approach—and to open the way for disabled persons to play a leading role in planning and implementing CBR programs—it was decided that the course include:

1. a substantial number of disabled participants (or family members), some of whom should be disabled organization leaders and activists;

2. home visits and discussions with willing, local disabled persons/families living in difficult circumstances, to get their views on needs, obstacles, wishes, and ideas for priorities;

3. hands-on, problem-solving activities with disabled children and their families, including making assistive devices with low-cost materials, designed for and with the individual child.

We felt that if the course could help rehabilitation professionals work together with communities, listen to disabled persons, and relate to them as partners and equals in the problem-solving process, much might be gained. The goal should be to encourage rehabilitation workers to EMPOWER, not merely to prescribe.

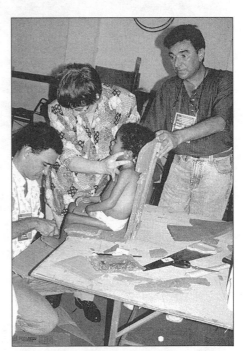

The course involved hands-on problem-solving activities, such as helping families to design and create assistive equipment. Here, participants use metal rods covered with cardboard to make a seat for a multiply-disabled child.

The CORDE staff did a good job of recruiting. Nearly one quarter of the course participants were either disabled themselves or were parents of disabled children. These disabled participants—who included leaders of disabled persons' associations, community service programs, and Brazil's budding Independent Living Movement—provided a key dynamic. They led discussions about needs and possibilities based on their own experiences.

COURSE PREPARATIONS. In preparation for the course, we facilitators visited a government-run hostel for abandoned, severely disabled children. Sixty children were cared for by an average of only 5 or 6 caretakers at any one time. Several of the most handicapped children appeared to be starving. Their wasted condition (marasmus) was apparently due, not to scarcity of food, but to a shortage of staff. Those children who had poor head-control and trouble swallowing could take only liquid foods in small sips. Getting enough food into them called for a lot of time and patience. With so many children to feed, clean, and care for, the few care-providers did not have time to adequately feed and mother those who needed extra help. As a result, these children were becoming more and more disabled. Apart from insufficient food, they got less hugging and stimulation than needed for their minds and bodies to grow.

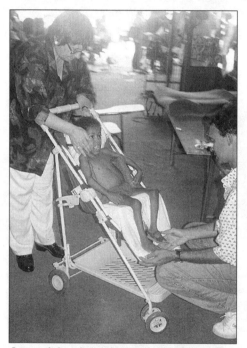

In a workshop during the course, participants improvised a seat-insert to help this child sit in a better position in his stroller.

On arriving at this hostel, we saw a dozen disabled children lined up on the porch, sitting in wheeled strollers. All the strollers were exactly the same—regardless of the size, spastic patterns, or individual needs of the children. Their canvas seats were held by metal-tube frames. The children sat passively in half-reclining positions, like sacks of potatoes.

The strollers neither provided good positioning nor stimulated head and body control. For many of the children, the awkward positioning was leading to increasing spasticity and deformity. A few of the less severely disabled children were able to take a few steps with assistance, but they had no walkers. The one walker we saw was broken.

Given these children's extensive unmet needs, it occurred to me that—with some guidance and the use of books (such as *Disabled Village Children*)—the participants in the training course might be able to make simple, individually-adapted seats, assistive devices, and stimulating play-things for some of the children. With the help of the staff, we chose 6 children whom they agreed to take to a workshop to be conducted during the course.

CHILD-TO-CHILD. One day of the course was spent on Child-to-Child activities. Participants watched a slide-show from Mexico to spark their imaginations. Then they practiced Child-to-Child activities among themselves—including simulation games, role-plays, and discussions to sensitize school-age children to the needs and potentials of children who are different.

That afternoon, participants went to a public school. Small groups visited different classrooms. After ice-breaking games, they facilitated activities with the children. At first, the children were shy. But when they discovered that the adults actually listened to them and took interest in their ideas, the kids warmed up. They expressed their doubts and fears concerning disability. They acted out role-plays, and asked perceptive questions.

At the end, participants asked the children if they had liked the activities, and what they had learned. **What they liked most, they said, was the chance to talk openly with the disabled members of our group,** some of whom were blind or paralyzed. One of our group, Geronimo—who has flipper-like arms and marked deformities—quickly won the children's respect with his friendliness, candor, and self-assurance. One of their lingering doubts was put to rest when Geronimo introduced his vivacious young wife and said they were expecting a baby. The students agreed that the activities and discussions helped them realize that disabled people are ordinary people like themselves, with the same needs, emotions, and dreams. *It is what we have in common that matters most.*

THE APPROPRIATE TECHNOLOGY WORKSHOP.

THE APPROPRIATE TECHNOLOGY WORKSHOP. Two days of the course were spent in a small wheelchair-making shop run by disabled youth in a poor neighborhood. We facilitators had visited the shop beforehand to talk with the workers and to ask them for their help. We had told them that we hoped to bring disabled children from the government hostel (described earlier) so that the course participants could evaluate their needs, and try to make them simple assistive devices. The disabled shop-workers were eager to assist.

I had feared that a workshop with 60 participants would be total chaos. The situation might be overwhelming for the disabled children, especially those who were in delicate health. But my fears were soon calmed. On arrival, the participants formed 6 groups, each with a bewildered child. Among the participants were educators, psychologists, physical and occupational therapists, technicians, disabled persons, and—most important—mothers of disabled children. The mothers, especially, tried to gain the children's confidence, talking gently to them, then tenderly beginning to touch them and take them into their arms. The children, starved for human contact, began to smile and respond. Three participants with experience in evaluating children's needs and in designing assistive equipment, circulated from group to group offering assistance. At first, some participants were afraid to rely on their own observations, or to innovate. But the children's needs were so enormous that the groups started to improvise. The disabled shop-workers—used to building wheelchairs and walkers—began enthusiastically working on innovative designs. They assisted the different groups when their skills were needed.

The results were impressive. Using cardboard, sticks, cloth, and bits of tubing, the groups created a variety of useful assistive devices. They made **special seats, wheelchair inserts, supports for improving body position and head control, a splint for better hand function, tray tables,** and **colorful toys to hang above a child to develop hand-eye coordination.** The children seemed to like both the attention and equipment. The staff from the hostel were thrilled with the creativity. They said they would make equipment for other children, and were delighted to receive a copy of *Disabled Village Children* (in Portuguese) to provide ideas and guidelines.

A survival seat for GUSTAVO. One of the children whose needs were most critical was Gustavo. Completely paralyzed by brain damage, the boy had been abandoned by his parents and ended up at the government hostel. Skin and bones, at age 14 he looked about 6 years old. Feeding him was hard, because his body and head were floppy and he had little mouth control. Although he could not to move or speak, his mental ability seemed intact. He could communicate only with his eyes. But he appeared to understand most questions. He would close his eyes to say no, and leave them open to say yes. At times, he almost smiled. Gustavo seemed to like both his new seat and all the attention. But sometimes when participants asked him questions, tears would roll down his cheeks—as if he were frustrated at not being able to communicate more effectively.

The participants realized that, although they were perhaps able to help Gustavo in a small way—such as a seat that would make feeding him easier—a lot remained undone. Gustavo needed a real home, a loving family, public assistance, and community support. "I never knew there were children like Gustavo in Brazil," said one rehabilitation center coordinator, tears in her eyes. "So starved! So neglected! And in our own institutions! How many more like him are there in Brazil?"

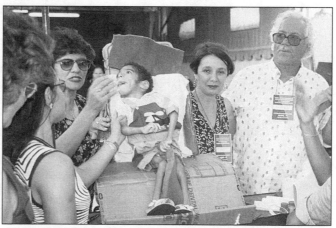

Sewing together layers of cardboard, participants made a special seat for Gustavo. One purpose of the seat was to make it easier to feed him.

JOÃO, the shop worker.

João, a young metal worker in the wheelchair shop, had one of his legs paralyzed by polio. He wanted to know if anything could be done so he could walk without having to push his thigh with his hand. A group of course participants tried to help João solve his problem. The group was encouraged to work with João as an equal in the problem-solving process, and not simply to design and make an assistive device for him. **"Work with him as a partner, not a patient!"**

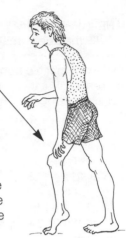

Examining João's leg, the group found that he had a knee contracture of about 25 degrees which, if possible, needed to be corrected before João tried to walk with a brace. They did a test to find out whether the contracture was primarily in the muscles or in the knee itself (see page 127). If the contracture is in the muscles, it can often be corrected with exercise, casting, or bracing, to slowly stretch the tight muscles. If the contracture is in the joint capsule, surgery may be necessary.

To explain all this to João, the group used a life-sized **plywood skeleton** made in Mexico (see Chapter 20), which I had taken with me to Brazil. João enjoyed the demonstration with the skeleton, and said it helped him to understand the functions of his knee.

The group decided that the first step toward improving João's walking was to make a **night brace to gradually correct his knee contracture.** Among the course participants was an orthotist (professional brace maker) who helped João's group design a simple leg brace which they could make from two long, flat metal bars joined by curved sections of metal tube (materials that were available in the wheelchair shop).

João was the only person in his group with the metal-working skills needed for making the brace. But when the group of professionals started working, the predictable thing happened. João was left sitting on the examining table, while the others began to cut, measure, and attempt to bend the pieces for the brace. João watched passively without comment. Then suddenly, one of the disabled participants woke up and said, "Hey! João is more skilled at metal-work than we are. And he knows more about his own leg. Rather than our making the brace for him, he should be making it himself, with our help. That way, if he has to adjust or re-make it after we are gone, he'll know how." Everyone agreed. With a grin, João climbed off the table and took charge.

João did an excellent job of making his brace. Everyone learned a great deal. But **the most important lesson they learned was to work with a disabled person as a partner and not a patient.** This is the key to enabling community rehabilitation.

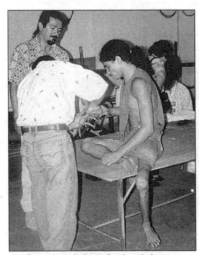

At first, the rehab professionals began to make João's metal leg-brace for him.

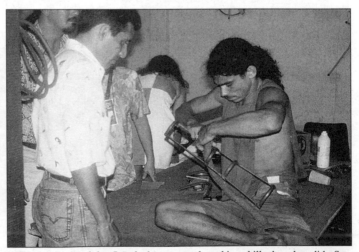

Later, they realized that João had more metal-working skills than they did. So they asked João to take the lead in making his own brace, which he proudly did.

CHILD-TO-CHILD: A MENTALLY HANDICAPPED GIRL LEARNS TO CARE FOR MULTIPLY-DISABLED CHILDREN

The course participants were deeply concerned about the inadequate care that disabled children at the hostel were receiving. They realized that the care-providers at the hostel were over-worked. "The hostel desperately needs more staff, more help! Children are starving because they don't have enough attendants to feed them! In the current economic climate, the government cuts back on budgets for public services, even as the need grows. *What can be done?*"

! *IDEA!* Then an idea came. Next-door to this hostel (part of the same institution) was a "home" for 50 abandoned mentally-handicapped girls. The girls were taught daily living skills, and many attended normal school (a big step forward). Some were also taught work skills. But as the girls got older, many had no place to go. So they stayed in the home with little direction or purpose in their lives.

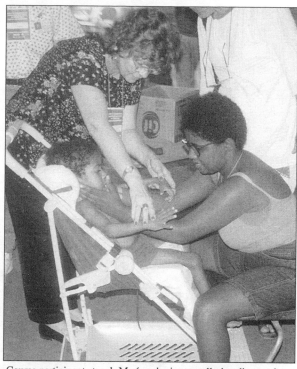

Course participants teach María, who is mentally handicapped, to help care for Ema, a profoundly disabled child. Here María learns simple activities to help the child gain better head control.

A possible solution to the needs of both hostels was evident. One hostel needed more staff to help hold, hug, feed, and mother the multiply-disabled children. The other hostel had mentally slow girls with motherly instincts, who needed worthwhile activities.

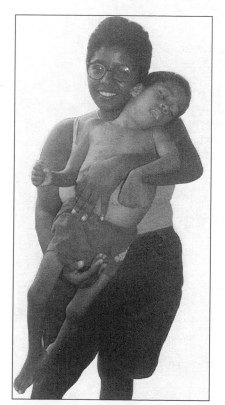

Then why not invite the older, more capable mentally-handicapped girls to help feed and care for the severely disabled children?

Following up on this suggestion, on the second day of the CBR workshop, caretakers from the government hostel brought one of the older, more capable mentally-handicapped girls along with the 5 multiply-disabled children. The girl, **MARÍA,** was eager to help. One of the course participants, herself a mother of a disabled child, showed María how to hold and handle **EMA,** a small girl with cerebral palsy who had almost no body control. María soon learned how to position and feed Eva in her new special seat (made by course participants). Another participant, a therapist, showed María how to help the child develop head control—by holding her upright and gently supporting the back of her head with her hands (see page 37).

Follow up. Everyone agreed that a big achievement of the course was the realization that a mentally slow girl like María could provide a vital service by caring for disabled children. Two course participants from Recife, a therapist and a priest, offered to visit the hostel regularly to help train María and other girls, and to assure that this Child-to-Child initiative is sustained.

Old Plastic Buckets Have Many Uses

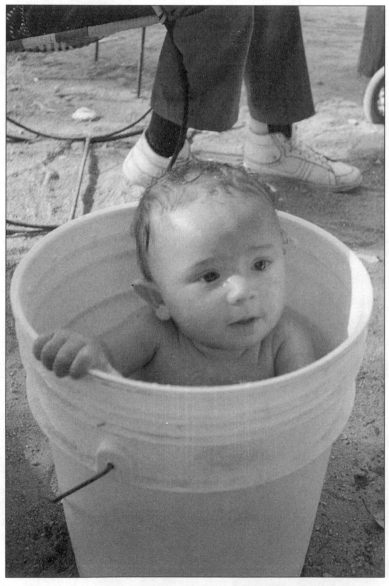

Davidcillo is the son of Magui, who has severe arthritis and runs the cooperative village store in the village of Ajoya. PROJIMO often provided child care for the baby while his mother tended the store. (See the photos of Martín holding and bathing Davidcillo on pages 22 and 236.) The baby was named after the author.

After-Thoughts:
Communication as if ALL People Matter

The Communications Age: Still a Need for Simple, Clear Alternatives

Some say we now live in The Age of Global Communications. The owners and decision-makers of our shrinking earth communicate with one another, world-wide, through computers, fax machines, and electronic mail (e-mail). They say that those who do not master the New Communication Technology will be left behind.

In fact, much of humanity has already been left behind. Today there are more hungry children in the world than ever before—not because of a lack of food and resources, but because of the growing inequality of distribution of resources. The model of global development based on *greed* rather than *need* has led to a brutal concentration of wealth. Today the world's 477 richest people (billionaires) have a total wealth greater than that of the poorest half of humanity. Most disabled people belong to this poorest half.

For the poorer half of humanity, communication tools remain basic. Most of the world's people—including most disabled people—have no access to computers, e-mail, or the Internet (a world-wide electronic information-sharing network). They still communicate with one another simply and directly, sharing information through spoken words, signs, pictures, gestures, and expressions.

This book has been written for disabled people and those concerned for their well-being. Most such persons lack costly communications equipment. They learn primarily through spoken and printed language, pictures, and direct hands-on experience.

One of my own biggest challenges as a health educator and disabled activist has been to **demystify medical and technical knowledge** and present it so that persons with little formal education can use it. The books that have grown out of this process include *Where There Is No Doctor, Helping Health Workers Learn, and Disabled Village Children.*

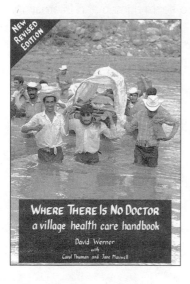

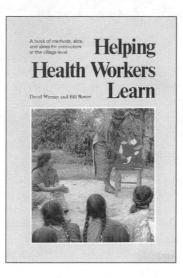

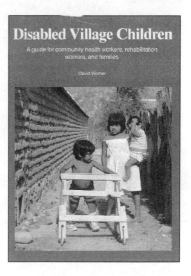

In preparing these books, my co-workers and I have tried to follow a few basic guidelines for making them readable, interesting, and useful, including for those who do not have a lot of practice reading. These guidelines are on the following page.

Suggestions For Effective Information-Sharing in Print

- *Use lots of pictures.* A picture is worth 1000 words.

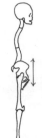

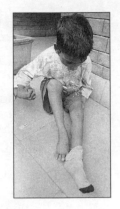

  - **Simple line drawings** are very useful for showing ways to do things. Try to make drawings of people realistic and attractive.

  - **Photographs** add life. They help to make messages and alternatives more believable.

  - To hold the attention of those who do not read much, try to use **pictures on almost every page.** Persons who are not used to using an index can flip through the pages, looking at the pictures to find the topic they want.

- *Keep language simple.* Avoid specialized terms and big words. Say things in the day-to-day language of ordinary people.

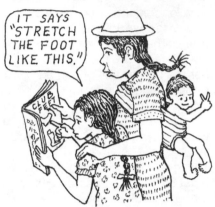

If you do use a less familiar term, explain it when you first use it. A list explaining difficult words may help.

- *Keep sentences and paragraphs short.* Try to limit sentences to about 20 words. Look for ways to break longer sentences into shorter pieces. Also break up long paragraphs.

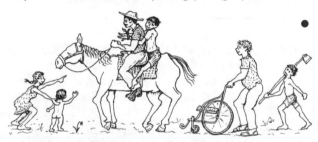

- *Add human interest. Use personal stories and real-life examples.* In presenting information and innovative approaches, give examples of how persons have used and adapted them. Include enough details so the persons described seem human and interesting.

- *Present information simply, but not simplistically.* People with little formal schooling are just as smart as anyone else. Often they have more skills for meeting basic needs (for example, producing food) than do scholars. Speak to them *IN* their terms and *ON* their terms, as equals. Do not talk down to them. They can understand complex ideas if you start with what they know, and build on that.

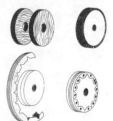

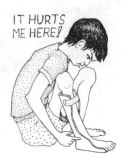

- *Develop and test the materials with a number of intended users.* Be sure to include users or readers who have little formal education, or know least about the subject matter. Ask them if they understand it, enjoy it, and find the information or ideas important and useful. Ask what they like most, and what they like least about it, and if they have any suggestions for making it better.

- Use **bolding,** BIG PRINT, *italics,* shading, and boxes to emphasize important points. Also use "bullets" and arrows.

Resource List 1
Programs and Organizations Promoting Innovative Technologies

This is a partial list of organizations and programs that help in developing assistive equipment at the community level. Included are programs that run training workshops or welcome apprentices who want to exchange ideas and explore "appropriate technologies." Some associations or parent organizations are listed that may be able to provide more local information and addresses in different countries. **Those that contributed to the information in this book are marked with an asterisk (*).**

Action on Disability and Development (ADD), 23 Lower Keyford, Frome, Somerset BAl 1 4AP, UK. Tel: (44-1373) 473064. Contact: Michael Albu, ADD Mobility Service. Community rehabilitation programs in several countries. Help in starting workshops for wheelchairs, tricycles and other equipment; advice on designs, training, administration.

African Medical and Research Foundation (AMREF), Wilson Airport, PO Box 30125, Nairobi, Kenya. Network of community health programs throughout Africa.

* Appropriate Health Resources and Technologies Action Group (AHRTAG), Farringdon Point, 29-35 Farringdon Road, London EC1M 3JB, UK. Tel: (44-171) 2420606. Contact: Ann Robins, Disability and Rehabilitation Unit. Information and resources on primary health care and rehabilitation in the Third World.

* Appropriate Mobility International, PO Box 3198, 2601 DD Delft, The Netherlands. Tel/Fax: (31-15) 2 12 22 70. Contact: Joep Verweij. Design and documentation of tricycles and other mobility aids.

* Appropriate Technology International, 1331 H Street NW, Washington DC 20005, USA. Advice on setting up workshops and training for Whirlwind wheelchairs.

Arigel's Haven Society, CPO Box 2840, Seoul, Korea. Contact: Roh Jae Dong. Walking and seating aids.

* CBR Centre, PPRBM, Jl Lu, Adisucipto Km7, Colomadu, Solo 57176, Indonesia

* Centre for the Rehabilitation of the Paralyzed, PO CRP, Chapain, Savar, Dhaka, 1343 Bangladesh. Tel: (880-2) 06226 464/465; Fax: (880-2) 837969. Contact: Valerie Taylor. Training of orthopedic technicians and setting up small workshops. Many innovations in wheelchairs, trollies, and other aids.

CEPRI (Center for the Promotion of Integrated Rehabilitation, Managua, Nicaragua), Apto 5765, Managua, Nicaragua. Tel: (505 2)663608. A program of families of disabled people. Good self-help manuals in Spanish for and by disabled, especially spinal-cord injured, persons.

* Christian Medical College, Rehabilitation Center, Vellore 632004, Tamilnadu, India. Contact: Dr. S. Bhattacharjee. Wide variety of innovative aids, wheelchairs, protective cushions for spinal-cord injured persons. Re-training in daily skills for rural life.

Christoffel Blindenmission, Nibelungenstrasse 124, D-6140 Bensheim 4, Germany. Africa Regional Office-East, PO Box 58004, Nairobi, Kenya. Low-cost treatment of eye disease, spectacle-making, and optical equipment.

* CISAS (Center for Health Information and Advisory Services) Apto. 3267, Managua, Nicaragua. Tel: (505-2) 661-662; Fax: (505-2) 224-098; e-mail: cisas @ibw.com.ni. Contacts: Maria Zuniga, Martín Reyes. Promotes community based health care and rehabilitation throughout Nicaragua. Also Child-to-Child involving disabled children in much of Latin America.

* Colombo Friend-in-Need Society, 171 Sir James Peiris Mawatha, Colombo 2, Sri Lanka. Contact: Mrs. Swarna Ferdinand, Project Manager, Jaipur Foot Programme. Artificial limbs.

The Disabled Living Centres Council, 380-384 Harrow Road, London W9 2HU. Contact: Tony Travis. Resource centre for information, and trials of equipment.

* Disabled People International, 101-7 Evergreen Place, Winnipeg, Manitoba, R3L 2T3, Canada. International association of national organizations of disabled persons. Tel. (204) 287-8010. Many country programs are involved in community based rehabilitation and some in innovative technologies.

* Economic and Social Commission for Asia and the Pacific (ESCAP), UN Building, Rajadaminern Ave. Bangkok 10200 Thailand. Tel. (662) 2881234; Fax: (662) 2881000. Contact: San Yuenwah. Workshops, documentation, and networking on assistive devices.

Guyana Community Based Rehabilitation Programme, c/o European Commission, PO Box 10847, Georgetown, Guyana. Tel: (592 2) 42249. Fax: (592 2) 62615. Contact: Brian O'Toole. International training programs in CBR and child development. Good teaching materials.

* Handicap International, Home office, 18 rue de Gerland, 69007 Lyon, France. Tel: (933 47) 861-1737. Contact: Jean-Baptiste Richardier. Orthopedic and rehabilitation equipment; designs, advice.

* Handicap International—India, No. 4 Ghandi Street, Colas Nagar, Pondicherry 605001, India. Contact: Xavier Mariadoss. Plastic-bucket braces.

Handicap International—Pakistan, Ahmadzai Colony, Sariab Road, Quetta, Pakistan. Contact: Pascal Simon. Limbs, wheelchairs, seating and walking aids.

* HealthWrights, P. O. Box 1344, Palo Alto, CA 94302, USA; E-mail: healthrights@igc.apc.org. Web site: http://www.healthwrights.org. Contact: David Werner. Development and publication of educational and self-help materials for community based health care and rehabilitation. Works with PROJIMO (see below) on innovative assistive equipment.

ILO, Center for International Cooperation and Appropriate Technology (CICAT/DUT). Stevinweg 1, PO Box 5048, 2600 GA Delft, Netherlands. Contact: Joep Verweij. Information on hand-power tricycles, worldwide. Detailed instructional materials with fine computer-drafted drawings.

* Institute of Child Health, Department of Growth and Development, 30 Guilford Street, London WCIN 1EH. Tel: (44-71) 242-9789. Information and research on planning health care. Course for trainers of Community Based Rehabilitation.

Intermediate Technology Information Ring, Nudestraat 4, 6701 CE Wageningen, The Netherlands. Information on assistive devices and opthalmologic instruments.

* Intermediate Technology Publications Ltd, 103-105 Southampton Row, London WC1 B 4HH, UK. Tel/Fax: (44-171) 436-2013. Publishing and supply of books on appropriate technology, tools, and workshop equipment.

* International Commission on Technology and Accessibility (ICTA) Information Center, Box 510, S-162 15 Vallingby, Sweden. Tel: (46 8) 620-1700. Contact: Tomas Lagerwall. Documents appropriate assistive technologies. Conducts seminars and hands-on workshops in Africa and Asia. Useful publications on assistive devices.

The Jairos Jiri Foundation, PO Box 1529, Bulawayo, Zimbabwe. Calipers,walking and sitting aids, wheelchairs, low-cost adaptations for children.

* Liliane Stichting Fonds, P.O. Box 75, 5250 Vlijmen, Holland, Tel: (31) 7351-19029; Fax: (31) 7351-17354. Contact: Kees van der Broeck. Helps cover disability-related costs for individual children in poor countries. Also helps cover some costs of community programs for disabled children.

* Mobility India, c/o The Association of the Physically Handicapped (APH), Hennur Road, St. Thomas Town, Lingarajapuram, Bangalore, 560084, Karnataka, India. Tel: (91-80) 5475165/or 5470390. Contact: Chapal Khasnabis (Mobility India), or N. S. Hema or D.M. Naidu (APH). Local production and training in high quality assistive and orthopedic aids.

* Mukti, 93 Loyds Road, Madras-600 014 India. Tel: (91-44) 477493. Contact: Meena Dadha. Runs mobile limb-making clinics to villages. Make low-cost "Mukti limbs" out of plastic pipe, with Jaipur feet.

Norwegian International Disability Alliance, P.O. Box 9218 Gronland, 0134 Oslo, Norway. Tel: 2217 4647; Fax: 2217 6177. email: srimapost@sbs.nida.msmail.telemax.no. Contact: Harald Lundqvist. Links with many disability groups and programs in Norway and beyond doing advocacy and innovative work.

* People Potential, Plum Cottage, Hattingley Road, Medstead, Alton, Hampshire, GU34 5NQ, UK. Tel. or Fax: (01420) 563741. Contact: Ken Westmacott. Design of aids for disabled persons; training in low-cost production of wide range of rehabilitation aids, including appropriate paper-based technology (APT).

* PROJIMO (Program of Rehabilitation Organized by Disabled Youth of Western Mexico). Apto. Postal 9, San Ignacio, Sinaloa, 82900, Mexico. Contact: Mari Picos and Conchita Lara. Community rehabilitation program. Disabled craftspersons design and make a wide range of assistive equipment. Peer counseling. Workshops and occasional short courses.

Rehabilitation and Limb Centre, K.G. Medical College, Lucknow, India. Contact: Prof. M.K. Goel. Limbs, appliances, walking and seating aids.

* Rehabilitation Centre, SMS Medical College, Jaipur 302004, Rajasthan, India. Jaipur Limb. Many other aids.

Relevant Technology Workshops, PMB 2174, Jos, Plateau State, Nigeria. Wheelchairs, tricycles, hospital equipment.

* RESCU, 21 Harare Street, PO Box 66044, Kopje, Harare, Zimbabwe. Contact: P. Gumete, Sheltered Workshop Manager. Wheelchair design, production and supply.

* Sarvodaya Economic Enterprises Development Services, 41 Lumbiri Avenue, Ratmalana, Sri Lanka. Wheelchair production. Community based rehabilitation.

* Spastics Society of Tamilnadu (SPASTN), Opposite TTTI, Taramani Road, Madras 600113, Tamilnadu, India. Tel & Fax: (91-44) 2350047. Contact: Aloka Guha. Wide variety of assistive aids and special seating. Karate for disabled children.

* Stichting Demotech—Design for Self-Reliance, Postbus 303, 6950 AH Dieren, The Netherlands. Contact: Reinder van Tijen. Innovative designs for energy-saving, simple living. Gravity-lift elevator. Communication tools.

* Tahanan Walang Hagdanang (House With No Stairs), 61 Banawe Street, Quezon City, Philippines. Tel (63 2) 695–2576. Wheelchairs built by wheelchair riders.

* Teaching Aids at Low Cost (TALC), P.O. Box 49, St Albans, Herts ALI 4AX. Tel: (44 1727) 853–869; Fax: 846–852. Supplier of training materials; books on health care and disability, including those by David Werner.

* Viklang Kendra Research Society, Rehabilitation Centre for the Handicapped 13, Lukerganj, Allahabad, 211001, India. Contact: Dr. Bhanerjee. Innovative appliances, limbs, and wheelchairs made from bamboo.

* Volunteer Health Association of India (VHAI), Tong Swasthya Bhawan, 40 Institutional Area (Behind Qutab Hotel), New Delhi 110016, India. Tel: (91-11) 6518071-72; Fax: (91 11)6953708. Contacts with many community rehabilitation programs throughout India. Many publications. Indian version of *Disabled Village Children*.

* Wheeled Mobility Center, School of Engineering, San Francisco State University, 1600 Holloway Avenue, San Francisco, CA 94132, USA. Tel: (415) 338-2878. Contact Ralf Hotchkiss or Peter Pfaelzer. World-wide network of wheelchair designers and builders. Hands-on courses in wheelchair building in many countries.

* World Health Organization (WHO), 20 Avenue Appia CH-1211 Geneva, Switzerland. Contact: Dr. Enrico Pupulin, Chief Medical Officer, Rehabilitation. Tel. (41 22) 791 3656. Fax. (41 22) 791 4874. WHO has promoted Community Based Rehabilitation in many counties, and produced many valuable resource materials.

* Worth Trust, 48 Thiruvalam Road, Katpadi 632007, Tamilnadu, India. Contact: Bos Cruz. Disabled workers produce a wide variety of assistive devices, from sophisticated to simple. Innovative research with carbon-fiber braces.

Resource List 2
Reading and Teaching Materials

This is a short list of writings and teaching materials about or relevant to innovative technologies for disabled persons. Many of these writings share the vision of self-determination and enablement that are encouraged in this book. For a more complete list of early writings (before 1987) on ideas and aids for community based rehabilitation, see the Reference List in Disabled Village Children *(see below). For more up-to-date lists, write to AHRTAG, TALC, Handicap International, or ICTA. Their addresses can be found below in the entries marked with an asterisk (*). The addresses are also in Resource List 1, pages 341-342.)*

* *Appropriate Paper-Based Technology.* Slide show. Available from Teaching Aids at Low Cost (**TALC**), PO Box 49, St. Albans, Herts, AL1 5TX, UK. Price 4.50 pounds for self-mounted slides, 6.20 pounds for mounted slides.

* *Appropriate Technology—an essential part of a CBR programme,* by Tomas Lagerwall. 1995. 21 pages, free. **ICTA** Information Center, Box 510, S-162 15, Vallingby, Sweden.

Asia-Pacific Disability Aids and Appliances Handbook. 1982. 84 pages. ACROD, P.O. Box 60, Curtin, A.C.T., 2605, Australia.

Behold Your Body: Anatomy and Physiology Anyone Can Enjoy, Volume One, by Charlene Penner. 1996. 400 pages. Rose Bud Publishing, 17126 Mt. Woodson Road, Ramona, CA 92065, USA. US$34.95.

"Build Yourself" Plastic Wheelchair. Directions for assembly available from Spinal Research Unit, Royal North Shore Hospital of Sydney, St. Leonards, NSW 2065, Australia.

* *Disabled Village Children: A guide for community health workers, rehabilitation workers and families,* by David Werner. 1987. 664 pages. Available in English and Spanish through HealthWrights, P. O. Box 1344, Palo Alto, CA 94302, USA., or through TALC, PO Box 49, St. Albans, Herts, AL 5TX, UK. Also available—from other sources—in French, Portuguese, and other languages. Write HealthWrights for information.

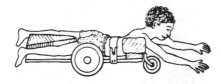

* *Essential CBR Information Resources: an international listing of publications.* 1996. 34 pages. **AHRTAG** (Appropriate Health Resources and Technologies Action Group), Farringdon Point, 29-35 Farringdon Road, London EC1M 3JB, UK.

AHRTAG also produces several basic books on low-cost aids. These include:
- ***Personal Transport for Disabled People***
- ***Alternative Limb Making***
- ***How to Make Simple Disability Aids***
- ***Low Cost Aids***

All these books are also available from TALC, PO Box 49, St. Albans, Herts, AL 5TX, UK.

Functional Aids for the Multiply Handicapped, by Isabel Robinault. Harper and Row, Hagerstown, MD, USA. (Mostly factory built examples, but some good design ideas.)

Guidlines for the Prevention of Deformities in Polio, World Health Organization, 1995. 1211 Geneva 27, Switzerland.

Handling the Young Cerebral Palsied Child at Home, by Nancy Finnie. Dutton Sunrise, 2 Park Ave., New York, NY 10016, USA, 1975. 337 pages. Excellent, very complete information for home care, with many simple, practical aids and devices.

Helping Health Workers Learn, by David Werner. 1982. 632 pages. Available through HealthWrights, P. O. Box 1344, Palo Alto, CA 94302, USA. People-centered methodologies. Useful section on Child-to-Child.

Independence through Mobility, A guide to the manufacture of the ATI-Hotchkiss Wheelchair, by Ralf Hotchkiss. 1985. 162 pages. Available through Wheeled Mobility Center, San Francisco State University, San Francisco, CA 94132, USA.

The Jaipur above-knee prosthetic systems: fabrication manual, by M.K. Mathur. 1989. 47 pages. SMS Medical Centre, Jaipur 302 004, India.

The Lever-Powered Tricycle, Manufactured in Burkina Faso. 1995. 100 pages. **Handicap International**, ERAC, 14, Avenue Berthelot, 69361 Lyon, cedex 07, France. Price 55 FF. Handicap International (HI) also has many excellent booklets and videos on appropriate technologies for disabled persons, including **artificial limbs, braces, wheelchairs, and crutches designs.** Write HI for a list.

Local Production of Appropriate Technical Aids for Disabled People, Report from a Rehabilitation International workshop in Kibwezi, Kenya. 1992. 32 pages. ICTA Information Center, Box 510, S-162 15, Vallingby, Sweden.

Making Health-Care Equipment: Ideas for local design and production, by Adam Platt and Nicola Carter. 1990. 80 pages. Intermediate Technology Productions. 103-105 Southampton Row, London WC1B 4HH, UK. (Good wheelchair, convertible wheelchair-tricycle, and many other designs.)

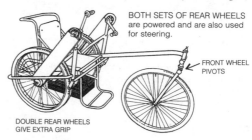

BOTH SETS OF REAR WHEELS are powered and are also used for steering.

FRONT WHEEL PIVOTS

DOUBLE REAR WHEELS GIVE EXTRA GRIP

A Manual: Appropriate Paper-Based Technology (APT), by Bevill Packer. Revised 1995. 120 pages. Intermediate Technology Publications, Ltd. 103-105 Southampton Row, London WC1B 4HH, UK.

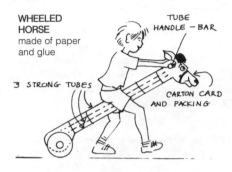

More With Less: Aids for Disabled People in Daily Life, by Gery van der Hulst and others. 1993. TOOL Publications, Sarphatistraat 650, 1018 AV Amsterdam, Netherlands.

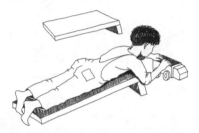

A Plastic Caliper for Children, by Handicap International staff at its Pondicherry, India branch. Available through Handicap International, or from ERAC, 14 avenue Berthelot, 69361 Lyon cedex 07, France.

Positioning the Client with Central Nervous System Deficits: The wheelchair and other adapted equipment. Andrienne Falk Bergen and others. Second edition 1985. 237 pages. Valhalla Rehabilitation Publications, PO Box 195, Valhalla, NY 10595, USA.

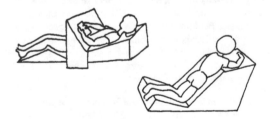

Promoting the Development of Young Children with Cerebral Palsy: A Guide for Mid-Level Rehabilitation Workers, World Health Organization, 1993. 20 Avenue Appia, 1211 Geneva 27, Switzerland.

Questioning the Solution: The Politics of Primary Health Care and Child Survival, by David Werner and David Sanders. 1997. 206 pages. HealthWrights, P. O. Box 1344, Palo Alto, CA 94302, USA.

Rehabilitation technology in community-based rehabilitation: a compendium, by S. Olney, T. Packe and U. Wyss. Kingston, 1994. 212 pages. Available from School of Rehabilitation Therapy, Queens University, Ontario K7L 3N6, Canada.

Special Seating, by Jean Anne Zollars. Second edition 1992. 92 pages. Otto Bock Orthopedic Industry, Inc., Rehab Publications, 3000 Xenium Lane, Minneapolis, MN 55441, USA.

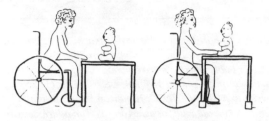

Teaching Yogasana to Mentally Retarded Persons, by Vijay Human Services. 1988. 120 pages. Krishnamacharya Yoga Maniram, 13 Fourth Cross Street, A.K. Nagar, Madras 600 028, India.

Training in the Community for People with Disabilities, by Einer Helander et al. 1989. 582 pages. Available in English, French, Portuguese and Spanish. World Health Organization, 20 Avenue Appia, CH-1211 Geneva 27, Switzerland.

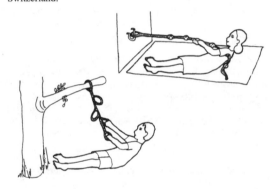

Tricycle Production Manual, by Annemiek van Boeijen, Joep Verweij, et al. 1996. 110 pages. CICAT/DUT Stevinweg 1, PO Box 5048, 2600 GA Delft, Netherlands. Joep Verweij and friends have also put together an excellent *Inventory of Tricycle Models* with examples and photos from around the world.

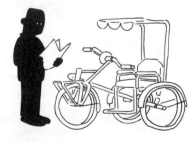

For additional tricycle design resources, see page 202.

UPKARAN: A manual of aids for the multiply handicapped. 106 pages. Spastics Society of India, Upper Colaba Road, Opposite Afghan Church, Colaba, Bombay, 400-005 India.

We can play and move: a manual to help disabled children learn to move by playing with others, by Sophie Levitt. 1992. 56 pages. Available from TALC, PO Box 49, St. Albans, Herts, AL 5TX, UK.

INDEX

This **INDEX** lists in **alphabetical order** most of the topics and names included in this book:

- Names of PERSONS who appear in the stories are listed in the Index like this:
  CARINA; CONCHITA LARA, EDGAR; MARI PICOS (first names first).

- Names of **assistive devices** and technologies appear like this:
  braces, communication boards, wheelchairs.

- Names of different *disabilities* or problems are listed like this:
  blindness; speech problems, spinal-cord injury.

- Names of *"books"* are listed like this: *"Handling the Cerebral Palsied Child at Home."*

- Names of *organizations* are listed like this: *Handicap International, People Potential.*

- All other entries are listed in ordinary letters, like this: India, land mines, women's rights.